PENGUIN BOOKS

INEQUALITIES IN HEALTH

The Black Report:

Peter Townsend is Professor of Social Policy at Bristol University and visiting Michael Harrington Professor of Social Science in City University, New York, 1991–2. He was Chairman of the Child Poverty Action Group from 1969 until 1989 and is now its President. He has been Chairman of the Disability Alliance since 1974, and was a member of the Government Working Group on Inequalities and Health from 1977 until 1980. His books include *The Family Life of Old People* (1957), *The Last Refuge* (1962), *The Social Minority* (1973), *Sociology and Social Policy* (1975), *Poverty in the United Kingdom* (1979) and, as co-author, *Disability in Britain* (1981), *Responses to Poverty: Lessons from Europe* (1984), *Poverty and Labour in London* (1987) and *Health and Deprivation: Inequality and the North* (1988).

Nick Davidson is a journalist, writer and award-winning documentary film maker who has written widely about the National Health Service and social policy. He is co-author of *Out of Our Hands* (1982) and author of *A Question of Care* (1987).

The Health Divide:

Margaret Whitehead is a biologist with a background in medical and health education research, having worked for the Medical Research Council in London and Edinburgh and the Scottish Health Education Group before becoming a freelance researcher and writer. Her particular interests encompass the issue of inequalities in health and the implementation of health promotion strategies. In relation to these subjects, her publications include *Swimming Upstream: Trends and Prospects in Education for Health* (1989) and *The Concepts and Principles of Equity in Health* (1990). She is also co-author of *Policies and Strategies to Promote Equity in Health* (1992) and co-editor of a new edition of *The Nation's Health: a Strategy for the 1990s* (1991).

Inequalities in Health

The Black Report
**Sir Douglas Black, Professor J. N. Morris,
Dr Cyril Smith, Professor Peter Townsend
Edited by Peter Townsend and Nick Davidson**

The Health Divide
Margaret Whitehead

PENGUIN BOOKS

PENGUIN BOOKS

Published by the Penguin Group
Penguin Books Ltd, 27 Wrights Lane, London W8 5TZ, England
Penguin Putnam Inc., 375 Hudson Street, New York, New York 10014, USA
Penguin Books Australia Ltd, Ringwood, Victoria, Australia
Penguin Books Canada Ltd, 10 Alcorn Avenue, Toronto, Ontario, Canada M4V 3B2
Penguin Books (NZ) Ltd, Private Bag 102902, NSMC, Auckland, New Zealand

Penguin Books Ltd, Registered Offices: Harmondsworth, Middlesex, England

First published in Pelican Books, containing *The Black Report* only 1982
This edition, comprising *The Black Report* and *The Health Divide*,
first published in Pelican Books 1988
Reprinted in Penguin Books 1990
Reprinted with revisions to *The Health Divide* 1992
10 9 8 7

Preface and Introduction copyright © Peter Townsend and Nick Davidson, 1982;
copyright © Peter Townsend, Nick Davidson and Margaret Whitehead, 1988, 1992
The Black Report copyright © Crown Copyright, 1980
The Health Divide copyright © Margaret Whitehead, 1988, 1992
All rights reserved

The moral right of the author of *The Health Divide* has been asserted

Typeset by DatIX International Limited, Bungay, Suffolk
Typeset in 9 on 11 pt Times
Printed in England by Clays Ltd, St Ives plc

Contents

Contents

List of Figures

List of Tables

The Health Divide

Preface

This publication brings together two major reports on inequalities in health, with an introduction which sets them both in context and spells out what needs to be done in the future.

The first is the 1980 Report of the Working Group on Inequalities in Health (known as the Black Report after its Chairman, Sir Douglas Black). A slightly slimmed-down version is presented here which has been read and approved in general terms by the original Working Group of four members: Sir Douglas Black (Chairman), Chief Scientist at the DHSS (to April 1978) and later President of the Royal College of Physicians; Professor J. N. Morris, Professor of Community Health in the University of London at the London School of Hygiene and Tropical Medicine; Dr Cyril Smith, Secretary of the Social Science Research Council; and Professor Peter Townsend, Professor of Sociology at the University of Essex, now Professor of Social Policy, University of Bristol. Dr Stuart Blume was Scientific Secretary to the Group, and the Administrative Secretary was Mr A. J. Forsdick. Dr Nicky Hart was seconded by the University of Essex to act as Research Fellow to the Group. Some statistical and technical details and elaborations of the text have been cut, but a large body of information remains in this version, which is nearly two-thirds of the length of the original report.

The terms of reference of the Working Group, which had been appointed in April 1977, were: (i) To assemble available information about the differences in health status among the social classes and about factors which might contribute to these, including relevant data from other industrial countries; (ii) To analyse this material in order to identify possible causal relationships, to examine the hypotheses that have been formulated and the testing of them, and to assess the implications for policy; and (iii) to suggest what further research should be initiated.

The second is a review of the studies on the same subject which have appeared since the Black Report was published in 1980. This review was originally published in 1987 by the Health Education Council under the title *The Health Divide: Inequalities in Health in the 1980s*. In this book the review has been substantially extended to expand the treatment of topics which attracted particular public interest, and this new edition adds evidence for the years up to and including 1992.

Acknowledgements

Peter Townsend and Nick Davidson would like to thank the Controller of Her Majesty's Stationery Office for permission to reproduce sections of the original Black Report. The Department of Health wish to make it clear that this permission in no way implies their authorization or approval of this book.

Margaret Whitehead expresses her thanks to the many people who have helped bring *The Health Divide* into the light of day, not least to David Player for identifying the need for the review and setting it in motion. Special thanks are due to the informal group who gave invaluable support and critical comment throughout, including Alex Scott-Samuel, Bobbie Jacobson, Peter Townsend, J. N. Morris, Madeleine Gantley, Pattie White and Richard Wilkinson. I am indebted to Anna Ritsatakis and Göran Dahlgren for sharing their insight on Europe with me. For the second edition, many people have been generous in sending me research material and putting up with my endless queries, including Peter Goldblatt, John Fox, Michael Marmot, Mildred Blaxter, Karen Dunnell, George Davey Smith, Alison Macfarlane, Shirley Goodwin, Denny Vågerö, David Leon and Sir Douglas Black. Fast and efficient back-up services were provided by Christina Coltart and her staff, Fiona Martin, Bron Jones and John Whitehead.

The author is grateful to the following for kindly giving permission to reproduce material from their publications in *The Health Divide*: the *Lancet* (fig. 6), the *British Medical Journal* (fig. 10), OPCS/HMSO (figs. 2, 7 and 11) and Peter Townsend (fig. 12).

Introduction to *Inequalities in Health*, 1992 Edition

Peter Townsend, Margaret Whitehead and Nick Davidson

The background to the Black Report

Inequalities in health are of concern to all countries and represent one of the biggest possible challenges to the conduct of government policy. This has become even more true in the extreme conditions of the 1990s than it was in the 1980s. The Black Report provides an example, which is rare anywhere in the world, of an attempt authorized by a government to explain trends in inequalities in health and to relate these to the policies intended to promote as well as restore health. Because it concentrates on Britain, the report also provides a commentary on the achievements of forty years of a National Health Service in reducing these inequalities, and, by the same token, a standard by which to judge the current attempts of the government to develop a new mixture of private and public services.

We begin with some necessary background to the preparation of the report. In its publications the Department of Health frequently acknowledged Britain's failure to match the improvement in health observed in some other countries and has admitted the relationship of this to persistent internal inequalities of health (for example, *Prevention and Health: Everybody's Business*, 1976, especially Chapters 1 and 4). In a speech on 27 March 1977, David Ennals, the Secretary of State for Social Services, stated:

... the crude differences in mortality rates between the various social classes are worrying. To take the extreme example, in 1971 the death rate for adult men in social class V (unskilled workers) was nearly twice that of adult men in social class I (professional workers) ... when you look at death rates for specific diseases the gap is even wider ... the first step towards remedial action is to put together what is already known about the problem ... it is a major challenge for the next ten or more years to try to narrow the gap in health standards between different social classes.

There were those like Sir John Brotherston, the Chief Medical Officer of Scotland, who in 1976 voiced the concern of many working in the health services and who had called the nation's attention to the social gulf in health which still existed and were calling for action. Many of those inside as well as outside the National Health Service were also aware that such inequalities might account for the failure of mortality rates in Britain to improve as far or as fast as in some other rich societies. Thus among the countries of the world having the lowest infant mortality Britain ranked eighth in 1960 but had slipped to fifteenth by 1978. In the latter year, the infant mortality rates for Hong Kong and Singapore were slightly lower than the rate for Britain (World Bank, 1981).

Accordingly, in 1977 the Secretary of State for Social Services of the Labour government appointed a Research Working Group to assess the national and international evidence and draw some of the implications for policy from the evidence on inequalities in health. The group consisted of Sir Douglas Black, formerly Chief Scientist at the Department of Health and at that time President of the Royal College of Physicians; Professor J. N. Morris of the Department of Community Health, London University; Dr Cyril Smith, Secretary of the Social Science Research Council; and Professor Peter Townsend, at that time Professor of Sociology at the University of Essex.

The Working Group completed its review in 1980. In essence it concluded that the poorer health experience of lower occupational groups applied at all stages of life. If the mortality rates of occupational class I (professional workers and members of their families) had applied to classes IV and V (partly skilled and unskilled manual workers and members of their families) during 1970–72, 74,000 lives of people aged under seventy-five would not have been lost. This estimate included nearly 10,000 children and 32,000 men aged 15 to 64. The class gradient seemed to be greater than in some comparable countries (though it must be said that the data for the United Kingdom almost invariably are fuller) and was becoming more marked. During the twenty years up to the early 1970s covered by the Black Report the mortality rates for both men and women aged 35 and over in occupational classes I and II had steadily diminished while those in IV and V changed very little or had even deteriorated.

What had gone wrong? The Working Group argued that much of the problem lay outside the scope of the NHS. Social and economic factors like income, work (or lack of it), environment, education, housing, transport and what are today called 'life-styles' all affect health and all favour the better-off. Yet they have largely remained outside the ambit of national health policy. The Group also found that those belonging to the manual classes made smaller use of the health care system in a number of different respects, yet needed it more. Its thirty-seven recommendations included giving effect to improvements in information, research and organization so that better plans might be drawn up, redressing the balance of the health care system so that more emphasis was given to prevention, primary care and community health, and, most important of all, radically improving the material conditions of life of poorer groups, especially children and people with disabilities, by increasing or introducing certain cash benefits, like child benefit, maternity grant and infant care allowance, and a comprehensive disablement allowance, and developing new schemes for day nurseries, ante-natal clinics, sheltered housing, home improvements, improved conditions at work and community services. So there were two policy thrusts:

(i) calling for a total and not merely a service-oriented approach to the problems of health;

(ii) calling for a radical overhaul of the balance of activity and proportionate distribution of resources within the health and associated services.

A frosty reception

In April 1980 the report was submitted to the Secretary of State of the new Conservative administration. But how were the findings received by the new government? Instead of being properly printed and published by the DHSS or HMSO, only 260 duplicated copies of the typescript were made available. No press release or press conference was arranged but a few copies were sent to selected journalists on the Friday before the August Bank Holiday – a date which virtually guaranteed the lowest possible level of publicity. However, this led to an unforeseen reaction when one of the journalists realized the significance of the report and persuaded the Working Group to call an alternative press conference which, because it was not allowed at the DHSS, was duly held at the Royal College of Physicians. Both the specialist and general press began to display a keen interest in the manner of the appearance of the report and its substance. The *Lancet* referred to the Secretary of State's reception as 'frosty', and pointed out that publicity for the report was 'in the lowest possible key' and that Ministers and officials gave the impression of being 'keen to reduce the report's impact to a minimum' (6 Septemper 1980, pp. 513 and 545). The *British Medical Journal* wrote angrily of the failure to take measured account of the work of experts and urged that the report 'should be examined more closely than Patrick Jenkin's foreword suggests that it has been' (6 September 1980, p. 690, and 20 September 1980, p. 763). It said that, like the Short Report of 1980, it had been discarded with 'shallow indifference' (20 December, p. 1663).

The Secretary of State's dismissal was brief. After stating in two short paragraphs the scope of the Working Group's task he went on:

> I must make it clear that additional expenditure on the scale which could result from the report's recommendations – the amount involved could be upwards of £2 billion a year – is quite unrealistic in present or any foreseeable economic circumstances, quite apart from any judgement that may be formed of the effectiveness of such expenditure in dealing with the problems identified. I cannot, therefore, endorse the Group's recommendations.

There followed vigorous correspondence within the pages of the medical journals. Interested trade unions, and the TUC itself, published summaries for their members (COHSE, 1980; TUC, 1981), and quite exceptional efforts were made by bodies connected with the health and welfare services to bring the evidence and arguments in the report to a wide audience (for example, Gray, 1981; Black, 1981a; Deitch, 1981; Watkins and Elton, 1981; Townsend, 1982; and Radical Community Medicine, 1980). In July 1981, following a special conference devoted to the report, the Association of Community Health Councils for England and Wales adopted a resolution which deplored 'the negative response of Her Majesty's Government ... We call upon the Secretary of State for Health and Social Services to present a report to Parliament and to allow a debate on the important issues raised. We call upon the Minister to press for the necessary resources to provide the services and to analyse and give guidance to health authorities on the many recommendations which have little or no revenue consequences.' Partly at the prompting of bodies like the Socialist Health Association, the Labour Party took an active interest in the report and a resolution passed in October at the annual conference called on the next Labour government to give priority to the implementation of its recommendations and, since many measures in the report could be introduced by local authorities, Labour representatives on councils and health authorities should 'do all in their power to ensure the implementation of these recommendations'. The General Secretary wrote to all Labour Groups accordingly (*Labour Weekly*, 4 December 1981).

By the spring of 1981 the Secretary of State found it necessary to elaborate on his first reaction and in a speech in Cardiff he drew attention to what he considered to be the report's three principal shortcomings. First, he claimed it did not adequately explain the causes of inequalities in health, and 'its enormously expensive' programme of recommendations could not therefore be accepted.

Secondly, Mr Jenkin argued that new evidence disproved the thesis that the working class suffered poorer access to the health services.

My department has looked at a whole lot more evidence. We have compared the total use of the health services and we have found that people with lower incomes, more of whom are likely to be elderly, tend to receive proportionately more services than the average for the population as a whole. Moreover, there is support for this finding from an independent source – a recent analysis by two researchers at Bath University who have used quite different data based on the General Household Survey. The widely held view, therefore, that the poor do not have a proper crack of the whip when it comes to using the National Health Service is simply not supported by the facts. This is a very encouraging finding. (Cardiff, 13 March 1981)

Thirdly, Mr Jenkin argued in his Cardiff speech, and elsewhere (Deitch, 1981, p. 159), that there was no evidence that more money would make any difference (so missing the main point of the report).

We have been spending money in ever-increasing amounts on the NHS for thirty years and it has not actually had much effect on increasing people's health. (Deitch, 1981, p. 159)

The first and third of these objections were reiterated by Sir George Young, the Under-Secretary of State for Health and Social Security, on 31 July, in a short adjournment debate in the House of Commons, when replying to Mr William Hamilton, MP for Fife Central, who had drawn attention to the report. He repeated the costs given in the report (for November 1979), but suggested that by November 1980 the costs would be up to £4.8 billion. He did, however, go on to say that the government agreed with some of the recommendations, particularly those on prevention. But, disappointingly, he did not seem to have recognized the gulf between the Working Group's concept of prevention and that of the government.

I see the progress being made by encouraging health education, personal responsibility for health, and encouraging voluntary organizations to help in the personal social services and helping to complement the NHS. That is the right way forward, given the difficult economic circumstances in which we find ourselves, rather than committing ourselves to the rather expensive solutions outlined by the Black Report, which we are not absolutely convinced would deliver the goods. (*British Medical Journal*, 22 August 1981)

All three objections raised by government Ministers – explanation, access and money – were strongly contested by the members of the Working Group in the early years after the initial publication, who not only reaffirmed the original findings, but called attention to new evidence that had become available since the publication of the report (Black, 1981a and 1981b; Morris, 1980a, 1980b and 1980c; Townsend, 1982).

Members of the Working Group were wary of claiming too much for their analysis of the *causes* of inequalities in health. Too little work of a wide-ranging kind on different age groups, and on the interrelationships between mortality or, even more, morbidity, and social and economic as well as biological and clinical factors has been carried out. But the Working Group were convinced that it was difficult to begin to explain the pattern of inequalities except by invoking material deprivation as a key concept. In looking at the causes of death for different age-groups where differences between the classes are at their greatest, it is particularly difficult to deny the relevance of socio-economic variables. While it is as yet often impossible to pinpoint exactly how poverty and socio-economic circumstances *cause* ill-health and death, there is little doubt about the kind of strategy which deserves to be pursued – a theme we shall return to later when policies are discussed.

The review of evidence on causes of inequalities and on access to the NHS has been brought up to date in the revised 1992 edition of *The Health Divide* in this volume, and such evidence clearly confirms the main conclusions drawn in the Black Report. The one study quoted by the Secretary of State to cast doubt on the health service findings has itself been severely criticized (see p. 282). *The Health Divide* also charts the progress of the Black Report's recommendations up to the present day, so let us now turn to the treatment that that report received at the hands of the media, the politicians and the professionals.

The reception to *The Health Divide*

To understand some of the responses to the publication of *The Health Divide* it is necessary to know something of the events leading up to it.

In January 1986 the Health Education Council's Director General, David Player, commissioned Margaret Whitehead to update the evidence on inequalities in health which had accumulated since 1980 and to assess the progress made on the thirty-seven recommendations of the Black Report. This update was prepared during 1986 and finally published in March 1987 as an HEC occasional report. But in the intervening months between commission and publication there were two unforeseen developments: plans were announced to disband the HEC from 31 March 1987, and many political commentators were convinced that an early General Election would be called.

The plans to disband the Health Education Council (which was theoretically an independent body funded by the DHSS) came as a complete surprise to almost everybody – staff, Council members and fellow professionals in the health services alike. The Secretary of State for Social Services, Norman Fowler, announced in November 1986 the plan to dissolve the HEC, which had been responsible for a wide range of health education programmes at a national level, and to reconstitute a special Health Education Authority within the NHS. Some members of staff would be transferred automatically to the new Authority, but senior members would be asked to re-apply for the top posts. The Authority was to carry on the responsibilities of the old HEC but also take over responsibility from the Department of Health for the national education programme on AIDS, with an extra £20 million budget earmarked for that purpose.

There was a very mixed reception to this announcement. Some saw it as a logical step identifying health education firmly as a proprity and also as a direct responsibility of the NHS, with the new body more likely to be responsive to the needs of the various health authorities within the service. However, grave doubts were expressed in other quarters, voiced most strongly by the medical press and Labour and Alliance MPs. There were fears that this move was another attempt to subdue independent criticism of official policies voiced by bodies like the HEC in the 1980s. Professional and consumer disquiet would have smaller influence and the commercial interests of big business, entrenched among parliamentary and ministerial representatives, would tend to dominate.

Alliance MPs suggested to the Health Minister that 'the termination of the HEC had far more to do than Ministers admitted with its high-profile campaigning on issues such as smoking, drinking, and diet, which had offended great interests the government preferred to keep sweet' (*Lancet*, 1987a).

The expected election, of course, heightened sensitivity to any report likely to pose difficult questions about the government's handling of policy.

History repeats itself

It was against this background that *The Health Divide* was launched on Tuesday, 24 March. Pre-publication copies were sent to Regional and District Health Authorities and Community Health Councils. The Academic and popular press were also circulated with the report over the previous weekend and were invited to a briefing on the afternoon of the 24th. A panel of distinguished experts in the field, some of whom had acted as scientific advisers in the preparation of the report, had agreed to take part and answer questions on aspects of their research featured in *The Health Divide*. The panel consisted of two of the original members of the Working Group for the Black Report – Sir Douglas Black and Professor Peter Townsend, together with Professor John Fox, Professor Michael Marmot, Dr David Player and Dr Alex Scott-Samuel, as well as the report's author.

Television, radio and national press representatives were already showing great interest and arranging interviews when the Chairman of the HEC, Sir Brian Bailey, decided to cancel the press briefing at the Council offices an hour before it was due to begin. Media interest was thereby heightened. Sir Brian was quoted by the *Independent* as saying the report was 'political dynamite in an election year', and he issued a statement explaining that it was necessary to postpone the briefing until the full Council was able to consider this 'important and possibly controversial document'.

Members of the panel, who had already assembled, decided to proceed with the press briefing at the nearby offices of the Disability Alliance. The Director General of the HEC and his staff, however, were instructed by Sir Brian not to attend. During the briefing some journalists who had also been present at the Black Report's alternative conference nearly seven years earlier admitted to experiencing a distinct feeling of *déjà vu* – in the event, both reports had been similarly treated. This helps to explain the huge media coverage. The report and the manner of its launch provided the leading story that evening on Channel 4 news and it was featured prominently on ITV and BBC television and radio news programmes. By the next morning the story was on the front pages of *The Times*, the *Guardian*, the *Independent* and the *Daily Mirror*, and virtually all the other national papers carried features or leaders on the report. The *Independent* even started a series of daily extracts from it. In the weeks that followed a wide range of regional newspapers took up the story, as did the medical and nursing journals and a variety of discussion and phone-in programmes from the BBC World Service to the Jimmy Young Show. But what exactly were they saying? The majority presented the cancellation of the press conference as an attempted cover-up of unpalatable information about the nation's health and duly brought the information to the attention of readers. Others, like *The Times*, saw the report more as a devastating 'final salvo' from David Player to the government as the HEC was about to be disbanded. The *News of the World* saw more sinister undertones in it and went so far as to suggest that the whole affair was part of a plot by an anti-government group to 'hijack' the HEC!

More controversy was generated when it was discovered that an official from the Department of Health had been in touch with the Chairman of the HEC about the report the night before the conference was cancelled. Attention was turned to possible intervention from the Department or even government Ministers. The Prime Minister was challenged in the House of Commons and denied any involvement by Ministers or officials. The Department agreed that there had been contact but 'there was no pressure'. Others argued that even if Sir Brian had acted entirely of his own accord, he could be accused of trying to blunt the report's political impact (*Lancet*, 1987b).

By 30 March all available copies of *The Health Divide* had been distributed and an uncharacteristic row broke out in the House of Lords because Members of the House could not obtain copies for a major debate on the NHS scheduled for 1 April. Baroness Seear argued that 'unless this report is published, we are all bound to assume that there are things that the government do not wish the public to see' (Seear, 1987). Viscount Whitelaw calmed the peers by promising to look into the whole matter of publication. A rush reprint was ordered and copies were also made available to the Lords for their debate. In the House of Commons a debate on 6 April on social and economic inequalities gave a great deal of prominence to health inequalities.

Political controversy about the reports

Because of the uproar created upon its publication, *The Health Divide* was read by a much wider audience than would otherwise have been expected, and the Black Report's findings were examined once again. Although there was much misquoting of the evidence, concern about the inequalities in health was expressed in many quarters. Twenty-six MPs put down a Commons motion calling for a programme recognizing the relationship between poverty and poor health.

In the House of Lords it was obvious that some peers had understood fully the fundamental issues involved. A common response of the government Ministers questioned about the action to be taken on inequalities in health was to divert attention to improvements in overall health in the United Kingdom, with rising life expectancy and falling infant mortality. These improvements were in fact acknowledged in both reports (pp. 57–62 and 264), but that is not the point at issue. Improvements in the health of the poor have failed to keep up with improvements enjoyed by the prosperous – a detail which is hidden when only overall health trends are quoted. Lord Kilmarnock seized on the significance of this and expressed it eloquently in the House of Lords debate:

'Just as the gap between the richest and the poorest has increased within an overall increased national income and the plight of the homeless has become worse within an overall pattern of increased home-ownership, so health inequalities have increased . . . It is all part of the same pattern.' (Kilmarnock, 1987)

We would argue that the improved health of the nation as a whole should not be used as an excuse for inaction on the health problems affecting substantial sections of, indeed many millions within, the population.

In the House of Commons attempts were made to discredit the reports by suggesting that they were biased and did not reflect mainstream scientific opinion. A former Under-Secretary of State for Health, Mr Ray Whitney, observed:

'These issues can be approached from a class bias, a fascination with a class division of society which is basically a Marxist approach . . . Marxism is entirely based on this class approach and is carefully reflected in the Black Report and *The Health Divide* . . . the answer is not to impose on society the socialism that everyone else has rejected, and seemingly only the few authors of these reports and a few left-behind diehards on the Opposition Benches still believe in.' (Whitney, 1987a)

Other MPs reminded this former Minister that the Archbishop of Canterbury's commission on 'Faith in the City' had likewise been labelled Marxist when it raised the issues of poverty and deprivation in the cities.

This illustrates one type of political reaction made throughout the decade to scientific conclusions which are found to be unpalatable. Two familiar points need to be made. Firstly, against the charge of bias can be set testimonies to the unbiased nature of the reports. In the Lords debate, for instance, much was made of the fairness of *The Health Divide*, referred to as 'scrupulously fair' (Lord Kilmarnock); 'a worthy successor to the Black Report, an objective account' (Lord Rea). A *Lancet* leader stressed that *The Health Divide* was not mere polemic but 'a critical scientific review . . . properly careful when inferring causation' (*Lancet*, 1987c). Secondly, against the suggestion that the reports are out of touch with scientific opinion can be set the hundreds of scientific and statistical studies listed on pages 401–37. As we shall emphasize later, recommendations stemming from the two reports are not exceptional or unrepresentative but very much in line with the strategies running through many other recent reports from a large number of independent sources, including those from the British Medical Association, the Faculty of Public Health Medicine and the World Health Organization, not to mention several stemming from the Department of Health itself. Many of the recommendations could be said to reflect the general consensus among specialists in the field of health promotion.

Another common response from Ministers was to accept that health differences exist but to suggest that these differences were due to individual behaviour patterns, like smoking, heavy drinking and lack of exercise, rather than to poverty or other forms of deprivation – an approach commonly referred to as 'victim-blaming' in the literature. For example, the former Under-Secretary of State for Health, Ray Whitney, suggested that both reports ignored the evidence on life-styles and concentrated on poverty. 'Those rates do not mean that those diseases are a function of poverty. Other reasons and issues are neglected by those who write these reports and those who pounce on them and seek to benefit politically from them' (Whitney, 1987b). Such a criticism requires detailed refutation.

First, inspection of pp. 110–15 of the Black Report and pp. 316–26 of *The Health Divide* will show that life-style factors are discussed in both reports. The evidence is illustrated in various tables and the influence of behaviour acknowledged: 'the evidence outlined above suggests that differences in life-style could indeed account for some of the class differential in health' (p. 323). However, the point is also made in both reports (which some politicians seem to have missed) that life-style factors, while explaining some of the health differences observed, cannot adequately explain them all. This can be said to be a continuing theme of scientific reports. Attention is drawn to all the causes of death showing a marked class gradient which do not appear to be linked to smoking, alcohol abuse or any other known risk factor. Studies are also quoted which control for life-style factors, yet the gradient in health remains marked. In the Whitehall study (p. 324), for example, the difference in mortality from coronary heart disease between grades of the Civil Service was reduced by less than a third when known risk factors were controlled for. The Alameda County study (p. 324) also showed a small reduction in the difference in the survival chances of rich and poor when thirteen risk factors were controlled for, yet most of the differential remained. While some of the links between deprivation and ill-health are still very poorly understood, life-style is clearly far from being the whole answer. Even where life-style is implicated it cannot be assumed that choice of life-style is completely voluntary in the way ordinarily believed. Groups and upbringing, but also commercial advertising and interventionist policies of the state, exert a major hold over individual behaviour. Evidence from in-depth studies (pp. 327–34) also suggests that some people have more freedom than others by virtue of their individual situation and circumstances to choose a healthy life-style, the unlucky ones being restrained from adopting a healthier life, even when they would wish to do so, by income, housing, work and other social constraints. Such evidence has led some observers to criticize certain health education campaigns for putting all the emphasis on individual responsibility while neglecting the government's responsibility to develop policies to support the desired life-style changes. For example, on the 1987 'Look after your Heart' campaign Dr Tim Lang of the London Food Commission was quoted as saying, 'instead of exhorting people to eat better, smoke less and exercise more, Ministers should make it easier for them to improve their health – that means tackling poverty by improving welfare benefits, improving the quality of food and making the industry tell people what it puts in their food' (*Guardian*, 22 April 1987).

Individual and state accountability

This problem of distinguishing between individual and corporate or government responsibility for health can be illustrated by one event in 1986. The publication by the Northern Regional Health Authority of a report about inequalities of health in the North (Townsend, Phillimore and Beattie, 1986) happened to coincide with a visit to Newcastle by a newly appointed junior Health Minister, Mrs Edwina Currie, who was quoted by the *Daily Telegraph*, the *Guardian* and other newspapers as having 'dismissed' or 'rejected' the report's link between ill-health and material deprivation or poverty: 'I honestly don't think it has anything to do with poverty. The problem very often for many people is just ignorance ... and failing to realize they do have some control over their own lives.' Her comments provoked widespread controversy, and the prevalence of unhealthy dietary practices and heavy smoking and drinking in the North were at the centre of that controversy for several weeks. Mrs Currie subsequently had second thoughts, but these attracted rather less attention. In an article in the *Evening Chronicle* (10 October 1986) she wrote: 'Nor would I ever deny the links between poverty, unemployment and ill-health ... What bothers me is that this is too simple an explanation. We may be ignoring the possibilities of improving people's health ... by encouraging a greater awareness of other links between smoking, heavy drinking and illness.' That is plainly a very different position, and equally carries profound implications for government interpretations of the problems of the nation's health and its sponsorship of scientific research.

No one would deny that individual options in life-style substantially affect outcomes in health – though they can of course be influenced in turn by education, family, the press, commerce and other institutions. The question is whether the scientific and political establishment may be said to be taking sufficiently seriously the evidence that material deprivation accounts for much the largest part of variations in health outcomes. The

Working Group under Sir Douglas Black had concluded that, while genetic and cultural or behavioural explanations played their part, the predominant or governing explanation for inequalities in health lay in material deprivation. For statisticians perhaps the most impressive finding of the study of 678 wards in the North was that 65 per cent of the variation in ill-health, as measured not only by deaths but also permanent sickness and low-weight births, could be 'explained' (in regression analyses) by indicators of material deprivation. That finding needs to be followed up in depth, using research strategies very different from those of the laboratory and the symptomatology of the individual, to pin down both the factors within 'material deprivation' which are most at issue for different forms of ill-health, and the specific policies which can reduce particular effects of deprivation. None the less, the finding helps to confirm what should be the government's first priority in any strategy designed to improve health, and puts into proportion the scope for complementary individual action with the same aim.

Majority and minority scientific opinion

In contrast to the hostile reception from government, the health professions and the research community have taken the findings of the two reports seriously. There is widespread agreement on three main premises in the reports: that in absolute terms the standards of health of the population as a whole have improved since the Second World War; that despite that improvement serious social inequalities in health have persisted; and that socio-economic factors have played an important part in maintaining and even increasing these differentials.

However, a few social scientists have questioned the finding that the health gap between the rich and poor has widened since the war. They have expressed to an undue extent reservations about the usefulness of occupational class as a social indicator when making comparisons of health over long time-spans. They have minimized the findings about the class differentials in health or the trends in those differentials on a variety of grounds and have put forward an alternative measure not of differences of ill-health or mortality between classes or rich and poor but of differences in the age of death of people dying in different years (LeGrand, 1985; LeGrand and Rabin, 1986; Illsley, 1986, 1987a, 1987b; Illsley and LeGrand, 1986; LeGrand, 1987). The problems of using occupational class in studies of health trends are widely appreciated and are set out in the Black Report (pp. 39–41) and *The Health Divide* (pp. 265–7). However, as there has recently been much confusion in reporting this issue, even in professional journals, some of the main arguments will be examined again here.

Occupational class has been used for many years as a convenient indicator of the standards of living and way of life of different groups and has been used to represent 'social' class. A person's named occupation is basically a pragmatic guide to that person's social position and his or her likely command over resources, and as such has its limitations. It is only an approximate indicator of family living standards or social position. Some objections to its use for measuring trends are related to the changes successive Registrars General have made in allocating occupations to different classes. Others are related to structural shifts in the pattern of employment over the past fifty years, which have led to more non-manual and fewer manual jobs. But these changes can be monitored and, by applying strict estimation procedures, generalizations about quantitative trends can reliably be made. Doubts have been raised particularly about studies which only compare classes I and V, the two extremes of the social range, covering a small proportion of the population. In the latest report on mortality, for example, by the Registrar General, attention was called to the uncertain classification of some occupations in class V. But, like some of the residual problems in measuring the national income, such problems have to be put into proportion, and can be controlled. These are legitimate reasons for concern, and *The Health Divide* specifies recent studies which have re-examined the figures with these problems in mind. The studies assess inequalities across all classes, not just between the extremes, and weight each according to its share of the population. To compensate for classification changes the analyses were also checked by following only those occupations which could be consistently traced throughout the time-span. Using such techniques, health inequality was found to have increased for adults of working age over the years from 1931 to 1971, confirming the original observations of the Black Report. A further study (Marmot and McDowall, 1986, quoted on p. 271) which reported a widening health gap between manual and non-manual classes from 1971–2 to 1979–83 also noted the measurement problems and re-evaluated the results accordingly. The authors concluded that neither changes in classification nor the 4 per cent shift in the population from manual to non-manual occupations during the decade could account for the widening of the health gap which they observed.

Illsley and LeGrand have also raised objections to studies based only on people aged under 65, partly because the proportion of deaths in this age range has changed over the past fifty years, making comparisons difficult, and partly because a large proportion of deaths now take place over the age of 65 and the results found in the under-65s may not apply to the older age-groups. Two responses have been made to this objection. Firstly, it is still very important to consider deaths under the age of 65. Even though they are a minority they are premature deaths, and in many cases they can also be regarded as the most preventable. It is customary in many areas of preventive medicine and health promotion to focus on premature deaths for this very reason. Secondly, new evidence available on the health of people aged over 65 tends to confirm the pattern of inequality found among younger people.

The familiar occupational class gradient in mortality has now been established securely for those aged 65–75 and even for those aged 75 plus (see p. 231). Rates of chronic sickness are higher in manual than in non-manual socio-economic groups at ages over 65 and the gap between the two widened significantly over the years 1974 to 1984. The 1986 Health and Life-Style Survey confirmed the social pattern of chronic disease and disability in older people in different socio-economic and income groups. Such evidence is in line with the findings at younger ages. There is certainly no evidence to suggest that the social pattern of health suddenly reverses after age 65.

Most confusion has arisen over the statistical methods for studying the health of populations. The method of measuring trends in the distribution of age at death which, following their critique of occupational class, Illsley and LeGrand have put forward has been widely misinterpreted in the press as an alternative way of measuring social inequalities in health. This statistical patterning of deaths by age appears to show a steady decrease in inequality since the 1920s, in contrast to the prevailing social or occupational class evidence. In fact it does not measure differences between social classes or between rich and poor at all. It measures only the variation in the age of death of individuals in the population. LeGrand makes it quite clear that he considers his approach to be complementary to that taken by the Black Working Group, rather than a competing or conflicting approach. Latterly the two authors have diverged in their interpretation of the 'age-at-death' methodology. Illsley still believes it challenges the thesis of a widening inequality in health (Illsley, 1987). However, LeGrand concludes that the techniques of measuring inequalities in age of death 'do not answer the same kinds of questions' as comparisons between social classes 'and therefore should be viewed as complements to them, not as substitutes'. Although this method shows that the variation in the age of death is decreasing over the population as a whole, it cannot help us with the question of whether social inequalities in death are changing too. As the British Medical Association comments, 'it makes no distinction between random variations in life-span and variations that are due to different people's experience of deprivation or social inequality' (BMA, 1987).

Some social scientists have countered the conclusions drawn from the 'age-at-death' methodology in specific terms (see, in particular, Wilkinson, 1986, 1987; Hart, 1987).

What has been happening since the 1920s is a dramatic decrease in the infectious and respiratory diseases which caused high mortality in child-hood and fell most heavily on the poor. The variation in the age of death would be expected to decrease as a result. But the diseases which predomin-ate today, the degenerative diseases of middle and old age, still affect the poor sections of society more than the rich, and some of them to an even greater extent proportionately than they did, though Illsley and LeGrand's calculations would not be able to detect this situation. In theory it would be possible for the variation in the age of death of *individuals* to decrease over the same period as *social* inequalities in death increased. In short, the research on life-span changes should not be regarded as challenging the conclusions of the Black Report and *The Health Divide* but treated on its own merits in addressing a limited and different set of questions. The debate has continued into the 1990s (Klein, 1988 and 1991; Townsend, 1990 and 1991; Strong 1990).

There are of course respects in which differences between the parties to the debate cannot be kept within the rational bounds of scientific discourse. Ideological and political investment in the outcomes, as well as the assump-tions, is very high. But there continue to be specialized discoveries and technical commentaries which add to the principal conclusions of the Black Report and the Health Divide. Thus, one commentary shows the Gini coefficient (used by those believing inequalities have not widened) is an inappropriate measure of social inequalities of health (Wagstaff et al., 1991, *The Health Divide*, Chapter 3).

Action: local, organizational and national

A leader in the *British Medical Journal* has likened the Black Report to the Bible: 'much quoted, occasionally read and largely ignored when it comes to action' (*British Medical Journal*, 1986). That may be true of government, but not in some other respects.

In *The Health Divide* the progress made on the thirty-seven recommenda-tions of the Black Report is assessed and a distinct lack of action at national and central level is apparent. However, activity was stimulated at the grass-roots level and in research as a result of the Black Report. Initiatives have been taken by people in the health services, local govern-ment, voluntary agencies and research units around the country. The professional bodies representing members in the health and social services have also undertaken a range of activities, as the accounts on pp. 357–64 and 391–2 show. Nevertheless, without a national commitment all this has, understandably, had piecemeal results.

With the publication of *The Health Divide*, inequalities in health were once again put firmly on the agenda. It has been the theme of numerous professional conferences, and meetings sponsored by community health councils throughout the country. The correspondence columns of the medical journals include many references, briefing papers on the issue have been prepared by many of the agencies, including new public health departments, and petitions to the Health Education Authority have been prepared.

Most discussion centres not on the evidence, which by and large is accepted, but what action would be appropriate. This is plainly of crucial importance and the rest of this introduction looks at economic options, at health care policy, and at the implications of a wider intersectoral strategy.

The economics of choosing health

Successive governments have argued that the country cannot afford to implement the Black Report's recommendations. This is a question of both priorities and scale. In a wealthy country like Britain money for health is only not there if it is being spent on something else – like defence, roads or the marketing of consumer goods. Underlying the Working Group's judgement of the measures which might be possible in the current political and economic climate there runs a powerful argument: that a positive health strategy depends on observing different political and economic priorities and determining to gradually reconstruct certain institutions. The choice of priorities is partly a question of arguing that health in the broadest sense deserves to have a higher place in the claims that can be made on a nation's resources, partly that this in turn will necessarily involve spreading wealth around more equally than has been customary in Britain, and partly that expenditure on health encourages national production and hence national wealth *and* welfare. Substantial expenditure on a programme for health represents necessary national investment in a thriving economy.

Successive governments seem disinclined to accept investment in health as a necessary assumption of planning. The welfare state was born at a time when public expenditure was seen as an aid or adjunct to economic growth, and the pioneers of the welfare state, in making a case for spending some public money on welfare, did so without any doubt that welfare expenditure was conditional on that growth taking place – a desirable spin-off. It was not seen, except in the most incidental sense, as laying the necessary basis for that growth. Welfare expenditure came to be regarded as something different from economic growth and efficiency – at best neutral, at worst a potential 'burden' on growth.

Since then, governments of all political persuasions have repeated the same message, over and over again. Yet that message depends on inadequate theory. According to orthodox neo-classical economic theory, economic growth is a measure of the increase in the value of the sum total of goods and services that are sold by either a company or a national economy. And that is all. Thus, every extra unit produced and sold from a factory is a contribution to the growth of that factory and, in as much as that factory is part of the national economy, to the growth of the national economy. But suppose that in increasing the number of units sold safety standards are reduced, thereby increasing the number of industrial injuries and also raising the levels of stress among the workforce, making work less 'fulfilling' for participating individuals and reducing work satisfaction (and *potential* productivity). This 'hidden cost', known as an 'externality' in mainstream economics, is not deducted or in any way connected with the increased aggregate 'wealth' generated by that factory. Yet the community as a whole will have to meet the cost of treating and caring for the casualties, as well as those regarded as incapable of, or prohibited from, entering the labour force, which must imply some decrease in overall well-being. The apparent wealth generated by an industrial unit and the actual wealth taking into account such externalities are therefore two very different measures.

More careful examination of the evidence for and against the traditional theory demonstrates the importance of basic public services in many societies with above average levels of economic growth. There is a lot of support in the 1990s for 'trickle-up' rather than for 'trickle-down' theories. (Newman and Thomson, 1989; Quick and Wilkinson, 1991). Richard Titmuss argued that social costs, 'if allowed to lie where they fall, may result in larger costs in the shape of physical or psychological handicaps, destitution, deprived children, ill-educated workers unable or unwilling to acquire new skills and a general slackening in the sense of social involvement'.

Economic and social development are intertwined in ways which still require analysis. Whether we consider the urban riots in Britain in the early 1980s and 1990s, underfunding of public housing and the homeless throughout the decades, or the millions of people who are unemployed, social costs can be very real costs, even if not easily measurable in cash. Cost-benefit analysis and output budgeting cannot be taken very far. It is hard to quantify social costs. The technical wizardry of accountants, actuaries, statisticians and econometricians is hard to apply to even a fraction of the daunting problems of measuring the costs of the ill-health and health of an entire population. It is difficult to put a cost on injury, pain, discomfort or dissatisfaction, as well as premature death, and to measure matters pertinent to 'positive' health, such as range of physical and mental activity, degree of social integration, the quality of the roles people play and their performance in the jobs they undertake, or extent of personal fulfilment. A population with health is one with abundant energies and powers of improvisation as well as one with high standards of skill, education and social experience. Qualitative judgements as well as quantitative measures of health have to be combined.

There is a sense in which the amount a nation can afford to spend on the pursuit of health is what it *chooses* to spend. This point is emphasized by developments resulting from changes in central and eastern Europe, leading to improvements in East–West relations. In 1991, the Stockholm Initiative on Global Security and Governance concluded that the trend towards disarmament in industrial countries could release as much as $1,000 billion to $2,000 billion during the course of the 1990s. Countries that have *chosen* to spend vast amounts on military expenditure can now *choose* to invest these savings in the promotion of health and social development, if they so wish.

Certainly, there is an impressive case to be made – whether by comparison with other equally rich societies, the demonstrated need in our own society, or the health benefits which accrue from reducing inequality – for a more generous national commitment of resources to lessening inequality.

Funding and planning health services

These arguments, however, are not in favour today. Recent governments have reiterated their belief in giving priority to economic growth as a prerequisite for spending anything more on health and welfare. One result of this is that funding for health and welfare services has continued to be tight. While successive governments have continued to insist that funding of the NHS is well ahead of inflation, a closer examination of the figures reveals a mixed story.

From Table A it can be seen that over the decade to 1991 the total spending on the NHS appeared to have increased by 43 per cent when general inflation alone is taken into account. However, as the costs of health care goods and services have risen faster than general inflation, allowance needs to be made for this, and the increase in spending over the

Table A: *Changes in total spending on the NHS, 1978–79 to 1990–91*

Estimated changes in real spending	*% change over decade*
1. Allowing for general inflation (RPI)	+43
2. Allowing for inflation as applied to NHS goods and services	+19
3. Allowing for demographic changes and new technology	+1

Source: Adapted from Radical Statistics Health Group (1992).

decade is thereby reduced to 19 per cent. When, in addition, demographic changes and the introduction of new technology are taken into account, the increase over the same period amounts to 1 per cent (Radical Statistics Health Group, 1992). The technical adjustments that can be made to reach some conclusions on the trends in real spending on the health services are of course incomplete. Table A summarizes what can be deduced from official statistics. What has to be remembered is that changes in need such as, for example, more in a population having severe ill-health or disability, are not taken into account. The extra expense of introducing successive NHS reforms and management initiatives are also not included. Allowing for all these factors, it would be difficult to sustain the argument that an increased commitment to services for patients had been made.

The second point that needs to be made is that the gross figures for total spending on the NHS ignore the fact that funds are unevenly distributed across the country. Since the mid 1970s, the DHSS has been engaged in an exercise designed to foster greater equality in health resources in the different regions of the country. This had its origins in the recommendations of the Resource Allocation Working Party (RAWP) which were designed to channel extra resources to those parts of the country which have been historically neglected, primarily the North and the Midlands. But in a period of virtually static growth the only way this redistribution can take place is if some areas gain *at the expense of others*. This is what has happened. The Thames regions in particular have suffered net falls in their budgets in order that the historically poorer regions, like Trent and Northern, can continue to grow. The National Association of Health Authorities (1986), in a profile of one of the Thames regions, recorded:

The RAWP allocation process has led to planned reductions in real resources of up to 0.3 per cent per year. However, by far the largest proportion of reductions in resources came from unplanned and therefore unanticipated factors. These unplanned reductions stemmed from the consequences of pay award shortfalls and the recurring loss of the 1983/4 public expenditure cuts. Therefore during the period 1982/3 to 1985/6, the real reduction in resources amounted to approximately 3 per cent of total resources.

It can be seen that, far from experiencing an increase in resources, some parts of the country have had a decrease. This situation continued to worsen throughout the 1980s and was set to come to crisis point with the introduction of the internal market in the latest NHS reforms. In anticipation of this, the King's Fund set up a London Commission in 1990, at a cost of £500,000, to examine the issue of the health care needs of the capital up to the year 2010. A year later, the Government announced a review with a similar remit, to report in 1992. The King's Fund Commission report, published in June 1992, has concluded that there would be a sharp decline in the number of patients referred to London hospitals with the internal market arrangements, and there was a real risk of indiscriminate attrition of hospital services: the excellent just as likely to go to the wall as the mediocre. At the same time, it found that there were great deficiencies in the provision of GP and community nursing services which would get even worse if present trends continued (King's Fund, 1992). What was needed, the report argued, was a long-term strategic approach, with the planned closure of selected hospital beds over many years, the reorganization of other specialist centres at appropriate sites, and a great expansion of community and primary health services.

However, although the proposals make sense, it is difficult to see how they could be implemented within the new market structures introduced into the NHS. How could hospital changes be planned, for instance, when several hospitals in the city had been allowed to become independent trusts, with freedom to go in their own direction? Would some agree to close themselves if necessary? The same problems arise with GP fundholders. Some of the market-oriented solutions adopted over the past five years would have to be halted or reversed for coherent planning on the necessary scale to take place. And these problems are not confined to London, but apply equally to other major cities.

Another potential problem with the King's Fund proposals is that history might repeat itself, and hospital beds will be closed long before the necessary services in the community are available, if at all. The experience with long-stay mental illness beds acts as a timely reminder of what could happen. For people with mental illness, the average number of beds available daily in long-stay hospitals in England fell by 27,000 from 1980 to 1990, whereas the number of places in local authority, private and voluntary hostels and homes increased by only 5840 during the same period

(Radical Statistics Health Group, 1992). It would be a disaster for Londoners if a similar pattern of events unfolded over the next decade in relation to all the health services in the capital. This is particularly important in the light of another King's Fund report on London which shows the close correlation between adverse material circumstances and all measures of poor health (Benzeval *et al.*, 1992).

What are needed for the NHS throughout the country are resource allocation arrangements that make allowance for equity considerations, and mechanisms in place to make it possible to plan strategically for the equitable distribution of services.

Efficiency and equity

One positive development in the NHS reforms – planning health care on the basis of an assessment of the health needs of a given population – has the potential to focus more attention on action to reduce inequalities in health. For instance, it could lead to the identification of groups in the population with poorer health than the average, who could be considered in need of extra attention and help to bring up their standard of health closer to the more favourable level of the rest of the population. This could lead to plans being drawn up to reduce the identified inequalities in health, with the action the local health services could take clearly specified, together with plans for awareness raising and co-operation with agencies outside the NHS. This positive development, however, is in danger of foundering if it gets tangled up in the growing business ethos which has permeated the NHS in recent years. It is worth looking at how this business ethos has developed within the service to understand its implications.

The year 1979 saw the election of a Conservative government strongly committed to the values of the market-place and private enterprise. It was simultaneously impressed and embarrassed by reports at the time which suggested that the public services in general, and the NHS in particular, were 'out of control'. The House of Commons Public Accounts Committee, for instance, published a highly critical report of the management and administration of the health service which questioned whether the service was susceptible to normal managerial controls.

As on other occasions the government turned to the private sector and the business community for advice, and invited Roy Griffiths, Managing Director of the Sainsbury supermarket chain, to review the entire administration of the NHS. The Griffiths team was struck by what it saw as an apparent lack of clearly identified leaders and lines of management authority. They argued that the absence of overall general managers meant that, 'there is no driving force seeking and accepting direct and personal responsibility for developing management plans, securing their implementation and monitoring actual achievement'. They said that, coming from a business environment, they were surprised to find that, 'rarely are precise management objectives set; there is little measurement of health output; clinical evaluation of particular practices is by no means common and economic evaluation of these practices is extremely rare'.

The result was a series of recommendations, the most important of which were the adoption of a management structure and management techniques common in the business and commercial world. The existing system of 'consensus management', whereby administrators and health care professionals shared the task of running the health service, would be replaced by a service of professional general managers who would not only assume overall control of the service, but would have the task of introducing clearer planning guidelines and performance targets and regularly monitoring progress towards these targets. The proposals were rapidly accepted by the government.

But perhaps more important than the detailed proposals themselves, the Griffiths Report represented the triumph of a set of beliefs about what was important and how things should be done. It thrust management and management preoccupations to the very centre of NHS thinking, pushing aside, or at least subordinating, the arguably less clearly formulated collection of ideas about service and the public good which had hitherto provided the dominant ethos.

The results are still working their way through the service, but already it is possible to discern a distinct shift in thinking. Modern management is about establishing procedures in which activity can be measured against clearly defined objectives. It involves breaking down an activity into inputs and outputs and developing procedures for monitoring the achievement of one against the other. But to do this it becomes essential to be able to measure activity, and in something as complex as health care this cannot be done without ignoring key aspects of treatment and recovery and oversimplifying measures of outcome. In an attempt to come to grips with the problems, the NHS has developed a series of indicators of its performance: how many people pass through a hospital bed in a year; how many operations are performed; and how much it costs to keep a patient in hospital for a day. There are now several thousand of these performance indicators, as they are called, covering almost every area of activity. They have been put on to computer disks so that a health authority can look up its own performance and, more importantly, can compare this with other districts.

But what exactly is being measured and what is being left out in this attempt to create a 'scientific' management ethos for the health service? The difficulty revolves around the fact that performance indicators as management tools have been developed in a business environment where inputs and outputs can be readily quantified and measured. It is by no means clear that they are so easily extended to something like health provision which, as much as anything else, is also about qualitative issues. It is of limited use to know how many patients are passing through a hospital bed each year if we don't also know the outcome of their treatment. Activity, in the case of health care, does not necessarily equal beneficial activity, and performance indicators put us in the difficult position of being unable to say whether an increase in activity is actually improving the nation's health.

It is easy to forget, in all the management jargon, what is implied. The significance of the new scientific, business, ethos is that it has shifted attention away from a concern with the overall quantity and quality of the service being provided to a preoccupation with how resources can best (most productively) be used. The objectives are changing. What counts are service outputs – so many extra operations, so many extra patients treated. In other words, as inputs become virtually static, the focus of attention has shifted from the adequacy of what is going into the NHS to how much can be squeezed out. Good management, business management, holds out the promise that the NHS can still flourish even when its budget is falling. But, as Sir Douglas Black aptly commented in 1989: 'I believe that what may be appropriate for a chain store is no way to run a health service.'

In the late 1980s, further major changes were introduced into the structure of the NHS (looking remarkably like advice from the United States; see for example Enthoven, 1991). District health authorities were given a duty to purchase a range of health care services. The duty of assessing need and *purchasing* services was partly separated from the *provision* of services. Step by step, hospitals and community units are being encouraged to adopt Trust status, independent of local health authority control, and take responsibilities for working within their budgets and adapting their services to attract purchasers. All hospitals and other service providers would be in competition with each other for contracts from the purchasers of services.

Groups of general practitioners are also being offered Fund-holder contracts, giving them responsibility for managing budgets and purchasing specialist services for their patients from competing provider units. These organizational changes are still at an early stage. They represent the development of an internal market in health care, about which there is passionate political controversy. Some take the view that although since

1948 inequalities in access to health care may not have been entirely removed, the objective of disconnecting care during ill-health from capacity to pay for services has been wonderfully achieved, and that Britain has been a model of both equity and economical provision of health care for the rest of the world to follow. Others have argued that competition will spur services to achieve higher standards and greater efficiency in terms of lower costs. Indeed, some fear that responsiveness to market innovation and general freedom from state bureaucracy will never be achieved if something as large as the NHS is allowed to exist at the heart of free enterprise. The risk of re-introducing a two-tier service has to be accepted to serve bigger political goals.

Some of the inherent problems of introducing this form of internal market into health services are discussed on pages 357–9 of *The Health Divide*, but the issue of the prevailing ethos of the service is particularly relevant here. With the new emphasis on basing decisions on an assessment of the health needs of a population, coupled with the narrow management conception of efficiency outlined above, there is a danger of concentrating resources on those with the most to *gain*, without consideration for those in greater *need* (Scott-Samuel, 1992). With rationing of services, it is not difficult to envisage situations where communities with very poor health are judged to be not worth spending resources on, and that would be a very dangerous development indeed. Health care services need to be built on the principles of efficiency *and* equity, and vigilance is needed to ensure that these principles are adhered to.

A policy for health development, not only health services

A genuine commitment to assess and respond to the health needs of a population leads to the necessity for a wider health policy going beyond the health care sector. In the public debate a preoccupation with the provision of traditional health services prevails, with hospital closures and the reduction of operation waiting-lists. Health is equated with more and better medical services. The 1987 and 1992 General Election campaigns were almost exclusively concerned with this theme. But, on the contrary, a new kind of health policy is required which takes account of the many and varied factors which influence health far beyond the specific elements of the health services themselves. Just as the NHS should not take all the blame for the present state of health inequalities in this country, neither should it be expected to reduce the problem single-handedly in the future. Those who suggest that the evidence on widening health inequalities undermines the achievements of the NHS have totally misunderstood this fundamental point. Just as certain improvements in medical treatment have assisted the recovery of individual patients, so the continuation or deepening of poverty and multiple deprivation have, for some sections of the population, lowered their resistance to ill-health or produced various impairments or disabilities.

A wide strategy encompassing co-ordinated action at local and national levels is required in addition to health service activity. This point is stressed time and time again throughout discussions in the Black Report and *The Health Divide*. Nowhere is this premise more evident than in the World Health Organization's 'Targets for Health for All by the Year 2000', with the theme of reducing inequalities in health by a broadly based strategy running right through the thirty-eight detailed targets. Recent policy developments on the issue and possible results from the WHO programme are discussed below (pp. 339–43). An international strategy is also discussed in Whitehead and Dahlgren (1991).

One pitfall to avoid in devising such a wider policy is concentration on the dangerous notion of an 'underclass'. Since the mid-1980s, first in America (Mincey et al., 1990; Wilson, 1987; Jencks, 1989; Kornblum, 1991) and then in Britain (Murray et al., 1990; Townsend, 1992), this concept has surfaced in various guises. It is a very vague concept used in differing ways to indicate groups of people who, because of a life-time of poverty, unemployment and exclusion from mainstream activities, have become alienated from society and no longer conform to community laws or share common values. It is a convenient concept for the better-off to invoke because 'the underclass' can then be seen as a discrete problem to be tackled without changing the ways of the more privileged majority. Policies proposed for addressing the problem usually involve cuts in welfare spending and stronger law and order measures to contain 'the underclass' in its ghettos. As a leader in the Lancet put it:

'The emotion of the well-heeled towards underclasses is fear, often voiced as blame and articulated in exhortation to uphold the family, obey the law, be industrious, and make use of the opportunities of the market. More appropriate emotions might be shame and indignation. One cannot walk about London – an exercise eschewed by Prime Ministers – without a strong measure of both.' (Lancet, 1990)

In fact, there is no evidence to suggest that any but a tiny minority of poor people reject the common values and hopes of the society in which they live (Lister, 1990). Instead of labelling poor people in general as 'the underclass', policies should be focusing on tackling the causes of the desperate plight in which too many of the country's citizens find themselves. And that involves accepting the challenge to develop a health strategy for the nation that accepts the importance of collective responsibility and includes all its citizens.

The beginning of the 1990s heralded the first tentative steps taken towards the development of a national health strategy. A draft strategy for England was published in the form of a Green Paper in June 1991 (Department of Health, 1991). In one sense the Green Paper was welcomed, because it recognized that the development of a health strategy was 'a new concept for England' and with the NHS reforms 'we can now think strategically about the future direction of health (page v). But it paid little attention to the identification of the causes of inequalities in health and failed therefore to underline the growing scientific argument for broad action, for example, to reduce material and social deprivation as a key strategy to save many lives and also promote good health. Thus no attempt is made in the plan to ask how the first target of the WHO strategy was to be achieved, namely, to reduce the differences in health status between groups within countries by at least 25 per cent by the year 2000.

In contrast, the Welsh strategy published in 1990 did acknowledge the importance of inequalities in health and set targets for reducing specific aspects of the problem (Health Promotion Authority for Wales, 1990). The final version of the English strategy was published as a Government White Paper in July 1992 (DOH, 1992). Although these first attempts are welcome, it is difficult to see them as policies for health development, not just for health education or health services. Above all, it is the link between growing inequality in living standards and inequalities in health which requires attention, and which the Government ignores in its July 1992 White Paper. New evidence from the DSS for the 10 years 1979 – 1988/89 confirms that average real incomes of the poorest 20 per cent of households, after housing costs, did not rise at all. Within that 20 per cent some sections, such as couples with children, experienced a fall. Yet the richest 20 per cent increased their average incomes by 40 per cent, or £5,304 per year (Parliamentary written answer, 16 July, 1992).

In our own view, a national health strategy that does not address the issue of the poorer health of the more disadvantaged sections of the population falls short of what is required on two counts. Firstly, on a matter of principle, it does not enter into the spirit of striving for 'Health for All' – the WHO strategy which Britain, along with all the other countries in Europe, has agreed to follow. Secondly, on a practical level, a strategy that ignores one of the major problems related to health in this country is hardly likely to be effective in its main aim of improving the health of the nation. During the course of the 1990s we have an opportunity to work together to put this right.

List of Abbreviations and Definitions

DoH: Department of Health.

DHSS: Department of Health and Social Security.

DSS: Department of Social Security.

GHS: General Household Survey. Carried out annually by the Office of Population Censuses and Surveys. Based on a sample of 15,000 households in the United Kingdom, it provides data on a range of topics including health, education, employment, housing and migration. It has been running annually since 1970.

HIPE: Hospital Inpatient Enquiry. An annual survey carried out jointly by the Department of Health and Social Security, the OPCS and the Welsh Office and designed to find out how fully hospitals are used and what for.

MRC: Medical Research Council.

Neonatal mortality: Deaths during the first four weeks of life.

OPCS: Office of Population Censuses and Surveys. A governmental department which is in charge of the national census and many other recurrent and occasional surveys and collection of statistics.

Perinatal mortality: Still-births and deaths in the first week of life.

Post-neonatal mortality: Deaths after the first month but before the end of the first year of life.

Registrar General: The head of the OPCS responsible for the collection of official statistics by that department.

Registrar General's Decennial Supplements: The OPCS gathers mortality and morbidity data annually. Every ten years it supplements these annual data with extra information from the ten-year census and publishes it as decennial supplements, one on occupational mortality and the other on area mortality.

SMR: Standardized Mortality Ratio. A method of comparing death rates between different sections of the population, holding other variables constant; e.g. comparing one area with another holding age, sex and occupation constant. Thus Merseyside has a higher SMR than East Anglia, even allowing for the different population structures of the two areas.

WHO: World Health Organization.

The Black Report

Foreword by Patrick Jenkin

The Working Group on Inequalities in Health was set up in 1977, on the initiative of my predecessor as Secretary of State, under the Chairmanship of Sir Douglas Black, to review information about differences in health status between the social classes; to consider possible causes and the implications for policy; and to suggest further research.

The Group was given a formidable task, and Sir Douglas and his colleagues deserve thanks for seeing the work through, and for the thoroughness with which they have surveyed the considerable literature on the subject. As they make clear, the influences at work in explaining the relative health experience of different parts of our society are many and interrelated; and, while it is disappointing that the Group were unable to make greater progress in disentangling the various causes of inequalities in health, the difficulties they experienced are perhaps no surprise given current measurement techniques.

It will come as a disappointment to many that over long periods since the inception of the NHS there is generally little sign of health inequalities in Britain actually diminishing and, in some cases, they may be increasing. It will be seen that the Group has reached the view that the causes of health inequalities are so deep-rooted that only a major and wide-ranging programme of public expenditure is capable of altering the pattern. I must make it clear that additional expenditure on the scale which could result from the report's recommendations – the amount involved could be upwards of £2 billion a year – is quite unrealistic in present or any foreseeable economic circumstances, quite apart from any judgement that may be formed of the effectiveness of such expenditure in dealing with the problems identified. I cannot, therefore, endorse the Group's recommendations. I am making the report available for discussion, but without any commitment by the government to its proposals.

PATRICK JENKIN
Secretary of State for
Social Services

August 1980

Chapter 1

Concepts of Health and Inequality

Throughout history different meanings have been given to the idea of 'health'. One is freedom from clinically ascertainable disease, which has been central to the development of medicine. In ancient Greece the followers of Asclepius believed that the chief role of the physician was to 'treat disease, to restore health by correcting any imperfections caused by the accidents of birth or life' (Dubos, 1960, p. 109). Beginning with primitive surgical intervention and herbal treatment, a tradition was established which was to prove extraordinarily powerful, accelerating in the eighteenth century with the rise of science and again in the twentieth century as a consequence of the massive resources provided for research and innovation in medical technologies. The Cartesian philosophy of the body conceived as a machine and the body controlled as a machine provided an impetus for scientific experiment and a stream of practical outcomes which for an increasing proportion of the population seemed to validate a mechanistic perspective.

There can be no doubt about the success with which such an 'engineering' approach in medicine has been applied. Medical education became concerned with the structure and functions of the body and with disease processes, and medical science became represented predominantly by the acute hospital with its concentration of technological resources (Abel-Smith, 1964). The relatively restricted and familiar use of the word 'health' is therefore associated with the belief systems and the practice of a medicine from which its origins can be traced. Health, which derives from a word meaning whole, is the object of the healing process. To heal is literally to make whole or to restore health. The structure of medicine and of the health services helps to sustain this meaning. Some (for example, McKeown, 1976) have argued however that this development in medicine has distorted our understanding of the problems of human health and well-being and that there are alternative or complementary approaches which it is increasingly important to clarify and properly finance.

Much wider meanings have been given to the word 'health', which hold major implications for the organization of society and the pattern upon which personal life may be modelled. To the followers of the ideas symbolized in ancient Greece by the goddess Hygeia, rational social organization and rational individual behaviour were all-important to the promotion of human health. It was an attribute to which men were entitled if they governed their lives wisely and is echoed in today's 'life-style' approaches to good health. According to them, 'the most important function of medicine is to discover and teach the natural laws which will ensure a man a healthy mind in a healthy body' (Dubos, 1960, p. 109). Implicit also are ideas of the good life: not just freedom from pain, discomfort, stress and boredom, which themselves extend beyond the competence of clinicians to diagnose or treat, but positive expression of vigour, well-being and engagement with one's environment or community. In some respects this more comprehensive approach reached its apogee in the definition of health adopted at the foundation of the World Health Organization at the end of the Second World War as a 'state of complete physical, mental and social well-being and not merely the absence of disease or infirmity'. Adherents of this more comprehensive approach, which is usually called 'social', have worked both within and outside medicine. In most countries there are movements for physical fitness and good diet. Immunization is a standard public health practice. And through direct and indirect 'health education' and counselling, higher standards of health are encouraged. In the case of children this wider conception of health directs concern not only to the presence or absence of disease, but to growth and development, physical, cognitive and emotional. (There is, anyway, abundant evidence for the interaction of disease and development in infants. Low-birth-weight babies show a higher mortality and also incidence of neurological and physical disorder·(Birch and Gussow, 1970, p. 52) and, later in life, there is evidence for the aetiological significance of even mild under-nutrition in inhibiting growth (Marshall, 1977, p. 118).) It becomes relevant to look at evidence relating to acuity of hearing and vision in children, and at heights, weights and age at the onset of puberty, even though none of these things is in any sense an aspect of 'disease'. Given the significance of this kind of thinking, we consider that the different meanings of 'health' and hence of national objectives in maintaining and promoting health are often not given as much attention as they might be, a point we shall return to. Plainly for our purposes the 'social model' of health is more relevant than the 'medical' and we have therefore in the main followed it.

The two models are not, of course, either exclusive or exhaustive. (Discussions based essentially on the 'medical model' are given by Black (1979) and by Dollery (1978).) Conceptions of health and illness vary among different groups within a single society and between societies, as well as in any single society over time (Morris, 1975). It is in part for this reason that 'illness behaviour' – the response to symptoms and the tendency or reluctance to define any symptom as a health problem and to seek medical care – varies between cultural and social groups (Mechanic, 1968). Conceptions are moreover in constant process of adaptation or revision. Changes occur by virtue of scientific discovery and innovation, and developments in professional judgements of needs and the status of different diseases and treatments. They also occur in response to the pressure of established interests, and the extent of public anxiety about illness or safety, as well as the current level of demand for health, environmental and social services. Thus one result of research on the elderly and disabled, and the heightening of public interest and concern about their problems, has been that pain, discomfort, debility and different forms of incapacity have come to play a more prominent part in social and medical conceptions. If we consider mental illness or mental handicap, or the history of 'fringe' medicine, to take very diverse examples, we can see how conceptions of health and illness have changed. And just as conceptions themselves may gradually change, elements within them are accorded different weight or priority. We make this point for two reasons. The first is that our understanding of 'health' will always be evolving, and we must be prepared to absorb new knowledge about changes in health and social conditions. The second is to make better judgements about the strengths and weaknesses of the present health care services.

Within for instance any general approach to the meaning of 'health', views are reached about the seriousness of certain states of health. The construction of the health care services and the priorities which are identified in their development reflect those views. To the extent that a mechanistic model of health holds sway, the health care services will give priority to such matters as surgery, the immunological response to transplanted organs, chemo-therapy and the molecular basis of inheritance. Medicine comes to be structured according to a scale of values associated with such a model. The most sought-after posts will be those at the heart of the model, and medical education and medical careers are similarly influenced. Medicine is not, we know, monolithic, as developments in paediatrics, obstetrics, psychiatry and rehabilitation, and research in the social aspects and in prevention, indicate. However, once a conception of disease finds embodiment in the structure of a service, major changes become more difficult to introduce. All professions tend to become over-committed to existing practice and their receptivity to the need for change is liable to become weak. The medical, nursing and other professions are no different in this respect. We have to face the uncomfortable fact that society cannot look to the professions working within the health services for an account of illness and health which is always as detached or as full as it might be. Indeed, particularized conceptions of health and illness (including their stages and severity) are already institutionalized in medical practice and the organization, sub-divisions and administration of services.

Therefore, while the knowledge, experience and views of the health care professions are bound to play a predominant part in the debate, the extension of knowledge about the problems of human health and illness depends also on sources outside the health professions. Under the auspices of the medical and social sciences there needs to be a determined search for evidence of a wide variety of health conditions and their social, environmental and psychological as well as physiological significance.

In the last hundred and fifty years it could be said 'that the pursuit of health has increasingly been acknowledged to be a social and not merely a technical enterprise. In part this is due to the success of medical science in reducing mortality from infectious disease and thus directing attention towards chronic diseases of complex aetiology, but it is also due to the development of public health services, statistical studies of health, the work of epidemiologists in demonstrating the importance of living standards, protection from hazards and population limitation in improving health, and latterly the work of sociologists on the complex effects of the economy and different forms of social organization, including the family, upon levels of health. (See for example Susser and Watson, 1971; Morris, 1975; McKeown, 1976; Tuckett, 1976.)

Nevertheless the shift in emphasis from a medical to a social model still has some way to go. Although bio-medical research will continue to be vital, there is, in the words of one commentator, a 'need for a shift in the balance of effort, from laboratory to epidemiology in recognition that improvement in health is likely to come in future, as in the past, from modification of the conditions which led to disease rather than from intervention in the mechanism of disease after it has occurred' (McKeown, 1976, p. 179). The sociological contribution is recognized to be, in part, to increase understanding of the social and socio-economic factors which play a part in the promotion of health and the causation of disease and in part to take the natural next step and relate these factors themselves to the broader social structure (see Brown and Harris, 1978).

Some working in medical sociology would emphasize a different perspective. They would argue that their contribution is not only like that of social medicine, to contribute to the understanding of the origins of health and disease in the way people live together in society. 'Disease', they would argue, is a medical, not a sociological concept. Sociology is concerned with the social production of understanding, meanings, knowledge; with social structure and process; and with the behaviour of people. Sociologists will try to understand the failure to seek medical attention for what to the physician is a serious disease episode not in terms of simple irrationality, but in terms of the individual's own (learned) coping mechanisms, social situation, and the meaning which he attaches to his symptoms. Hence there is a lot of interest in the social production of conceptions of health, in inconsistencies between lay and professional conceptions, and in conditions which are generated by different forms of social organization.

While the perspectives adopted in the three fields – medicine, epidemiology and sociology – tend to be different, they are subject to mutual influence and some of the most creative practitioners acknowledge the need to absorb or combine their strengths. Thus, nearly forty years ago Sigerist, a famous American medical historian (following Virchow, a German pathologist, long before), argued that 'The task of medicine is to promote health, to prevent disease, to treat the sick when prevention is broken down and to rehabilitate the people after they have been cured. These are highly social functions and we must look at medicine as basically a social science' (Sigerist, 1943, p. 241).

Choice of indicators of health and ill-health

Conceptions of health may vary in time and according to place, but science demands precision, and different aspects of the meaning of health and ill-health have to be translated into operational terms and applied systematically.

Measures of the 'health' of populations can take many different forms. Among the most familiar are mortality rates, prevalence or incidence of morbidity rates, sickness-absence rates and restricted-activity rates. Each of these indicators poses problems of measurement and has its limitations. For example, undue dependence on mortality rates can induce comparative indifference towards problems of chronic illness. Undue dependence on morbidity rates can discourage interest in congenital and other permanently incapacitating conditions, as well as conditions affecting human well-being which fall outside the conventional classification of 'morbidity'.

Partly because of the problems of measurement, but also because of the need for time-series statistics, we have given precedence to mortality rates. But we wish to call attention to the need for measures of health which combine several factors and which allow the real experiences among the population to be captured. For instance a combined indicator of pain and restricted activity has been proposed (Culyer *et al.*, 1972) and in current Canadian work indicators reflecting social, emotional and physical functioning are being developed (Sackett *et al.*, 1977). Again, the need to relate rather complex indicators of depression to the measure of life events was felt to apply to the community generally and not just those selected for psychiatric treatment (Brown and Harris, 1978).

A distinction is often drawn between acute and chronic sickness, and attempts have been made to relate the utilization of health services to these conditions. But it is clear from GHS reports over the years that the choice of terminology in 'indicator' questions can considerably affect the percentage of the population identifying themselves as having 'short-term' or 'chronic' health problems. Moreover, whatever method is adopted for distinguishing acute from chronic sickness we would also want to call attention to the dangers of treating any two sets of people so identified as distinct (Morris, 1975). Acute and chronic conditions in some patients are difficult to distinguish. Since the evidence suggests that the poorer groups are at greater risk of chronic sickness and disablement, there are dangers of distorting conclusions being reached about the characteristics of the 'acute' sick if all those with chronic sickness are first excluded from any analysis.

Disablement is also an important related concept. While interpretation of the concept of disability varies, it has been identified increasingly in recent years (as in the GHS surveys) with restriction of activity, which includes self-care, household management, and occupational and social activities. Parallel with this trend has been a greater emphasis on treating severity of disablement irrespective of cause or sex or age. Most local authorities have made returns since 1975 which have sought to distinguish the numbers of the physically handicapped according to severity of handicap. Non-statutory bodies are pressing for even wider application of this principle. 'All disabled people: the old, young adults and children; the mentally and physically handicapped, those disabled at home as well as at work or in war; and those disabled from birth, after an accident, or a long illness must be treated alike. It is not the origins or type of disablement or age which should count.' This statement is made on behalf of a large number of organizations of and for disabled people (*Disability Rights Handbook for 1980*, 1979, p. 48) which are concerned to call public attention to the consequences for individuals of the effects of disablement rather than its origins or type. Surveys of public opinion seem to endorse such statements (*Help for the Disabled*, 1974).

Concepts of inequality

The distribution of health or ill-health among and between populations has for many years been expressed most forcefully in terms of ideas on 'inequality'. These ideas are not just 'differences'. There may be differences between species, races, the sexes and people of different age, but the focus of interest is not so much natural physiological constitution or process as outcomes which have been socially or economically determined. This may seem to be straightforward, but the lengthy literature, and widespread public interest in the subject of inequality, show that factors which are recognizably or discernibly man-made are not so easy to disentangle from the complex physical and social structure in which man finds himself. Differences between people are accepted all too readily as eternal and unalterable. The institutions of society are very complex and exert their influence indirectly and subtly as well as directly and self-evidently. For some the concept of inequality also carries a moral reinforcement, as a fact which is undesirable or avoidable. For others the moral issue is relatively inconsequential. For them differences in riches or work conditions are an inevitable and hence 'natural' outcome of the history of attempts by man to build society, and they conclude that the scope for modification is small and, besides other matters, of little importance.

Central to the development of work on inequality has been the development of concepts of 'social class': that is *segments of the population sharing broadly similar types and levels of resources, with broadly similar styles of living and* (for some sociologists) *some shared perception of their collective condition*. This too has been controversial and there remains considerable controversy within sociology about the origins and relative importance of class in relation to social inequalities and social change.

The problems of choosing indicators of inequality

Traditionally inequalities have been portrayed through a characterization of class obtained by ranking occupations according to their social status or prestige. Of course, a variety of other factors may be said to play a part in determining class: income, wealth, type of housing tenure, education, style of consumption, mode of behaviour, social origins and family and local connections. They are interrelated and none of them should be regarded as sufficient in itself. But historically occupation has been selected as the principal indicator, partly because it has been regarded as more potent than some alternatives, but partly because it was the most convenient for statistical measurement and analysis. Occupation not simply designates type of work but tends also to show broadly how strenuous or unhealthy it is, what are the likely working conditions – for example whether it is indoors or outdoors and whether there is exposure to noise, dust or vibration – and what amenities and facilities are available, as well as level of remuneration and likely access to various fringe benefits. Pay will also determine family living standards and, while members of a family will not be exposed to some features of the working conditions experienced, there are others which may affect them indirectly, like the risk of intermittent unemployment, or the stress of disablement and of shift work.

Throughout this report we shall employ occupation as a basis of class because of its convenience. In particular we shall use the Registrar General's categories as follows:

I. Professional (for example accountant, doctor, lawyer) (5 per cent)*

II. Intermediate (for example manager, nurse, schoolteacher) (18 per cent)

IIIN. Skilled non-manual (for example clerical worker, secretary, shop assistant) (12 per cent)

IIIM. Skilled manual (for example bus driver, butcher, carpenter, coal face worker) (38 per cent)

IV. Partly skilled (for example agricultural worker, bus conductor, postman) (18 per cent)

V. Unskilled (for example cleaner, dock worker, labourer) (9 per cent).

But in doing this we should also be aware of its limitations. *We believe an effort should be made to make this classification in the rankings of occupations as objective as possible, by taking into account current and lifetime earnings, fringe benefits, security, working conditions and amenities.* Our intention is to shift attention from the more elusive subjective rating of 'prestige' or 'general standing' of occupations that have been traditionally used, to their material or environmental (and more measurable) properties. *Second, it would be desirable for the term 'occupational class' to be used rather than 'social class' when the current occupation of the individual is used as the basis of the classification* (and we shall do this throughout the report when we use this definition of class). *Third, it will become increasingly important to use the married man's occupation in combination with the married woman's occupation in analysing various health conditions and experiences,* for example infant and child mortality. *Fourth, the need for a 'social class' measure for analysis of the health of the family unit as a whole or of individual members of the family unit will become increasingly important.* One possibility is using the current occupations of both parents, together with information, where it can be obtained, about the main occupations of the husband's father and the wife's father. We return to these possibilities in Chapter 7.

* The percentages are of the total number of economically active and retired males

Finally, use of occupation as an indicator of social class has become so widespread in Britain in recent decades that the pre-occupations of some pioneer health statisticians have been forgotten. Some, however, were particularly concerned to relate health experience to riches or poverty (for example, Stevenson, 1928). Efforts should be made to restore this tradition, and not only because of the difficulties of taking occupation as a reliable indicator of a family's social class. The growth of absolute levels of resources, the spread of employer welfare benefits in kind and of social service benefits, and the increase of owner-occupation among the working classes makes a measure of 'resources' all the more important. The term 'resources' seems to be more appropriate than 'income' because of the present-day impact of wealth and both employer welfare and social service benefits-in-kind upon living standards. Considerable sums are spent each year on official annual surveys – including the Family Expenditure Survey (FES), the General Household Survey (GHS) and the National Food Survey. The FES provides the best measure of income, and although some information is collected about employer welfare and social service benefits it is incomplete and rather rough. Valuable data about the distribution of health are collected in the GHS, and although the information collected about income has, since 1979, been the same as in the FES, it is not supplemented by information on other resources. The development of a more adequate measure will not be easy, and the Royal Commission on the Distribution of Income and Wealth took a very cautious view in some of its reports about the possibilities of linking income and wealth in surveys (see especially Reports Nos. 1, 4 and 5). However, its Seventh Report took a more positive view about the need to develop joint distributions of income and wealth as a priority (p. 160) and about the desirability of sample surveys of personal wealth holdings.

We recommend that in the General Household Survey steps should be taken (not necessarily in every year) to develop a more comprehensive measure of income, or command over resources, through either (a) a means of modifying such a measure with estimates of total wealth or at least some of the most prevalent forms of wealth, such as housing and savings, or (b) the integration of income and wealth, employing a method of, for example, annuitization. (Questions of improvements in our knowledge about health in relation to inequalities are also taken up in Chapter 7.)

Summary

In examining the state of health of a population it is necessary to remember there are different meanings of 'health' which have different implications for action to improve health. On the one hand 'health' can be conceived as the outcome of freeing man from disease or disorder, as identified throughout history by medicine. On the other hand, it can be conceived as man's vigorous, creative and even joyous involvement in environment and community, of which presence or absence of disease is only a part. While there are many indicators of health and ill-health, including mortality rates, morbidity rates, sickness-absence rates and restricted activity rates, we concentrate most attention in this report, mainly for practical reasons, on mortality rates.

Different meanings are also given to the term 'inequality'. Interest tends to be concentrated on those (substantial) differences in condition or experience among populations which have been brought about by social or industrial organization and which tend to be regarded as undesirable or of doubtful validity by groups in society. Inequality is difficult to measure and trends in inequalities in the distribution of income and wealth, for example, cannot yet be related to indicators of health, except indirectly. Partly for reasons of convenience, therefore, occupational status or class (which is correlated closely with various other measures of inequality) is used as the principal indicator of social inequality in this report.

Chapter 2

The Pattern of Present Health Inequalities

Inequalities in health take a number of distinctive forms in Britain today. This chapter examines the pattern of inequalities according to a number of criteria: the relationships between gender and mortality, race and mortality, regional background and mortality, plus a range of measures of ill-health. But undoubtedly the clearest and most unequivocal – if only because there is more evidence to go on – is the relationship between occupational class and mortality. This will be the main theme of the next chapter.

Occupational class and mortality

Every death in Britain is a registered and certified event in which both the cause and the occupation of the deceased or his or her next of kin are recorded. By taking the actual incidence of death among members of the Registrar General's occupational classes and dividing this by the total in each occupational class it is possible to derive an estimate of class differences in mortality. This shows that on the basis of figures drawn from the early 1970s, when the most recent decennial survey was conducted, men and women in occupational class V had a two-and-a-half times greater chance of dying before reaching retirement age than their professional counterparts in occupational class I (Table 1, p. 49). Even when allowance is made for the fact that there are more older people in unskilled than professional work, the probability of death before retirement is still double.

What lies behind this gross statistic? Where do we begin to look for an explanation? If we break it down by age we find that class differences in mortality are a constant feature of the entire human life-span (see Fig. 1). They are found at birth, during the first year of life, in childhood, adolescence and adult life. At *any* age people in occupational class V have a higher rate of death than their better-off counterparts. This is not to say that the differences are uniform; in general they are more marked at the start of life and, less obviously, in early adulthood.

At birth and during the first month of life the risk of death in families of unskilled workers is double that of professional families. Children of

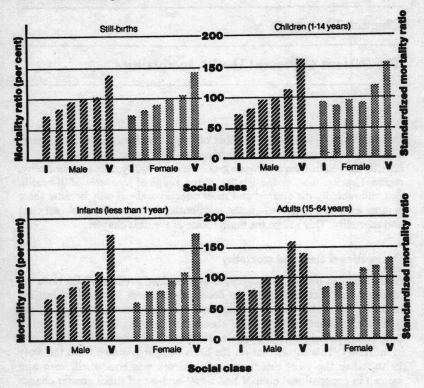

Figure 1. *Mortality by occupational class and age. Relative mortality (%) is the ratio of rates for the occupational class to the rate for all males (or females). (Source:* Occupational Mortality 1970–72, *HMSO, 1978, p. 196)*

skilled manual fathers (occupational class IIIM) run a 1.5 times greater risk.

For the next eleven months of a child's life this ratio widens still further. For the death of every one male infant of professional parents, we can expect almost two among children of skilled manual workers and three among children of unskilled manual workers. Among females the ratios are even greater.

If we measure this against different causes of death – Fig. 2 – we find that the most marked class gradients are for deaths from accidents and respiratory disease, two causes which we will show later to be closely related to the socio-economic environment (see Chapter 6). Other causes, associated

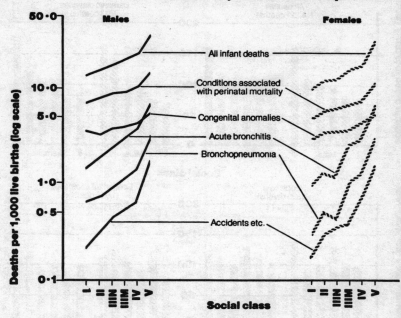

Figure 2. *Infant mortality by sex, occupational class and cause of death.* (*Source: Occupational Mortality 1970–72, HMSO, 1978, p. 158.*)

with birth itself and with congenital disabilities, have significantly less steep class gradients.

Between the ages of 1 and 14 relative class death rates narrow, but are still clearly visible. Among boys the ratio of mortality in occupational class V as compared with I is of the order of 2 to 1, while among girls it varies between 1.5 and 1.9 to 1.

Once again the causes of these differences can be traced largely to environmental factors. Accidents, which are by far the biggest single cause of childhood deaths (30 per cent of the total), continue to show the sharpest class gradient. Boys in class V have a ten times greater chance of dying from fire, falls or drowning than those in class I. The corresponding ratio of deaths caused to youthful pedestrians by motor vehicles is more than 7 to 1. Trailing somewhere behind this, but also with a marked class gradient, are infectious and parasitic diseases, responsible for 5 per cent of all childhood deaths, and pneumonia, responsible for 8 per cent of the total. Most other causes of death show less clear evidence of class disadvantage (Fig. 3).

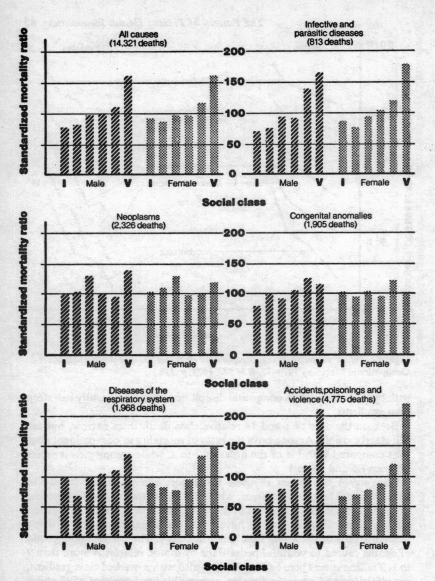

Figure 3. *Class and mortality in childhood (males and females 0–14). (Source: Occupational Mortality 1970–72, H M S O, 1978, p. 160.)*

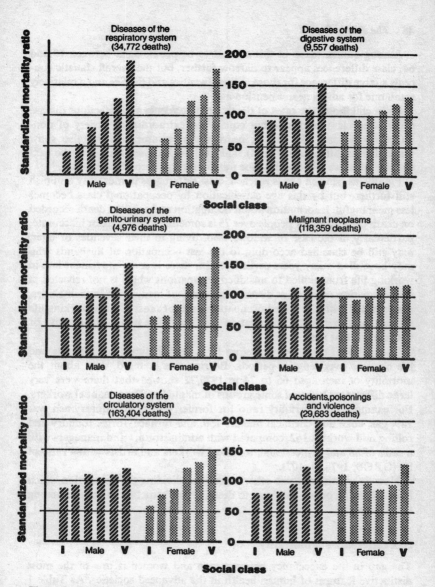

Figure 4. *Occupational class and mortality in adult life (men and married women 15–64), by husband's occupation. (Source: Occupational Mortality 1970–72, HMSO, 1978.)*

Among adults, taken in this context to be people aged between 15 and 64, class differences appear to narrow further, but the overall statistic conceals a large difference for those in their twenties and thirties and a relatively small one for adults nearer pension age.

As in childhood the rates of death from accidents and infectious disease show steep class gradients, but equally an extraordinary variety of non-infectious diseases like cancer, heart and respiratory disease also show marked class differences (Fig. 4). This will be discussed further in the next chapter when we come to describe *trends* in the pattern of death rates.

Finally, as pension age is reached, class differences in mortality diminish still further, but by this age classification by occupational class becomes less meaningful. Information about occupation and cause of death recorded on death certificates for people over 75 is sometimes imprecise or inaccurate, particularly in the case of widows who, dying in their seventies or later, may still be classified according to the last occupation of husbands who may have died many years earlier. Again, there is some movement late in working life from skilled to unskilled occupations which is not reflected in the occupation reported at death. A minority of men, dying in their sixties, are recorded with the skilled occupation held for most of their working life rather than the unskilled occupation they may have had in the last five or ten years of that life.

Occupational class may therefore be a weak indicator of life-style and life chances over lengthy periods. Bearing this in mind, data about the mortality of men aged 65 to 74 in 1970/72 showed that there were very large differences between some groups of manual and non-manual workers. For example, the mortality ratio for former miners and quarrymen was 149, gas, coke and chemical makers 150, and furnace, forge, foundry and rolling mill workers 162, compared with administrators and managers with a ratio of 88 and professional, technical workers and artists with a ratio of 89 (OPCS, 1978, p. 107).

Now let us look at some other criteria for dividing the population which have a bearing on any attempt to describe the 'structure' of health among the population.

Sex differences in mortality

The gap in life expectancy between men and women is one of the most distinctive features of human health in the advanced societies. As Table 1 indicates, the risk of death for men in each occupational class is almost twice that of women, the cumulative product of health inequalities between the sexes during the whole lifetime. It suggests that gender and class exert

Table 1: *Death rates by sex and social (occupational) class (15–64 years) (rates per 1,000 population, England and Wales, 1971)*

Social (occupational) class	Males	Females*	Ratio M/F
I (Professional)	3.98	2.15	1.85
II (Intermediate)	5.54	2.85	1.94
IIIN (Skilled non-manual)	5.80	2.76	1.96
IIIM (Skilled manual)	6.08	3.41	1.78
IV (Partly skilled)	7.96	4.27	1.87
V (Unskilled)	9.88	5.31	1.86
Ratio V/I	2.5	2.5	

* In this table women with husbands have been classified by their husband's occupation, women of other marital statuses are attributed to their *own* occupational class.
Source: *Occupational Mortality 1970–72* (microfiches and 1978, p. 37).

highly significant but different influences on the quality and duration of life in modern society.

It is also a gap in life expectancy which carries important implications for all spheres of social policy, but especially health, since old age is a time when demand for health care is at its greatest and the dominant pattern of premature male mortality adds the exacerbating problem of isolation for many women.

Although attempts have been made to explain the differences between the sexes, comparatively little systematic work exists on the aetiology of the mortality and morbidity differences between men and women and much remains to be disentangled. Women suffer uniquely from some diseases and it would be wrong, for example, to assume too readily that all wives share the same living conditions or even standards as their husbands. Some men have the advantage, for instance, not only of a preferential diet at home but subsidized meals at work. Where both husband and wife are in paid employment, the meals they get in the day, as well as working conditions and the nature of the work, may be radically different. There is a great deal more research to be undertaken to sort out these various influences.

Regional differences in mortality

Mortality rates also vary considerably between the regions which make up the United Kingdom. Using them as an indicator of health, the healthiest part of Britain appears to be the southern belt below a line drawn across

Table 2: *Regional variations in mortality*

Standard region	SMR: standardized for	
	Age	Age and class
Northern, Yorkshire and Humberside	113	113
North-west	106	105
East Midlands	116	116
West Midlands	96	94
East Anglia	105	104
South-east	90	90
South-west	93	93
Wales I (South)	114	117
Wales II (North and West)	110	113
England and Wales	100	100

Source: *Occupational Mortality 1970–72*, p. 180.

the country from the Wash to the Bristol Channel (see Table 2). This has not always been true. In the middle of the nineteenth century, the south-east of England recorded comparatively high rates of death, while other regions like Wales and the far north had a rather healthier profile.

Race, ethnicity and health

Another important dimension of inequality in contemporary Britain is race. Immigrants to this country from the so-called New Commonwealth, whose ethnic identity is clearly visible in the colour of their skin, are known to experience greater difficulty in finding work and adequate housing (Smith, 1976). Given these disabilities it is to be expected that they might also record rather higher than average rates of mortality and morbidity.

This hypothesis is difficult to test from official statistics, since 'race' has rarely been assessed in official censuses and surveys. Moreover it is far from clear what indicator should be utilized in any such assessment – skin colour, place of birth, nationality – and the most significant may depend on the precise issue of interest.

The pattern of social and economic disadvantage experienced by black Britons is connected with occupational class and is reflected in the working of the labour market. But other factors may also be important, and at least amongst adult males the variables of occupational class and race do not compound one another in a linear fashion as far as health is concerned, when place of birth is used as a means of measuring race. The age standardized mortality ratios of immigrant males compares favourably with their British-born equivalents in occupational classes IV and V, but less so higher up the scale in classes I and II (see Table 3). The interpretation of these ratios is made difficult at the higher end of the occupational scale because they are based on small numbers.

In the poorer occupational classes, where the standardized mortality ratio is based on larger numbers of deaths, men born in India, Pakistan or the West Indies seem to live longer than their British-born counterparts. It should be remembered, however, that the percentage of workers in class V among the British-born is less than 7 while the equivalent percentage of those born in, for example, India and Pakistan is 16. In addition, of course, the average British-born male classified as an unskilled manual worker is likely to be older than his foreign-born counterpart and is more likely to have acquired this low occupational status after a process of downward social mobility associated with failing health.

This rather favourable comparison between immigrant and British-born males may also reflect the underlying tendency for migrants to select themselves on the grounds of health and fitness. Men and women prepared to cross oceans and continents in order to seek new occupational opportunities or a new way of life do not represent a random cross-section of humanity. A better comparison for exploring health inequality would ideally involve second- or third-generation immigrants, but these are the very groups that are difficult to trace for statistical purposes. What little evidence that has

Table 3: *Mortality by country of birth and occupational class (SMR) (males 15–64)*

Country of birth	I	II	IIIN	IIIM	IV	V	All
India and Pakistan	122	127	114	105	93	73	98
West Indies	267	163	135	87	71	75	84
Europe (including UK and Eire)	121	109	98	83	81	82	89
UK and Eire (including England and Wales)	118	112	111	118	115	110	114
England and Wales	97	99	99	99	99	100	100
All birth places	100	100	100	100	100	100	100

Source: *Occupational Mortality, 1970–72*, pp. 186–7.

been accumulated, however, does suggest that the children of immigrants do suffer from certain specific health disabilities related to cultural factors such as diet or to their lack of natural immunity to certain infectious diseases (Thomas, 1968; Oppé, 1967; Gans, 1966). Studies based on small samples of immigrant children have pointed to the possibility of higher-than-average morbidity associated with material deprivation, but the evidence is scarce and somewhat inconclusive and needs to be augmented by further research (Hood *et al.*, 1970).

Housing tenure and mortality

Because of its bearing on our discussion in Chapter 6 of explanations for inequalities in health, it should also be noted that when the population is divided into housing tenure groups – owner-occupiers, private tenants and local-authority tenants – class gradients vary considerably (Table 4). People who live in houses which they own have lower rates of mortality than those who rent their homes from private landlords who in turn have lower rates than those who are tenants of local authorities. Housing tenure is, of course, one possible measure of the accumulation by an individual or family of fixed property or assets; it also says something about familial attitudes and priorities. Here it can be shown that this variable shows a very close relationship with the risk of premature death.

Table 4: *Mortality by tenure and class (SMR) (males 15–64 years)*

Class	Tenure		
	Owner-occupied	*Privately rented*	*Local-authority tenancy*
I	79	93	99
II	74	104	99
IIIN	79	112	121
IIIM	83	99	104
IV	83	100	106
V	98	126	123

Source: Unpublished data, Medical Statistics Division, OPCS, preliminary results of the LS 1970–75.

Illness and class

Morbidity data provide a second way of looking at the pattern of class inequalities in health. Moreover there is a sense in which the extent of ill-health in a social group is a better indicator of its health vis-à-vis another group than is the relative mortality rate. Morbidity data are available from a variety of studies and *ad hoc* surveys and are of two kinds, though both are scant at the national level. The first is based on examination of, or symptom identification in, the social group as a whole or in a properly selected sample. An approach of this kind has sometimes been used in the attempt to assess the prevalence of specific diseases within research studies. Social or occupational class is sometimes noted.

The second kind of data derives from analysis of medical consultation and hospital admission rates. But not only do we have few data of this kind by occupational class, there is the disadvantage that rates reflect not only the incidence of disease but also the process by which an individual defines himself (or herself) as ill, seeks medical attention and has his (or her) definition confirmed or legitimated by medical authority. Since we know that there are class-related differences in the propensity of an individual with a given set of symptoms to go for treatment or attention, as well as in the subsequent medical response (Chapter 4), we recognize that data of this kind cannot be interpreted clearly.

Nevertheless data from both these sources confirms, broadly speaking, the picture which mortality data has already indicated.

An example of the first sort of morbidity data is provided by a survey of the prevalence of chronic bronchitis in Great Britain. Ninety-two GPs, distributed throughout the country, were asked to select similarly sized age/sex-stratified random samples from their practice lists. All were to be aged between 40 and 64. In terms of GP diagnosis, the percentage suffering from chronic bronchitis rose with descending class from 6 per cent in class I to 26 per cent in class V. Bronchitis is diagnosed from symptoms and these can vary from doctor to doctor, but even when a more rigorous 'standard diagnosis' was used, the picture was broadly the same.

GPs have also recorded details of consultations. Results from one study showed that consultation rates for each of a wide range of conditions for males, females and children, classified according to occupational class, are of considerable interest though not easy to interpret (Logan and Cushion, 1960, p. 21). The findings were summarized in the following scheme, where + indicates morbidity above and − below average.

	agricultural occupations	*non-manual occupations*	*manual occupations*
psychoneurotic disorders	−	+	−
cardio-vascular disorders	−	+	−
respiratory disorders	−	−	+
gastric disorders	−	−	+
arthritis/rheumatism	−	−	+
injuries	−	−	+

Table 5: *Comparison of distribution of standardized patient consultation ratios (males 15–64, May 1955–April 1956) and standardized mortality ratios (males 20–64, 1949–53) by class: selected conditions*

	SPCR class					SMR class				
	I	II	III	IV	V	I	II	III	IV	V
Respiratory tuberculosis	102	85	105	102	91	58	63	102	95	143
Malignant neoplasms	75	111	94	91	111	94	86	104	95	113
Diabetes mellitus	89	123	100	108	74	134	100	99	85	105
Coronary disease/angina	89	108	102	89	93	147	110	105	79	89
Hypertension	120	127	99	70	89	123	106	103	83	101
Influenza	83	82	103	113	107	58	70	97	102	139
Pneumonia	70	87	90	121	132	53	64	92	105	150
Bronchitis	49	70	99	118	146	34	53	98	101	171
Gastric and duodenal ulcer	48	78	99	88	116	68	76	101	99	134

Source: Logan and Cushion, 1960, p. 16.

Another way of looking at the results is by comparing mortality ratios (by class and disease) with consultation ratios, as in Table 5. If we compare the class gradients on the left-hand side of the table with those on the right-hand side we find that with some exceptions (for instance coronary disease and diabetes) the gradients on the right-hand side are steeper. This suggests more severe sickness or smaller likelihood of treatment with declining class.

This tends to be brought out too in more recent national studies of self-reported illness, like the General Household Survey. Thus, the rates of 'limiting long-standing illness' (as defined in the GHS) rise with falling socio-economic status and are three times as high among unskilled manual males and females as they are among their professional counterparts (see Table 6). Further details are given on pp. 64–5 and 69–71. It will be

Table 6: *Sickness and medical consultation in early adulthood (average rates per 1,000 population 1971–1976)**

Socio-economic group	Limiting long-standing illness		Restricted activity (in two-week period)		Consultations	
	males	females	males	females	males	females†
Professional	79	81	78	89	105	134
Managerial	119	115	74	83	113	137
Intermediate	143	140	83	95	116	155
Skilled manual	141	135	87	86	123	147
Semi-skilled manual	168	203	87	102	131	160
Unskilled manual	236	257	101	103	153	158
Ratio unskilled manual to professional	3.0	3.2	1.3	1.2	1.5	1.2

* England and Wales for 1971–2.
† 1972–6.

Source: *General Household Survey, 1976*, HMSO, 1978.

seen however that the comparable ratios for 'restricted activity' or acute illness are much smaller, and generally resemble the ratios for consultation rates. However, inequalities are smaller in childhood and larger in middle age. Rates of sickness absence from work are also widely unequal. Thus, a special inquiry into the incidence of incapacity for work found marked class gradients for a number of diseases. When the number of employed males beginning a spell of incapacity was expressed per 1,000 in each occupational class, standardized for age, there were, for disease of the respiratory system, 91 in combined classes I and II and 177 in class V. For influenza the figures were 39 and 70, bronchitis 15 and 57 and arthritis and rheumatism 7 and 40 (Ministry of Pensions, 1965).

Summary

There are marked inequalities in health between the social classes in Britain. In this chapter mortality rates are taken as the best available indicator of the health of different social, or more strictly occupational classes and socio-economic groups. Mortality tends to rise inversely with falling occupational rank or status, for both sexes and at all ages. At birth and in the first month of life twice as many babies of unskilled manual parents as of professional parents die, and in the next eleven months of life nearly three times as many boys and more than three times as many girls, respectively, die. In later years of childhood the ratio of deaths in the poorest class falls to between one and a half and two times that of the wealthiest class, but increases again in early adulthood before falling again in middle and old age.

A class 'gradient' can be observed for most causes of death and is particularly steep for both sexes in the case of diseases of the respiratory system and infective and parasitic diseases.

Other aspects of class than merely occupational category have an impact on health, although few data relating mortality to education and income, for example, are available. This is however illustrated by evidence that in all classes owner-occupiers have lighter mortality than those paying rent.

Available data on (self-reported) morbidity tend to reflect those on mortality, though inequalities between occupational classes are more pronounced, and the gradients more uniform, in the case of chronic sickness than in the case of acute or short-term ill-health.

Chapter 3

Trends in Inequality of Health

For about 100 years mortality rates for both sexes, taken one decade with the next, have declined, even after discounting changes that have taken place in the age structure of the population (Fig. 5). At the same time rates for males have remained markedly higher than for females, and in recent decades the difference has become relatively greater (Fig. 6). In fact since 1946 the excess of male over female deaths has increased at all ages and

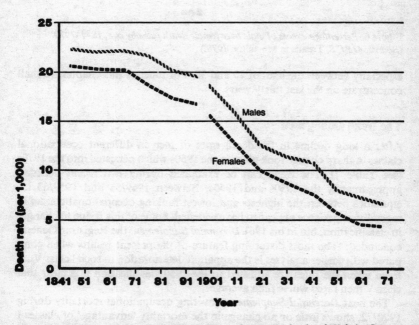

Figure 5. Death rates. standardized to 1901 population (England and Wales). (Source: T. McKeown, The Role of Medicine. Nuffield Provincial Hospitals Trust, 1976, p. 30.)

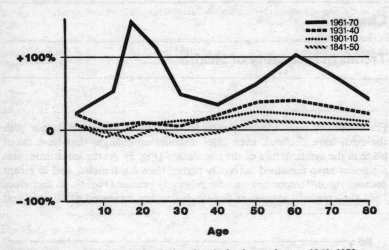

Figure 6. *Percentage excess of male over female death rates by age, 1841–1970.*
(*Source: OPCS*, Trends in Mortality, *1978*.)

especially between the ages of 10 and 30. For most of this chapter we shall
concentrate on the last thirty years.

The trend among men

After a long decline in the death rates of men in different occupational
classes, a sharp change took place in the 1950s which persisted into the 1970s
(see Table 7). The trend can be examined during two recent decades,
approximately the 1950s and 1960s. Between 1949/53 and 1959/63 inequalities between the highest- and lowest-ranking occupational classes in
mortality experience appear to have widened. Some of this is due to changes
in classification, but in his 1961 *Decennial Supplement* the Registrar General
concluded: 'The most disturbing feature of the present results when compared with earlier analyses is the apparent deterioration in social class V ...
Even when the rates are adjusted to the 1950 classification it is clear that
class V men fared worse than average.'

The next *Decennial Supplement*, covering occupational mortality during
1970/72, shows little or no change in the mortality 'advantage' of classes I
and II, but although there was an improvement in the mortality of social
class V relative to other classes, this improvement fell short of restoring the
position the class had reached in 1949/53 (OPCS, *Occupational Mortality*,

Table 7: *Mortality of men by occupational class (1930s–1970s) (standardized mortality ratios)*

Occupational class			Men aged 15–64			
			1959–63 unadjusted		1970–72 unadjusted	
	1930–32	1949–53*		adjusted †		adjusted
I Professional	90	86	76	75	77	75
II Managerial	94	92	81	—	81	—
III Skilled manual and non-manual	97	101	100	—	104	—
IV Partly skilled	102	104	103	—	114	—
V Unskilled	111	118	143	127	137	121

*Corrected figures as published in *Registrar General's Decennial Supplement England and Wales, 1961: Occupational Mortality Tables*, London, HMSO, 1971, p. 22.

†Occupations in 1959–63 and 1970–72 have been reclassified according to the 1950 classification.

Source: *Registrar General's Decennial Supplement* and *Occupational Mortality Tables* (see above).

Decennial Supplement, 1970–72, England and Wales, 1978, p. 174), and compared with 1959/63 the mortality of class IV relative to other classes had deteriorated.

Behind these relative changes in position (and those looked at in Chapter 2) lie absolute changes in mortality rates for the different classes. If we break the trends down by age group (Table 8) we see that mortality rates for younger men of all occupational classes declined throughout the 1950s and 1960s, but that for men in different ten-year age groups between 35 and 65 in occupational classes III, IV and V, the mortality rate actually increased or stood still, while rates for men in occupational class I and II continued to fall. The inequality between the classes was therefore greater by the beginning of the 1970s, as the bottom half of Table 8 demonstrates, by virtue of changes in the pattern of mortality rates for older men. (The trends among married women revealed by the table are discussed below.)

As before, one way of trying to understand this is to look at the changing causes of death. In 1959/63 more class V men died at every age than in 1949/53 from cancer of the lung, vascular lesions of the central nervous system, arteriosclerotic and degenerative heart disease and motor vehicle

Table 8: *Mortality rates per 100,000 and as percentage of rates for occupational classes I and II (1951–71, England and Wales, men and married women)*

Occupational class	*Age*	*Men: rates per 100,000*			*Married women: rates per 100,000*		
		1949–53	*1959–63*	*1970–72*	*1949–53*	*1959–63*	*1970–72*
I and II	25–34	124	81	72	85	51	42
III		148	100	90	114	64	51
IV and V		180	143	141	141	77	68
I and II	35–44	226	175	169	170	123	118
III		276	234	256	201	160	154
IV and V		331	300	305	226	186	193
I and II	45–54	712	544	554	427	323	337
III		812	708	733	480	402	431
IV and V		895	842	894	513	455	510
I and II	55–64	2,097	1,804	1,710	1,098	818	837
III		2,396	2,218	2,213	1,202	1,001	1,059
IV and V		2,339	2,433	2,409	1,226	1,129	1,131
		as per cent I and II			*as per cent I and II*		
I and II	25–34	100	100	100	100	100	100
III		119	123	125	134	125	121
IV and V		145	177	196	166	151	162
I and II	35–44	100	100	100	100	100	100
III		122	134	151	118	130	131
IV and V		146	171	180	133	151	164
I and II	45–54	100	100	100	100	100	100
III		114	130	132	112	124	128
IV and V		126	155	161	120	141	151
I and II	55–64	100	100	100	100	100	100
III		114	123	129	109	122	127
IV and V		112	135	141	112	138	135

Source: OPCS.

and other accidents. Some diseases, like lung cancer and duodenal ulcer, which forty to fifty years ago showed no trend with social class or, like coronary disease, an inverse trend, were by the 1960s producing higher mortality among social class IV and V than I and II. Indeed by 1959/63, forty-nine of the eighty-five observed causes of male death showed higher SMRs for classes IV and V than I and II. (And fifty-four out of eighty-seven applying to women.) For only four causes of death among men, and four among married women, was the class gradient reversed. (See *Registrar General's Decennial Supplement*, 1959/63, op. cit.)

By 1970/72 this position had grown still more marked. For ninety-two causes of death which were picked out for men aged 15 to 64 in the latest OPCS report, the mortality ratios for both classes IV and V were higher than for I and II in as many as sixty-eight, a proportionate increase compared with ten years earlier. For only four causes were mortality ratios for I and II higher than IV and V: accidents to motor vehicle drivers, malignant neoplasm of the skin, malignant neoplasm of the brain and polyarteritis nodosa and allied conditions (OPCS, 1978, op. cit., Table 4A). The question of course is why should there have been this proportionate increase in the number of causes of death showing a class gradient, a question we shall return to in Chapter 6.

The trend among women

With the exception of the youngest group, the 'spread' of inequality among women has been narrower than for men, as an examination of the lower half of Table 8 illustrates. But between 1949/53 and 1970/72, the 'spread' increased among married women aged 35 to 64, as Table 8 also illustrates. The trend for single and married women aged 15 to 64 in the second of the two decades is given for each occupational class in Table 9. The numbers in class I are small and the figures in the table have been placed in brackets on that account. There are also relatively small numbers of women, especially married women, in class V. With these reservations, it can be seen that the relative mortality of both married and single women in class IV, and of single women at least in class V, deteriorated between 1959/63 and 1970/72.

When causes of death are divided into thirteen broad groups for women aged 15 to 64, there is markedly higher mortality among the partly skilled and unskilled classes (whether defined by their own or a husband's occupation) in the case of infective and parasitic diseases, circulatory diseases, respiratory diseases, diseases of the genito-urinary sytem and, though less markedly, congenital anomalies, diseases of the blood, endocrine and nutritional diseases and diseases of the digestive system.

Table 9: *Mortality of women by occupational class (1961–71) (England and Wales) (standardized mortality ratios)*

| | Women aged 15–64 | | | |
| | Married | | Single | |
	1959–63	1970–72	1959–63	1970–72
I	(77)	(82)	(83)	(110)
II	83	87	88	79
III non-manual	}103{	92	}90{	92
III manual		115		108
IV	105	119	108	114
V	141	135	121	138

Sources: *Registrar General's Decennial Supplement: 1961*, pp. 91, 503; OPCS, *Decennial Supplement*, 1970–72, p. 211.

In the case of benign neoplasms there is no trend by class, but in mental disorders, diseases of the nervous system, malignant neoplasms and accidents, and poisoning and violence, there was a higher mortality in 1970/72 among classes I and II.

Throughout the 1960s maternal mortality fell by more than a third, but mortality among women in class V was still nearly double that of class I and II.

Infants and childhood mortality

Inequalities in mortality among infants reflect those among adults. Since the 1930s deaths per 1,000 live births have diminished among all classes, but in 1975 inequality was still marked. As the Court Committee (appointed by the government to examine the development of child health services) commented in its report in 1977, between 1950 and 1973 the perinatal mortality rate declined by 45 per cent for those of professional and 49 per cent for those of managerial class, but by only 34 per cent for those of unskilled manual class (Table 10).

Among children (1 year old and above) trends during the 1960s and early 1970s varied with age. There was a small reduction in the class difference between 1 and 4 years of age, especially for girls, little or no change between the ages of 5 to 9 and an increase in the difference between the ages of 10 and 14. For boys aged 1 to 14, mortality ratios for classes IV and V

Table 10: *Trends in infant mortality by occupational class (England and Wales)*

| | Ratios of actual to expected deaths of infants | | | |
	1930–32	1949–53	1959–63*	1970–72†
I	53	63 ⎫	73	74 ⎧ 66
II	73	73 ⎭		⎩ 77
III	94	97	98	94
IV	108	114 ⎫	119	128 ⎧ 111
V	125	138 ⎭		⎩ 175

	Infant deaths per 1,000 legitimate live births			
I	32	19	—	12
II	46	22	—	14
III	59	28	—	16
IV	63	35	—	20
V	80	42	—	31

*For 1959–63, estimates calculated from C. C. Spicer, and L. Lipworth, *Regional and Social Factors in Infant Mortality*, GRO, Studies on Medical and Population Subjects No. 19, London, HMSO, 1966, by J. Tudor Hart, 'Data on Occupational Mortality 1959–63'. *Lancet*, 22 January 1972, p. 192.

† For 1970–72, estimated from OPCS, *Occupational Mortality, Decennial Supplement*, 1970–72, England and Wales, pp. 168 and 216.

in 1970/72 were both higher than for classes I and II for twenty-three of thirty-eight observed causes of death, compared with only one cause (asthma) where the ratios were lower. For girls the corresponding figures were twenty-two and nought respectively (OPCS, 1978, op. cit., Table 7E).

The elderly

By 1970/72 the mortality ratios for several groups of manual occupations, including former miners and quarrymen, gas, coke and chemical makers and furnace, forge, foundry and rolling mill workers, had deteriorated relative to the death rate for all men. But we should bear in mind the qualification made in Chapter 2 about the value of occupational class as an indicator of life chances among older people.

Morbidity

It is difficult to trace morbidity data by class for any span of years. The General Household Survey has now been running since 1971, but it is still too early to distinguish reliable trends in health from that source. For example, Table 11, drawn from GHS data, shows that absence from work because of sickness or injury is sharply related to class, but that the precise rates are liable to fluctuation from year to year. The average number of days lost through illness or accident among unskilled manual men was 4.5 times that among professional men in 1971 and 1972 (the data are not given for 1977).

Table 12 is also drawn from GHS data and also shows a class gradient during the 1970s for restricted activity, this time measured in terms of acute sickness, long-stay (chronic) sickness and GP consultations, but the rates are even more uneven from year to year and in some years, for some age groups, there is no perceptible gradient. (However, information published since the report was submitted shows that in 1979 the gradient was marked.)

Table 11: *Working males absent from work owing to illness or injury*
(*England and Wales 1971*)

Socio-economic group	Absent from work due to illness or injury in a two week reference period – rate per 1,000			Average number of work days lost per person per year	
	1971	1972	1977*	1971	1972
Professional	37	21	20	3.9	3.1
Employers and managers	37	39	20	7.2	6.2
Intermediate and junior non-manual	44	48	50	7.6	6.0
Skilled manual	57	56	60	9.3	9.4
Semi-skilled manual	56	68	70	11.5	10.5
Unskilled manual	88	99	60	18.4	17.6
All groups	52	54	40	9.1	8.4

* Rate given only to nearest 10.

Sources: OPCS, *The General Household Survey, Introductory Report*, HMSO, 1973, p. 304; OPCS, *The General Household Survey, 1972*, HMSO, 1975, p. 207; OPCS, *General Household Survey, 1977*, HMSO, 1979, p. 65.

The figures illustrate the problem of drawing conclusions about trends

Table 12: *Rates of long-standing and acute illness and consultations per 1,000 of occupational classes IV and V, as a percentage of class I (1971–6, Britain)*

Sex/class/health indicator	1971	1972	1973	1974	1975	1976
Males class IV						
Long-standing illness	—	158	163	157	160	157
acute sickness	126	133	110	134	102	80
GP consultations	133	132	125	146	129	91
Males class V						
Long-standing illness	—	196	213	218	197	196
acute sickness	155	181	129	150	85	102
GP consultations	143	175	164	147	121	125
Females class IV						
Long-standing illness	—	274	214	182	197	176
acute sickness	105	128	115	115	134	95
GP consultations	—	108	150	110	123	114
Females class V						
Long-standing illness	—	320	276	204	253	246
acute sickness	107	141	113	122	128	94
GP consultations	—	117	150	120	107	102

Source: Reports of the General Household Survey.

in self-reported sickness for some major sex/age groups, if not for the population as a whole, during a short span of years.

Conclusion

When examining indicators of health for different occupational or socio-economic classes for a span of years, any changes that may be taking place in the relative size of particular classes may be as important as any changes in the inequality between classes in assessing trends in the overall health of the population. Some commentators have pointed out that while inequalities in health between the unskilled manual class and other classes may not have diminished, or may even have increased, that class has become smaller and therefore there has still been an 'improvement' in the distribution of health. This change has been regarded as compensation for the lack of any closing of the gap *between* classes.

Two comments should be made. The first is that changes in occupational classification have caused commentators to believe that the reduction of class V since 1931 has been greater than it has. (See Appendix, Tables 1 and 2.) In fact, as attempts to adjust census findings show, the fall in the proportion of men in class V has been small since 1961 and in absolute numbers has not fallen at all.

The second is that relatively poor health experience applies to other manual classes and especially class IV and that though this class too has fallen in proportion to the population, it continues to make up, together with class V, more than a quarter of the economically active male population. Mortality indicators for class IV, relative to other classes, have shown some deterioration between the early 1960s and the early 1970s, but perhaps the most important general finding is the lack of improvement, and in some respects deterioration, of the health experience of *both* class V and IV relative to class I, as judged by mortality indicators, during the 1960s and early 1970s.

The more specific conclusions, underlying this finding, are as follows. (These conclusions apply to England and Wales. Scottish experience has been rather similar, though certain differences are noted in the text.)

1. Mortality rates of males are higher at every age than of females and in recent decades the difference between the sexes has become relatively greater.

2. For men of economically active age there was greater inequality of mortality between occupational classes I and V both in 1970–72 and 1959–63 than in 1949–53.

3. For economically active men the mortality rates of occupational class III and combined classes IV and V for age groups over 35 either deteriorated or showed little or no improvement between 1959–63 and 1970–72. Relative to the mortality rates of occupational classes I and II they worsened.

4. For women aged 15–64 the standardized mortality ratios of combined classes IV and V deteriorated. For married and single women in class IV (the most numerous class) they deteriorated at all ages.

5. Although deaths per thousand live births in England and Wales have diminished among all classes, the relative excess in combined classes IV and V over I and II increased between 1959–63 and 1970–72.

6. During a period of less than a decade maternal mortality fell by more than a third. Although that of class I fell less sharply than other classes inequality between the more numerous class II and classes IV and V remained about the same.

7. Among children between 1 and 4 years of age, there has been a small reduction in the class differential (especially for girls), for children aged 5 to 9 little or no change, but for children aged 10 to 14 an increase in the differential. For boys aged 1–14, mortality ratios for classes IV and V in 1970–72 were *both* higher than for classes I and II for twenty-three of thirty-eight causes of death, compared with only one cause (asthma) where the ratios were lower. For girls the corresponding figures were twenty-two and nought respectively. There is evidence that as rates of child death from a specific condition decline to very low levels class gradients do disappear. The gradual elimination of death from rheumatic heart disease over the post-war period provides evidence of this (Morris, 1959).

Chapter 4

Inequality in the Availability and Use of the Health Service

One of the fundamental principles of the NHS is to 'divorce the care of health from questions of personal means or other factors irrelevant to it' (Cartwright and O'Brien, 1976). Yet a number of studies have revealed significant social inequalities in the availability and use of health services. In 1968 Richard Titmuss argued, on the basis of evidence then available, that: 'Higher income groups know how to make better use of the Service: they tend to receive more specialist attention; occupy more of the beds in better equipped and staffed hospitals...' Subsequent studies, many of which we shall refer to, have cast further light on the issue and added to the evidence.

Unequal usage will never be more than a partial explanation of the overall inequalities in standards of health. Several commentators have shown, and we shall go on to show this later, that differences in health between sections of the population may be far more a function of 'variations in the socio-demographic circumstances of the population than the amount and type of medical care provided and/or available' (Martini, Allan, Davison and Backett, 1977). Nevertheless, any inequality in the availability and use of health services in relation to need is in itself socially unjust and requires alleviation. This remains true whatever the relative importance of health care in comparison with other areas of social policy.

Moreover, since equal access has always been a fundamental principle of the NHS, the extent to which it has been achieved is a matter of considerable interest. In sorting out the evidence we have found it useful to look separately at GP consultation rates, hospital care, preventive services and services for the disabled and infirm. This is partly because such a distinction reflects the availability of information and the foci of research, and also because, as we shall show, while some uncertainty remains as to the existence of inequalities in the first two cases, there are no grounds for doubt in the case of preventive services in particular.

GP consultations

There is no simple interpretation of the evidence linking class with rates of consultation with general practitioners. The GHS is the best source of information, but the trend, while clear enough for the sample of males and females in general, does not apply to males aged 0 to 14 or females aged 0 to 14, and is uneven for some other age groups. GHS results have fluctuated from year to year and the consulting rate (and even more the average number of consultations) has not generally shown as marked a class gradient, as have the measures of morbidity discussed in earlier chapters. (See table on p. 55 above.)

For most years covered by the GHS the number of people consulting a doctor, and the average number of consultations, has tended to increase with falling class. However, for some years the figures are uneven and the rate for classes III, IV and V is lower than for classes I and II. This may partially miss the point. It may be that the proper basis for comparing rates of consultation is not one of simple population but of the *need* for care. One study, for example, using the GHS data, divided the number of GP consultations by the number of restricted activity days, each in a two-week reference period, for each occupational group (defined a little differently from the occupational classification referred to earlier). The 'use/need ratios' clearly declined in going from socio-economic class I to class V (Brotherston, 1976). Table 13 shows use/need ratios calculated on the basis of the GHS for 1974/6 which similarly show an overall pattern of decline from socio-economic group 1 to group 6. The table shows that the observation that the poor use GP services more is reversed once 'usage' is corrected for 'need'.

Another study used aggregated 1971 and 1972 GHS data and also found statistically significant trends in consultation rates/morbidity, where the 'morbidity' measure was rate of chronic sickness or rate of sickness absence

Table 13: *'Use/need ratios' by social group (Great Britain, 1974–6)*

Socio-economic group	Males	Females
1	0.23	0.23
2	0.21	0.24
3	0.20	0.22
4	0.18	0.22
5	0.20	0.20
6	0.17	0.19
All	0.19	0.22

from work or school, but a non-significant trend in the case of acute sickness (Forester, 1976). The study showed that in proportion to reported sickness and sickness absence from work, the semi-skilled and unskilled in fact made less use of GP services than did other groups.

A weakness of this method of relating use to need derives from the fact that many of those with restricted activity may not visit a GP but may visit a hospital out-patients' department, whereas others may visit a GP for reasons different from restricted activity. In other words, comparison of these rates may be purely indicative of differences in receipt of care when sick.

At the same time, comparison of *rates* of consultation, even when related to need as shown by mortality or morbidity data, is not a wholly adequate conceptualization of inequality in care. Several studies have shown that middle-class patients tend to have longer consultations than working-class

Table 14: *Morbidity and GP attendance indicators for socio-economic groups: semi-skilled and unskilled as a percentage of professional*

	Males					
	1971	1972	1973	1974	1975	1976
Long-standing illness						
semi-skilled	—	158	163	157	160	157
unskilled	—	196	213	218	197	196
Limiting long-standing illness						
semi-skilled	272	203	233	179	174	222
unskilled	371	290	333	274	244	292
Acute sickness (restricted activity)						
semi-skilled	126	133	110—	134—	102—	80—
unskilled	155	181	129—	150	85—	102—
Acute sickness (days per person)						
semi-skilled	—	169	168	169	130	122
unskilled	—	268	206	215	121	196
GP consultations:						
persons consulting (rate per 1,000)						
semi-skilled	122	132	121	146	122	91
unskilled	128	157	145	141	111	111
GP consultations (rate per 1,000)						
semi-skilled	133	132	125	146	129	91
unskilled	143	175	164	147	121	125

Females					
Long-standing illness					
semi-skilled	—	274	214	182	197	176
unskilled	—	320	276	204	253	246
Limiting long-standing illness					
semi-skilled	245	303	257	213	259	248
unskilled	298	355	332	246	346	348
Acute sickness (restricted activity)					
semi-skilled	105	128	115—	115	134	95—
unskilled	107	141	113—	122	128	94—
Acute sickness (days per person)					
semi-skilled	—	205	137—	117	136	127
unskilled	—	238	148	122	129	133
GP consultations:					
persons consulting (rate per 1,000)					
semi-skilled	—	113	147	110	118	116
unskilled	—	112	141	123	111	115
GP consultations (rate per 1,000)					
semi-skilled	—	108	150	110	123	114
unskilled	—	117	150	120	107	102

Source: Reports of the GHS 1971–6.

patients and that more problems are discussed during this period. One study also found that middle-class patients were able to make better use of the consultation time, as measured by the number of items of information communicated and the number of questions asked (Cartwright and O'Brien, 1976). Moreover, even though working-class patients tended to have been with the same practice for longer, the doctors seemed to have more knowledge of the personal and domestic circumstances of their middle-class patients. An earlier study found, for example, that middle-class patients were more likely to be visited by their GP when in hospital than were working-class patients (Cartwright, 1964). For cultural reasons, then, and also because there is a tendency for the 'better' doctors to work in middle-class areas (as we shall see), the suggestion must be that middle-class patients appear to receive a better service when they do present themselves than their working-class contemporaries.

The data are limited and further analyses remain to be carried out, but what is available suggests that the level of consultation among partly skilled and unskilled manual workers does not appear to match their need for health care (see Table 14). With certain exceptions,* the socio-economic or class differences in ill-health are larger than the corresponding class differences in GP attendance (rates for persons consulting and total number of consultations). If we were to combine different measures of chronic and acute ill-health and compare 'need' with 'care received' (on the basis of some principle of weighting), there would be no exceptions for any year.

Hospital services

There is no regular source of class-related information on use of hospital services comparable with that obtained on GP consultation rates, even though questions on hospital attendance are asked in the GHS. In the case of hospital in-patients, the percentage concerned (about 2 per cent) is too small for any class breakdown of GHS data to be statistically meaningful. Attendance at out-patients is higher, and although since 1972 these rates have not been published on a class basis, some information is available. This suggests that there are no systematic class gradients in out-patient attendance for either males or females.

Data given in the 1972 GHS report does however seem to suggest that men in occupational class V aged 15–64 do have particularly high rates of attendance, which drop off after retirement. Referring to this 'relatively much greater use of "out-patients" by unskilled males than by males of other groups', the report indicated that it did not distinguish between attendance at out-patient casualty departments and other ancillary services. But the decline in rate at retirement at least suggests that 'the higher rates amongst unskilled males of working age than amongst males of other groups may reflect a rather particular use of out-patient facilities related to their greater risk of exposure to accident or injury compared with other groups'. Though later data do not show this discontinuity at retirement, the possibility of this special use of hospital out-patients is a matter of interest.

Such little evidence as is available on hospital in-patient care describes not the proportions of various social groups spending time in hospital but the social composition of the groups admitted. For England and Wales admission rates on an occupational basis are available only prior to 1963 (from HIPE), after which date they ceased to be centrally collected (mainly owing to doubts about their quality). The older data, however, suggest that the rate of usage of hospital beds rises with declining class. In Scotland, an analysis of hospital admission rates and duration of stay found clear

---

* The relative consultation rates of semi-skilled and unskilled groups exceed the relative rates of restricted activity in the cases in the table marked with a dash, though in most of those instances they no longer do so when *days* of restricted activity are taken.

upwards trends in both with declining class. Moreover SHIPS (Scottish Hospitals In-Patient Survey) does continue to code social class and more recent figures confirm this class gradient, both in admission rates (given by SDR in Table 15) and length of stay (given by SBDR).

Table 15: *Hospital standardized discharge ratios (SDR)*
and standardized bed-day ratios (SBDR) by occupational class (Scotland, 1971)

Class	SDR		SBDR	
	Males	Females	Males	Females
I	79.5	95.9	63.7	92.5
II	80.9	98.0	73.3	93.6
III	94.0	90.4	93.9	91.0
IV	115.1	107.4	116.4	106.7
V	141.4	161.1	151.7	153.9

Source: Scottish Hospitals In-Patient Survey.

Preventive and promotive services

Although neither administrative returns nor the GHS provide information on the utilization of community health and preventive services by social or occupational class, there is a substantial body of research on which to draw, and it is well established that those in the manual classes make considerably less use of them than do those higher up the occupational scale. Moreover, the ambiguity which surrounds the relation of utilization to 'need' in the case of GP consultations is not encountered here. Assessment of morbidity, or need for care, is not at issue in comparing rates of attendance for ante-natal care (though this may be more essential for those put at risk by social factors), cervical screening, radiography or immunization of children.

In the case of family planning and maternity services substantial evidence shows that those social groups in greatest need make least use of services and (in the case of ante-natal care) are least likely to come early to the notice of the service. A study published in 1970 found clear class gradients in the proportion of mothers having an ante-natal examination, attending a family planning clinic and discussing birth control with their GP (Cartwright, 1970). Unintended pregnancies were also more common among working-class women. A second study, in 1973, appears to confirm these findings (Bone, 1973). It found that women from the non-manual classes make more use of family planning services than those from the manual classes. This is true both for married and unmarried women. Scottish data also show that late ante-natal booking is more common in poorer social groups, although the situation seems to be improving in all classes (Table 16). (They further suggest that late attendance for ante-natal care is an effective predictor of subsequent infant morbidity and mortality within families (Brotherston, 1976).)

Table 16: *Late ante-natal booking. Percentage of married women in each occupational class making an ante-natal booking after more than twenty weeks of gestation (Scotland 1971–3)*

Occupational class	1971	1972	1973
I	28.4	27.2	27.0
II	35.3	32.3	29.8
III	36.3	33.4	30.6
IV	39.3	37.8	35.3
V	47.1	44.2	40.5

Source: Brotherston, 1976. Data from Scottish Information Services Division.

Similar class differences have been found in attendance at post-natal examinations (Douglas and Rowntree, 1949), and immunization, ante-natal and post-natal supervision and uptake of vitamin foods (Gordon, 1951). Among slightly older children the National Child Development Study (1958 birth cohort) found substantial differences in immunization rates in children aged 7, as well as in attendance at the dentist (Table 17).

These patterns are further confirmed in studies of screening for cervical cancer, even though working-class women are much more likely to die from it. A study in Greater Manchester, for instance, showed that while women from classes IV and V accounted for over one third of all women living in the study area, they made up only about one sixth of women who had a smear test done.

Further studies show that working-class people make less use of dental services (Gray *et al.*, 1970; Bulman *et al.*, 1968) and of chiropody (Clarke, 1969) and receive inferior dental care (Sheiham and Hobdell, 1969). Many of these studies are admittedly old, and their findings cannot necessarily be accepted as still valid. Nevertheless, taken together, and in the absence of later evidence to the contrary, a clear relationship between social class and use of preventive services seems to have been demonstrated.

Table 17: *Use of health services by children under 7 by occupational class of father (Great Britain, 1965).*

	I	II	IIIN	IIIM	IV	V
Per cent who had never visited a dentist	16	20	19	24	27	31
Per cent not immunized against						
smallpox	6	14	16	25	29	33
polio	1	3	3	4	6	10
diphtheria	1	3	3	6	8	11

Source: Second Report of the NCDS.

Table 18: *Percentage of old persons of different occupational class who receive or feel the need for chiropody treatment (Great Britain, 1962)*

Source of chiropody treatment	Occupational class					
	I	II	IIIN	IIIM	IV	V
	%	%	%	%	%	%
Public or voluntary service	2	6	6	9	8	8
Privately paid	20	18	14	8	9	8
Non-professional or none, need felt	6	8	13	11	13	10
Non-professional or none, no need felt	72	68	67	72	71	74
Total	100	100	100	100	100	100
Number	82	557	396	1,193	1,040	457

Note: A further 42 persons were classed in armed services occupations, 10 had no occupation and 290 were unclassifiable.

Source: Townsend and Wedderburn, 1965.

Care of the infirm and disabled

There is little information on class inequalities in the care received by the infirm and disabled, though we now enter that awkward and neglected area where health care shades into the variety of other forms of social service provision. That is, to make comparisons of the care or services received by those who are disabled or infirm (including the aged infirm and the long-term chronic sick) would necessarily be to consider not only health care in the strict sense, but social work support, delivery of meals, home help, sheltered housing, mobility aids, sheltered work and rehabilitation etc., all or many of which may be crucial to the well-being of an infirm or disabled person.

But the slight, and unfortunately somewhat old, empirical evidence available does indicate that class inequalities are to be found here. A study of the elderly in residential homes and in geriatric and psychiatric hospitals carried out some years ago found not only that the manual and non-manual elderly were likely to be in different kinds of institution (the latter less commonly in hospital), but a gap in the standard of living and care available in institutions catering principally for one or the other group (Townsend, 1962). A second national study of people aged 65 and over found disparities

Table 19: *Percentage of old persons of different occupational class who were receiving public or private domestic help, or who said help was needed (Great Britain, 1962)*

Source of domestic help	Occupational class					
	I	*II*	*IIIN*	*IIIM*	*IV*	*V*
	%	%	%	%	%	%
Local authority	1	2	4	6	4	4
Privately paid	42	27	12	5	3	2
Other (e.g. family) or none, but need felt	10	7	6	6	6	4
Other (e.g. family) or none, no need felt	47	64	78	83	87	90
Total	100	100	100	100	100	100
Number	81	555	396	1,188	1,033	447

Source: Townsend and Wedderburn, 1965.

in receipt of a number of services. Both publicly provided chiropody services and domestic help, for instance, fail fully to compensate for unequal ability to purchase such services (Townsend and Wedderburn, 1965). (See Tables 18 and 19.)

Of equal concern is the difference in attitude between old people of different social classes. Table 19 shows that 90 per cent of those in class V neither receive domestic help (from outside their family) nor feel the need of it. Among the elderly who are incapacitated 'nearly half those in Social Classes I and II ... already had privately paid or local authority domestic help, and nearly half the others said they needed help. But only a sixth of those in Social Class V who were severely incapacitated had such help already and only a fifth of the remainder felt the need for it' (Townsend and Wedderburn, 1965, p. 46). While we cannot tell if these differences still exist, the study shows all too clearly the way in which norms and values associated with class may influence subjective perceptions of need.

In considering the needs of the disabled, aged infirm and chronic sick, not only is it difficult clearly to distinguish needs for strictly medical services from needs for other supportive services, but it is similarly difficult to distinguish needs related to the condition 'itself' (i.e. medically defined) from those relating to its social and economic consequences. In this context it may be helpful to look at the circumstances of the long-term sick, that is those receiving sickness, invalidity and industrial injury benefits for periods of between a month and a year (Martin and Morgan, 1975). This shows not only that the sample of benefit recipients as a whole contained a much higher proportion of semi-skilled and unskilled manual workers, which is to have been expected, but that the longer the spell of sickness, the higher the proportion of unskilled workers. Moreover, the longer the period of incapacity the less likely the sick person is to be able to return to the same type of work with the same employer as before, though skilled manual workers are more likely to have their jobs kept open for them than are semi-skilled or unskilled workers. Unsurprisingly also, receipt of sick pay from the employer is also related to duration of invalidity and to level of job (defined by occupational group).

Clearly therefore in considering the needs of the disabled, long-term sick and aged infirm, financial problems and (in some cases) problems of subsequent re-employment are both pertinent and class-related. The implication of this for policy (which we take up in Chapter 9) is that the equalization of provision of health and social services is not justifiably separable from the equalization of the social and economic consequences of long-term invalidity or sickness.

The interaction of geographic and social disparities

It has been known for a long time that there are differences in the health services available in well-to-do and poor areas. In 1957 a study of the social aspects of prescribing found that the average total cost of drugs per prescription was higher in wealthier areas (Martin, 1957). More recently an analysis of health expenditure at the regional level also found a positive correlation between the percentage of the population in professional and managerial socio-economic groups and both community health expenditure and hospital revenue expenditure, and a negative correlation between expenditure and proportion of population in unskilled and semi-skilled occupations (Noyce, Snaith and Trickey, 1974). The authors concluded: 'There are no regions of above-average spending which are not also high socio-economic status regions. Indeed, if one knew no other facts it would be possible to explain two thirds of the variation in community health expenditure by a knowledge of what proportion of the population in each region were managers, employers, or professional workers.'

In 1971 Tudor Hart (a general practitioner working in a poor area of Wales) contrasted the availability of medical care in poor industrial areas of high need and affluent salubrious areas of lower need in memorable terms. He wrote:

> In areas with most sickness and death, general practitioners have more work, larger lists, less hospital support and inherit more clinically ineffective traditions of consultation than in the healthiest areas; and hospital doctors shoulder heavier case-loads with less staff and equipment, more obsolete buildings and suffer recurrent crises in the availability of beds and replacement staff. These trends can be summed up as the inverse care law: that the availability of good medical care tends to vary inversely with the need of the population served. (Tudor Hart, 1971)

An analysis of data in 1976 on need for and provision of child health services for each of the fifteen pre-1974 hospital board regions of England and Wales showed how, in particular, regional provision of GPs and health visitors is negatively correlated with a number of indicators of need (including still-birth rate, level of infant mortality and birth rate to teenage mothers) (West and Lowe, 1976). There are indeed very few positive correlations; midwives alone seemed to be relatively well distributed throughout the regions. The authors go on to suggest: 'When data becomes available for area health authorities even greater differences between need and provision will probably be uncovered between areas than between regions' (cf. Morris, 1975, pp. 53, 77). In the meantime it has at least been established that *variations* in expenditure (Rickard, 1976) and in the provision of services

(Buxton and Klein, 1975; Jones and Masterman, 1976) are greater at the sub-regional than at the regional level. This, of course, is the level at which it matters to people. It is extremely difficult to know for sure what this means for small typically working-class areas in comparison with typically middle-class areas. One recent study does give some indications though. It looked at three areas of council housing, one in Newham (east London) and two in the Midlands, one solidly middle class, the other a council estate with a history of social problems. Unlike Newham, which has long suffered from severe deprivation of the environment, both Midlands areas were situated in 'a socially mixed county, with a teaching hospital, and an attractive environment: a highly desirable county in which to work, with no reputation for recruitment problems in general practice.' Questions covered morbidity (GHS questions were used) and experiences in seeking help from the GP. Although much was found to be common to the two working-class areas, differentiating their inhabitants from the middle-class residents of the third area, this was not the whole picture. Indeed, the principal conclusion of the study is as follows:

The provision of health care and the subjective experience of seeking that care are all partly determined by the socio-economic structure of society on an area basis, so that *a working-class person is at a greater disadvantage if he lives in a predominantly working-class area than if he lives in a socially mixed area.* The data ... are consistent with a theory of structural determination of need and demand for health care from an area, operating both through environmental and social conditions on the level of health, and through the social pressures and life experiences that further affect demand, particularly in the case of childhood illness. The level and quality of available medical manpower, relative to need and demand, is likely also to be strongly affected by the environment and social class composition of an area through the operation of the market for recruitment. (Skrimshire, 1978)

It is likely that similar conclusions would follow from a consideration of race or ethnicity. However, information on use of services by ethnic groups is sparse. One study has referred to hesitation in seeking ante-natal care among immigrants and their difficulties in securing adequate dietary information (Coombe, 1976), and there is evidence of some lack of appreciation among health services staff of the special needs of some immigrant groups, as well as a clear lack of adequate facilities in some of the areas in which they have been obliged to concentrate.

Conclusion

Generalization about inequality of utilization is made difficult partly because of sampling errors in the case of national surveys and of partial information in the case of local studies, and because of the (as yet unresolved) problem of relating utilization to need.

Inequalities appear to be greatest (and most worrying) in the case of the preventive services. Severe under-utilization by the working classes is a complex result of under-provision, of costs (financial, psychological) of attendance, and perhaps of a life-style which profoundly inhibits any attempt at rational action in the interests of *future* well-being. Such factors are not, in this case, outweighed by the costs of present disruption of normal social functioning. We have also seen, however, how services provided on an 'outreach' basis can serve to reduce at least some of the costs of attendance, with beneficial results.

The situation is not clear-cut in the case of GP attendance, partly because attendance rates cannot be compared with any precise measure of need. Excepting, for some years, children, more of those in lower than in higher socio-economic groups consult a doctor, and their total consultations are, relatively, greater. But on most of the health indicators their need for care is greater still. It is hard not to conclude that poorer groups make relatively low use of GP services, irrespective of the separate question of the *adequacy* of the services to which they typically have access.

Middle-class parents are, however, more likely than working-class parents to seek medical attention for their children. Since the (direct) costs of attendance may be presumed similar, this may imply that working-class *adults* are likely to be typically *more* sick than are middle-class ones before help is sought. Moreover, we have seen also that middle-class patients typically receive better care from their GP – a consequence, once more, of both interpersonal and ecological factors.

Hospital out-patient departments are used more by the working class than by the middle class. In the case of Accident and Emergency departments there is evidence of some use in place of the GP, access (as to the GP) being on the basis of self- (or 'lay') referral. It has been suggested that this preferred use of out-patients in treatment of 'traumatic' conditions (suffered at work or in the home) is principally a result of their greater availability: they are open twenty-four hours a day, no appointment is needed and availability of diagnostic aids is certain.

In the case of in-patient departments too, evidence suggests greater use by the working class. It may be noted that, since admission is generally on the basis of GP referral, a higher proportion of working-class patients than of middle-class patients consulting a GP must be subsequently admitted to hospital. This in turn must imply that more working-class patients have illnesses requiring hospital admission, or that the working-class patient seeing his GP is *typically* sicker and/or that he or she is seen as less likely to receive adequate care at home. And indeed, evidence from a survey of the elderly suggests that this is so: public provision of domiciliary services seems not fully to compensate for differential ability to purchase such services.

It is hard to resist the conclusion that this pattern of unequal use is explicable not in terms of non-rational response to sickness by working-class people, but of a rational weighting of the perceived costs and benefits to them of attendance and compliance with the prescribed regime. These costs and benefits differ between the social classes both on account of differences in way of life, constraints and resources, and of the fact that costs to the working class are actually increased by the lower levels and perhaps poorer quality of provision to which many have access.

Class differentials in the use of the various services which we have considered derive from the interaction of social and ecological factors. Differences in sheer availability and, at least to some extent, in the quality of care available in different *localities* provide one channel by which social inequality permeates the NHS. Reduced provision implied greater journeys, longer waiting lists, longer waiting times, difficulties in obtaining an appointment, shortage of space and so on. A second channel is provided by the structuring of health care *institutions* in accordance with the values, assumptions and preferences of the sophisticated middle-class 'consumer'. Inadequate attention may be paid to the different problems and needs of those who are less able to express themselves in acceptable terms and who suffer from lack of command over resources both of time and of money. In all cases, for an individual to seek medical care, his (or her) perception of his (or her) need for care will have to outweigh the perceived costs (financial and other) both of seeking care and of the regime which may be prescribed. These costs are class-related.

It is the interaction of these two sets of factors which produces the inequalities documented in this chapter

Chapter 5

International Comparisons

The success or otherwise of comparable developed countries in altering patterns of health inequality is an inevitable yardstick against which to measure the British performance and is also a possible pointer to what should or should not be done here. Accordingly we shall now attempt to set the British experience in an international context and in a limited way to explore what has been happening elsewhere. We start by looking at overall national levels and trends and go on to look at the different experiences of inequalities in health. Inevitably there are cultural and social (structural) variables which make any such comparisons complex and subject to a variety of interpretations. Nevertheless the success of some countries in raising health standards makes it an essential input into our analysis of the British experience. Once again mortality data are the most available indicator of relative levels of health, and in particular infant mortality, because infancy remains one of the most vulnerable periods of human life and infant mortality has long-term consequences, has been accepted as an important index of a country's achievements in the health field.

Levels of health and changes over time

International comparisons over the last two decades highlight a number of points about the relative success or otherwise of British health policy (see Tables 20 and 21).

1. In 1975 England, Wales and Scotland (in particular) experienced significantly higher perinatal mortality rates than those of the four Nordic countries and the Netherlands. France and Germany had broadly similar rates to the British.*

2. The overall decreases in perinatal mortality rates between 1960 and 1975

* More recent data show that by 1978 Scotland had caught up with England but that the conclusion otherwise holds. Rates of perinatal mortality in 1978: England 15.4; Wales 16.8; Scotland 15.4; Sweden (1977) 10.1; Norway (1977) 13.2; Denmark (1977) 10.6; Finland (1977) 11.0; Netherlands (1977 provisional) 12.9; France (provisional) 14.7; W. Germany (1977) 14.9.

Table 20: Perinatal and infant mortality in Europe

	Perinatal mortality per 1,000 live births				Infant mortality per 1,000 live births			
	1960	1975	% Decrease 1960–75	Annual % decrease 1971–5	1960	1975	% Decrease 1960–75	Annual % decrease 1972–5
England & Wales	33.5	17.9*	46.5‡	4.1	21.8	14.2*	34.3‡	4.5
Scotland	38.1	18.5*	51.3‡	5.1	26.4	14.8*	44.0‡	5.4
Sweden	26.2	11.1	57.7	7.3	16.6	8.3	50.0	7.7
Norway	24.0	14.2	40.8	5.1	18.9	11.1	41.3	2.0
Denmark	26.5	12.7‡	52.1‡	5.5	21.5	10.3*	52.0‡	3.9
Finland	25.3	13.9†	45.0§	5.9	21.0	11.0†	47.6§	1.4
Netherlands	25.6	14.0	45.3	4.3	16.5	10.6	35.7	3.1
France	31.8	19.5†	38.7§	4.8	27.4	11.1	59.8	10.2
W. Germany	36.3	19.4	46.5	4.8	33.8	19.7	41.6	4.5
(E. Germany)	—	(17.6)	—	—	—	(15.9)	—	(3.4)
USA	29.4	20.7	29.2	—	26.0	16.1	38.1	4.3

* 1976 † 1974 ‡ 1960–76 § 1960–74

Sources: 1960–72 data: Health Care – the Growing Dilemma; 1975 data: WHO and World Health Statistics, 1978, Vol. 1; 1975, France: Eurohealth Handbook, 1978.

Table 21: *Adult mortality in Europe: deaths per million*

	Men				Women			
	35–44		45–54		35–44		45–54	
	1964	1975	1964	1975	1964	1975	1964	1975
England and Wales	2,471	2,095*	7,330	6,985*	1,778	1,468*	4,382	4,298*
Scotland	3,245	2,817*	9,322	8,876*	2,029	1,896*	5,473	5,412
Sweden	2,205	2,343*	5,223	5,736*	1,444	1,372*	3,546	3,056*
Norway	2,327	2,012*	5,664	6,009*	1,299	947†	2,938	2,955*
Denmark	2,128	2,420*	6,126	6,865*	1,695	1,579*	4,000	4,529*
Finland	4,427	4,171†	?	10,748†	1,746	1,430†	4,413	3,537†
Netherlands	2,043	1,859*	5,811	5,897*	1,356	1,159*	3,421	3,159*
France	3,400	3,388†	8,200	8,288†	1,830	1,552†	4,145	3,681†
W. Germany	2,919	3,016	7,724	7,504	1,942	1,601	4,461	4,164
USA	3,836	3,469	9,643	8,563	2,315	1,908	5,227	4,563

*1976 †1974

Sources: 1966–9 data: McKinsey, *Health Care*; 1975 data: *World Health Statistics, 1978*, Vol. 1.

show that as a percentage of the 1960 rate, England and Wales, and Scotland in particular, performed more than averagely well. However, if we then look at the annual percentage decrease over the more recent period (1971–5) it appears that the result for England and Wales at least was no longer satisfactory, and improvements were not up to those being achieved in any of the other countries.*

3. Infant mortality rates (deaths in the first year of life) reflect socio-environmental factors to a greater degree than perinatal rates. In 1975 the Nordic countries and the Netherlands once again showed the lowest rates, but France had also joined them. There is then a significant jump to England, Wales, Scotland, Germany (East and West, the former being substantially lower than the latter) and the USA.

4. The decreases in infant mortality recorded between 1960 and 1975, as a percentage of the 1960 rates, show England and Wales to have done substantially less well than Scotland and, indeed, than any other country. By far the highest rate of improvement was obtained in France. In contrast to the perinatal rates, however, the relative performance of England and Wales, and Scotland in particular, was more creditable in the more recent period. Between 1972 and 1975 only France and Sweden recorded higher average annual rates of decrease.

5. The picture for adult mortality is somewhat less clear. Certainly so far as younger men are concerned, the 1975 rate for England and Wales compares favourably with several other countries and even with three of the four Nordic ones. Moreover the general improvement recorded over the period 1964 to 1975 (or 1976) was not paralleled in some of the countries with the lowest rates (Sweden, for example, showing rising mortality among men). In the case particularly of women aged 45–54, however, the data offer little comfort.

How are we to explain the differences? One way is through comparison of the relative importance of causes of death. If Sweden is compared with England and Wales, taking rates of infant death for a number of major causes, it becomes apparent that perinatal factors and respiratory conditions are major contributors to the poorer British rate.

If the difference between the two national rates is 5.9 per 1,000 live births, 2.8 of these are accounted for by various perinatal factors and 1.4 by respiratory conditions and pneumonia (Table 22). In other words it is not

---

*This conclusion does not hold for the most recent period. Rates of improvement since 1975 have been similar to those of, for example, Finland, France and W. Germany.

difficult to see how both factors impacting before and during birth *and* those which relate principally to the environment and care of the infant have their effect. The difference in death due to congenital abnormality is relatively slight and the fact that in Sweden, with its excellent record in perinatal and infant death, the congenital abnormality death rate remains comparable with the situation in England and Wales has led some commentators to the view that there may here be an 'irreducible minimum' beyond which progress is, given present knowledge, unlikely on this particular front (see for example Pharaoh and Morris, 1979).

Table 22: *Mortality rates under 1 year per 1,000 live births, for selected causes* *(1976)*

	Sweden	England and Wales	difference
Infections	0.26	0.43	0.17
Acute respiratory conditions	0.04	0.57	0.53
Pneumonia	0.13	1.02	0.89
Accidents	0.08	0.35	0.27
Various anoxic and hypoxic conditions of pregnancy	1.43	2.96	1.53
Other causes of perinatal mortality	1.07	2.30	1.23
Congenital abnormality	3.03	3.45	0.42

Another approach to an explanation might be through a comparison of levels of provision of health care in different countries (Table 23). Differences in numbers of doctors per head of population are not, however, extreme, and West Germany, which throughout the 1960s and early 1970s was the most generously endowed, shows up relatively poorly in the mortality tables. The supply of nurses accords a little better with mortality. But the importance of medical care provision, however expressed, has to be considered in relation to socio-environmental variables which are the principal determinants of relative levels of, and changes in, the health of nations.

For instance a comparison of health services in England, Sweden and the USA found that although Sweden put greater emphasis on child health and the USA on the health of old people (both spent similar proportions of GNP on health care) and that there were differences in access between income groups, the main conclusion was that: 'The dominant reason why

Table 23: *Availability of health care: physicians, nurses and hospital beds in Europe per 10,000 population*

	Physicians			Nurses		General (non-psychiatric) hospital beds	
	1960	1971	1975	1960	1975*	1960	1971
England and Wales	10.5	12.7⎫	11.0	20.8†	37.5	46.0	40.7
Scotland	11.8	15.6⎭		22.0	48.2	47.8	49.4
Sweden	9.5	13.9	16.2§	28.6	71.1	—	69.4
Norway	11.8	14.6	18.3¶	28.1	73.6	55.8	46.1
Denmark	12.3	—	17.9‡	37.7	80.4	59.7†	60.1
Finland	6.4	11.1	13.3§	33.8	81.9	41.9	46.8
Netherlands	11.2	13.2	15.9¶	—	32.2	45.0†	53.6
France	10.0	13.9	14.6	18.6	50.2	55.5†	60.5
W. Germany	14.9	17.8	19.2	22.0	35.9	65.3	66.8
USA	13.4	15.4	—	27.9	63.7	41.4	46.7

* breaks in series: data not comparable around break † 1959 ‡ 1968 § 1974 ¶ 1976

Sources: McKinsey, *Health – The Growing Dilemma*, New York, 1974; 1975 physicians' data: *Eurohealth Handbook*; 1975 nurses' data: WHO *World Health Statistics*, 1978, Vol. III.

the Swedish mortality rates are lower than in any state in the United States is a high minimum standard of living for everyone and a cultural homogeneity ... Health services are, of course, also a factor in the low mortality rates, but the elimination of poverty in the United States in the sense true for Sweden would be more likely to bring mortality rates closer to Sweden than a policy limited to health services only' (Anderson, 1972, p. 158).

One factor which can probably be eliminated as an explanation of the relatively poor British showing is the degree of regional disparity in medical services. Indeed, in so far as broadly aggregated data give an accurate picture, the regional disparity of physicians is more equitable in England (Table 24).

Inequalities in health: the international experience

While in the UK mortality and morbidity statistics are routinely presented by social class, the same is not true of other countries. It may be that social class is a less politically salient dimension of social stratification than in

Table 24: *Regional variations in number of physicians per thousand population: highest and lowest areas*

	England		France		Germany		Netherlands	
Average		1.06		1.47		1.74		1.36
Highest (H)	(N.W. Thames)	1.31	(Paris)	2.18	(W. Berlin)	2.97	(Utrecht)	2.10
Lowest (L)	(Trent)	0.91	(Basse Normandie)	0.98	(Nieder-Sachsen)	1.41	(Friesland)	0.92
Ratio H/L		1.4		2.2		2.1		2.3

Sources: England, France, Germany: A. Maynard in *Social and Economic Administration*, 12, 1, 1978; Netherlands: Compendium Gezondheitsstatistiek Nederland, Centraal Bureau voor de Statistiek, 1974.

the UK and other dimensions are more important, but whatever the reason, health inequality data are more commonly presented on a geographic or, as in the USA, ethnic basis. Certainly in those Nordic countries made up of industrialized densely populated southern regions and cold rural northern regions with sparse and declining populations this is not surprising. One result, though, is that international data expressing the extent of health inequalities are not readily presented on a comparable basis. Moreover, where social or occupational groupings are used these are not strictly comparable with the groupings used in Britain by the Registrar General. Additionally, the overall social class compositions of countries are far from identical. Nevertheless, though the data we have collected relate variously to regional, industrial, occupational or income groups, they do permit some attempt at answering the question: are the health inequalities in England and Wales which we have illustrated encountered also in Europe and the USA? The best way of dealing with our somewhat disparate data is to make country-by-country comparisons with England and Wales.

Denmark

Denmark has lower perinatal and infant mortality rates than England and Wales and has succeeded in reducing the latter but not the former by more than we have. Their rate is also more evenly divided among the social groups. While in England and Wales neonatal mortality rates in class V are twice those in class I, with regular class increments in between, in Denmark the difference is significantly less: 5.7 neonatal deaths per 1,000 live births in 1974 in the top social group against 9 per 1,000 in the bottom (Table 25). The neonatal mortality rate for unskilled workers in Denmark has also fallen by the same percentage as for the country as a whole, which it has not in Britain.

Table 25: *Denmark: neonatal mortality rate by occupation per 1,000 live births*

	1970	1972	1974
Self-employed	10.9	8.1	5.7
Salaried employee	9.9	9.8	7.5
Skilled worker	10.1	8.9	8.1
Unskilled worker	13.5	11.3	9.0
Other/unknown	11.1	10.2	8.8
All	11.0	9.7	8.0

Source: *Medicinisk Fødselssatistisk*, Copenhagen, 1974.

Table 26: *Finland: age-adjusted mortality indices (1970) by social group per 10,000 adults*

		Male	Female
I	Higher administrative or clerical employees, comparable employers, and people with academic degrees	78	95
II	Lower administrative or clerical employees, and comparable employers	95	100
III	Skilled and specialized workers	92	102
IV	Unskilled workers	148	103
V	Farmers	87	96

Source: S. Naytia, 'Social Group and Mortality in Finland', *British Journal of Preventive and Social Medicine*, 31, 4, 1977, p. 23.

Table 27: *France: rates of infant, neonatal and post-neonatal death by socio-professional group of father (per 1,000 legitimate live births)*

	1956–60			1970–72		
	Infant	Neo-natal	Post-neonatal	Infant	Neo-natal	Post-neonatal
Liberal professions; higher and middle cadres	17.0	12.4	4.6	11.6	8.7	2.9
Employees	24.9	19.7	8.2	14.7	10.8	3.9
Industrial and commercial proprietors	25.4	17.4	8.0	15.0	11.2	3.8
Skilled workers	28.1	17.7	10.4	26.2	11.4	4.8
Farmers	31.2	20.8	10.4	15.2	11.4	3.8
Specialized workers	32.9	19.6	13.3	19.0	13.2	5.8
Agricultural workers	35.3	21.0	14.3	19.8	14.0	5.8
Labourers	44.8	23.1	21.7	25.7	16.5	9.2
All	29.6	18.4	11.2	15.9	11.4	4.6

Note: Certain categories of workers, which fall within the range shown, are not given.

Source: Dinh Quang Chĩ and S. Hemery, 'Disparités régionales de la mortalité infantile', *Économie et statistique*, 1977, 85, pp. 3–12.

Finland

Finland is a country which, though enjoying low rates of perinatal and infant mortality, suffers from very high rates of adult mortality, far above those of England and Wales. The existence of regional disparities in adult Finnish mortality is well known, but there are also differences between social groups (Table 26).

France

The classification system in France suggests at first glance greater inequalities than in Britain, but in fact it seems the relativities are broadly comparable. There are pronounced differences in infant mortality rates both between social groups and regions. During the period 1956/60 and 1970/72,

Table 28: *France 1968: mortality rates among economically active men aged 45–64 (unstandardized) (per 100,000)*

I	Higher cadres (administrators etc.)	699
II	Industrialists, liberal professions, large commercial proprietors	919
III	Middle cadres (including teachers, medical/social service personnel, army, police)	928
IV	Artisans and small shopkeepers	1,225
V	Farmers	1,117
VI	Employees (including service workers, clergy)	1,392
VII	Qualified workers	1,589
VIII	Agricultural workers	1,520
IX	Other workers (including miners)	1,169
	All	1,189

Note: The French data shown in Table 28 refer to men aged 45–64 (unstandardized for age), excluding those classified in the census as 'inactive' (16 per cent of the total, and with a very much higher mortality rate) and excluding three regions of France in which a very high proportion of deaths are attributed to unspecified or inadequately specified causes. If those classified as 'inactive' are included, the overall rate rises from 1,189 to 1,443. Thus, though the classifications within I, II and III on the one hand and VII, VIII and IX on the other do not correspond to those in Great Britain, the picture of distinctly higher mortality rates in the latter group is comparable with the British.

Source: Derrienic *et al.*, 1977.

the ratio between infant mortality in the most favoured group (liberal professions) and the least favoured (labourers) fell slightly from 2.6 to 2.2 (Table 27). There was no change in the ratio of neonatal rates (first month), which remained at about 1.9. In the case of post-neonatal death rates, however, the least favoured social group has improved its relative standing very strikingly, the ratio falling from 4.7 to 3.2. This latter change is in marked contrast to Britain and seems to imply a greater levelling of socio-environmental factors closely implicated in post-neonatal death than has taken place here.

Among adults the difference between the most and least favoured social groups in terms of mortality is slightly more than a factor of two, a figure roughly comparable with the UK (Table 28).

From a regional point of view a factor of two separated the area of France enjoying the lowest infant mortality rates in 1970/72 from the highest. While Île de France, including Paris, had a figure of 13 per 1,000 legitimate live births, Corsica had a figure of 24.6 per 1,000. In 1956/60 these two regions also ran first and last and in the intervening years there has been no change in the ratios separating them.

The interaction between socio-economic and regional disparities can be shown by the cross-tabulation of infant mortality rates by occupation and region simultaneously. One study showed that for the group 'liberal professions and higher and middle cadres', the infant mortality rate in 1970–72 ranged from 10.2 in Haute-Normandie and Rhône-Alpes, to 17.6 in Corsica; but that in two areas (Franche-Comté, Languedoc-Roussillon) 'industrial and commercial proprietors' actually had lower rates. Similarly, for 'labourers', the range was from 18.3 (Pays de la Loire) to 33.4 (Franche-Comté); but once more in two areas (Corsica and Aquitaine) the group 'specialized workers' showed up less well. In terms of the ratio mortality rates between 'labourers' and 'liberal professions . . .' there was also a considerable range, from 1.4 (Corsica and Aquitaine) to 2.7 (Brittany).

West Germany

In the German case it is necessary to use regional disparities as an indicator of the existence of health inequalities. On this basis, and using infant and neonatal mortality as an indicator, the German experience shows up as being less favourable than that in England and Wales (Table 29).

Both rates, but particularly the infant mortality rate, show substantial variation. The same is true for England and Wales. The range in infant mortality rates for the German *Länder* is from 17.9 (Baden-Württemberg) to 25.9 (Bremen): a difference of 8.0 or 40 per cent of the lower figure. The comparison may be made with the RHAs of England and Wales. The lowest infant mortality rate here (1975) is Oxford (12.68 per 1,000 live births), the highest Yorkshire (17.93) – a difference of 5.2 or about 40 per cent of the lower figure (OPCS, DH3, no. 2, 1977).

Table 29: *West Germany 1974: infant mortality and early neonatal mortality rates, by Land*

Land	Infant mortality rate	Early neonatal mortality rate
		per 1,000 live births
Schleswig-Holstein	18.0	10.5
Hamburg	19.0	11.2
Niedersachsen	21.9	13.5
Bremen	25.9	12.1
Nordrhein-Westfalen	23.2	14.3
Hessen	21.5	13.3
Rheinland-Pfalz	22.3	12.6
Baden-Württemberg	17.9	11.4
Bayern	20.4	13.2
Saarland	25.6	15.7
W. Berlin	18.7	9.3
All	21.1	13.0

Source: Statistisches Bundesamt, 1974.

Netherlands

Here too social class or occupation categories do not seem to be employed in analyses of inequalities in health: provincial differences are, however, available. Table 30 shows variation in adult mortality rates between the Dutch provinces, standardized for age.

Once more, comparison may be made with OPCS statistics giving SMRs by English and Welsh RHAs (OPCS, DH5, no. 2, 1977). The range in SMRs among males is from 87 (Oxford), 88 (East Anglia) to 113 (North-West) and 111 (Northern); for females the range is distinctly smaller, from 92 (Wessex) and 93 (East Anglia) to 108 (Northern) and 110 (North-West). Allowing for the different bases on which the two sets of figures are given, the ranges from lowest to highest do not seem very different. The superior performance of the Netherlands seems, rather, to be reflected in the distribution of provinces within this range. There are more nearer the lower end than the higher.

Table 30: *Netherlands 1971: age-standardized adult mortality per 10,000 population*

Province	Males	Females
Groningen	88.8	71.6
Friesland	84.9	71.9
Drenthe	88.0	76.8
Overjssel	89.7	73.1
Gelderland	93.6	77.4
Utrecht	93.8	70.5
Noord Holland	94.5	73.0
Zuid Holland	92.4	71.4
Zeeland	80.9	68.5
Noord Brabant	95.5	79.4
Limburg	101.4	82.7
All Netherlands	92.8	74.3

Source: Centraal Bureau voor de Statistiek, 1974.

Norway

Like the Netherlands, Norway distinctly surpasses England and Wales in its rates of perinatal, infant and adult mortality. Norwegian statistics give standardized mortality rates for the twenty Norwegian counties, in relation to the national average, for adult males and females. The picture differs somewhat between the two groups. In both cases, however, the highest rates are found in Finnmark (the most northerly and very sparsely populated part of the country): 122 for men and 118 for women (1969–72). In the case of men the next highest rate is found in the Oslo area (the industrialized capital in which over 10 per cent of the population live); whereas in the case of women it is in Troms (a county also many hundreds of miles into the Arctic circle). These rates are 111 and 110 respectively. The southern regions of more moderate climate which are not industrialized have much lower mortality rates. Leaving aside Finnmark, the range for men is 85–111 and for women 95–110. However, if Troms also is omitted, the range for women falls to 95–104, the figure for Oslo being 99 (less than the national average). Clearly, in the case of Norway climatic factors render such comparisons of uncertain value.

Also available are morbidity data, more or less comparable with those given in the GHS, on an income basis. These data suggest something of an income gradient in morbidity among single persons and among the older members of multi-person households, though not among 16–49-year-olds.

Table 31: *Norway 1975: morbidity* by age and income: percentage of all in each group*

annual income	persons in multi-person households						single persons, ages over 16
	Age						
	0–6	*7–15*	*16–30*	*30–49*	*50–66*	*67+*	
under 15,000 kr	35	31	36	52	74	80	78
15,000–29,999 kr	29	30	44	54	76	78	75
30,000–49,999 kr	33	36	45	54	72	78	58
50,000–79,999 kr	31	34	42	52	65	77	58
over 80,000 kr	24	32	39	48	60	67	—

* 'Morbidity' is defined as persons sick on 1 October and/or at least one day of restricted activity in the period 1–15 October.

Source: Central Bureau of Statistics, Oslo, 1977.

Sweden

Sweden has the lowest perinatal and infant mortality rates in the world and, moreover, is succeeding in continuing to reduce them. The Swedish situation in this respect is of particular interest.

Early in the century Sweden suffered from substantial differentials in infant death rates, on both a geographical and an income basis. Thus, among legitimate infants born in Stockholm between 1918 and 1922, the infant mortality rate in families with an income over 10,000 S Kr was 14.3 per 1,000, in families with an income of less than 4,000 S Kr it was 48.9 per 1,000.* Professor Sjolin of Uppsala University writes of this differential: 'Today the difference is probably completely erased, but there are no recent studies to confirm it' (Sjolin, 1975). The decline in regional differentials is shown by Fig. 7, which compares rates for the three most northern and relatively poor counties with two southern counties (Uppsala, Göteborg). By 1971, Sjolin writes, the northern county of Vasternorrland had the lowest rate of infant mortality among all the Swedish counties (8.2).

Moreover, Sweden seems also to have eliminated socio-economic differ-

* Rietz Acta Paediat, 9, quoted by Sjolin.

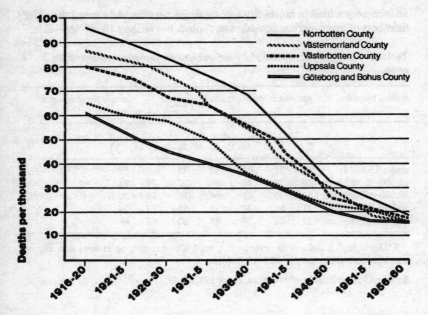

Figure 7. *Infant mortality in five Swedish counties, 1916–60. (Source: Sjolin, 1975.)*

ences in height and age of maturity among children. A study in 1976 found no such differences in a sample of 740 Swedish urban school children followed from age 9–17 (Lindgren, 1976). (By contrast, Rona, Swan and Altman (1978) found that social class remains an important determinant of children's height – between ages 5 and 11.5 years – in England and Scotland. Moreover, within each of the class-groups children with *unemployed* fathers were shorter.)

The reduction of inequalities

Several recent studies in the USA have attempted to focus on the question of *changing* inequalities. In particular there have been attempts to assess the effect of the poverty programmes of the 1960s on health inequalities, measured by adult and infant mortality rates and morbidity/utilization of the health services rates (Lerner and Stutz, 1977; Chase, 1977; and Wilson and White, 1977).

Taken together they indicate that the medico-social programmes of that period were associated (since causality cannot be assumed) with reductions in infant mortality differentials, though not adult mortality differentials, and with improved utilization of medical services by the poor relative to the non-poor, but again not with reductions in differentials in morbidity. In so far as this is an accurate picture, it might conceivably be seen as indicative of the feasibility of influencing the various indicators of 'health inequality' with which we are concerned.

So far as policies designed specifically to reduce the overall incidence of perinatal and infant mortality (and the associated morbidity among survivors) are concerned, the experience of France and Finland is particularly significant.

A study in France has attempted an analysis of the effect of laws promulgated in 1970/71 requiring all pregnant women to attend at least four pre-natal consultations (at three, six, eight and nine months) and requiring examination of all newborn infants by a doctor in the first week of life. The law also recommended pre-natal consultation with a doctor qualified in obstetrics and additional consultations for those assessed as 'at risk' (Rumeau-Rouquette *et al.*, 1977). The study took a representative sample of about 1,000 pregnancies in the Rhône-Alpes region in July 1972 and in June 1975, and looked at both the effect on the patterns of usage of services and the outcome. Overall, the proportion of women having less than four consultations fell from 14.4 per cent to 10.6 per cent, and the number with an obstetrician responsible for pre-natal surveillance rose from 56.6 per cent to 69.3 per cent. At the same time, however, there was a rise in the average educational level of the mothers, in the standard of housing, in the use of contraception and in the percentage of mothers working, and a fall in the percentage of mothers who already had two or more children. So far as outcome was concerned, it was found that the distribution of birth-weights was unchanged, but the rate of 'anomalies or pathologies at birth' fell from 23.8 to 15.6 per cent.

The adequacy of pre-natal surveillance as a function of various 'class' factors showed a complex pattern of change. In 1972 inadequate surveillance (a total of less than four consultations or first consultation after three months) was associated with immigrant status (mother or father), no post-primary education (mother or father), number of children and manual employment of father. By 1975 the association with educational level of mother and number of children had both fallen considerably. There was no clear change on the basis of manual/non-manual employment of the father.

In Finland success in reducing perinatal and infant mortality rates has been attributed in particular to a reduction in the hazards of child-birth for larger babies (over 2,500g birth-weight) and a reduction in the proportion of babies born at below 2,500g, even though there has been no improvement in the survival chances of the reduced number of fragile babies (Wynn and Wynn, 1974). A study of perinatal mortality in Sweden reaches similar conclusions (Geijerstam, 1969). In reducing the incidence of low birth-weight, nutrition seems to be crucial, and it is perhaps worth noting that ante-natal clinics in Finland typically recommend the consumption of 1–1½ litres of milk per day by the pregnant woman – considerably more than is recommended in England. There is, of course, a typically large difference in the consumption of dairy products between England and Finland – among all income groups – a fact which may show up both in perinatal and adult mortality rates (though in opposite senses).

High rates of attendance for ante-natal care are also characteristic of the Nordic countries and are generally agreed to be importantly related to low rates of mortality and morbidity. In Finland, a 1944 law required the establishment of at least one maternal health centre in each local authority area. At that time, according to the Wynns, 31.3 per cent of pregnant women who subsequently gave birth were registered: by 1968, 99.3 per cent were registered at one of the health centres. (The figure for Sweden is also over 95 per cent.) Moreover, by 1968 91.2 per cent were attending for first examination by the end of the fourth month of pregnancy. By contrast, it seems likely that only about 50 per cent of women have registered by this stage in England and Wales, and in some areas the figure is undoubtedly very much lower.

In addition in Finland all women deemed to be at risk by virtue of, for example, a previous failed pregnancy or hypertension are referred from the health centre to the ante-natal department of a major central hospital, for either one or more consultations. This accounts for about one quarter of all the women. It is part of a broader policy of disbanding domestic deliveries and concentrating child-birth in major specialized centres.

In emphasizing the importance of surveillance from an early stage of pregnancy, both Finland and France have made use of financial incentives to improve ante-natal take-up.

In Finland, only mothers who go for examination to a doctor, midwife or maternal health centre within the first four months of their pregnancy can receive the maternity grant. In 1974 this could be taken as a cash grant of 80 FMK (£10) or in the form of a baby 'kit' (which the Wynns estimated to be worth double) which most took. The view is that this relatively modest grant served as the necessary inducement at times and among groups of low income. Attendance now is simply taken for granted by all. It might also be noted that travel to the health centres is subsidized.

In France, maternity grants were initially seen as an instrument of population policy. Between 1946 and 1975 they were paid only where (1) a baby was conceived within two years of marriage, or (2) the mother was less than 25 years old, or (3) the interval between births was not more than three years (Doguet, 1978). Today, the grants, which form part of a rather complex French 'family policy', are seen specifically as a means of reducing perinatal mortality and birth handicap. To this end the total grant of 1,620 francs (£190) is paid in three instalments: at the end of three, six months and eight months of pregnancy, dates judged to be of significance for the detection of anomalies, and with proof of attendance at ante-natal examinations necessary. A fourth examination, in the ninth month, is also required according to a law of 1971.

A recent secondary analysis of survey data relating to 11,000 1972 births shows that among French-born mothers (where the father also was born in France) 14 per cent had three or less ante-natal examinations and 9 per cent attended for their first examination after three months of pregnancy. These figures rose to 27 per cent and 16 per cent for non-French (migrants) (and to 35 per cent and 16 per cent for the North African-born in the migrant group). However when those mothers who were French-born but were *also* both married to a manual worker and had received no post-primary education were considered alone, they also rose to 20 per cent and 12 per cent (Kaminski *et al.*, 1978). Thus, although there are both class and ethnic differences in this respect in France, like those in Britain, the overall rate of attendance seems to be distinctly better.

In both France and Finland financial incentives also play a part in ensuring post-natal medical examination. In Finland, the maternity health centres are informed of all births to mothers registered with them. Within forty-eight hours of returning home, the mother is visited by a midwife, who has the duty of ensuring that the child is registered at a child health centre. Today, over 90 per cent of children are registered within one month of birth. The proportion of those registered within the first year rose from 84.7 per cent in 1957 to 94.2 per cent in 1969.* Each child is seen ten to eleven times in the first year (twice by a doctor), and then twice a year between the ages of one and six by health centre staff. The Wynns point to the important contribution made by these staff beyond the assessment of purely medical well-being. They teach parents about nutrition, the care of minor ailments,

* This is higher than in Britain, where the National Child Development Survey found a figure of about 80 per cent. Official statistics show that of children born in England in 1974 90.1 per cent attended a child health clinic in 1976. However, in some AHAs the figure is very much lower: for example, Birmingham 71.2 per cent, Camden/Islington 70.6 per cent, Salford 68.2 per cent, Cornwall 62.4 per cent.

dealing with behaviour problems and the importance of mental stimulation of the child. It appears that parents increasingly go there for advice on all aspects of child behaviour. The third maternity allowance instalment is only paid after attendance at the post-natal medical examination.

In France, there exists a post-natal allowance of 2,130 francs (about £240), paid in three instalments. For the first, the child must be examined within the first week of life, for the second within the ninth month and for the third within the twenty-fourth month.

As well as these incentives, it is important to note that in Finland, when an appointment at the health centre is missed, a midwife or health visitor visits the home. This is felt to be very important and is, of course, made possible by very much more generous staffing levels. Also regarded as important to Finnish practice is the accountability for coverage required of Finnish public health services.

Today it is clear from the experience of both of these countries that a deliberate policy of attempting to ensure that ante-natal and child health services have a 100 per cent take-up yields major benefits for perinatal and infant mortality rates. It is not possible unambiguously to conclude that the financial incentives used in Finland and France are themselves directly responsible for the improved rates of attendance and consequent reduction in death and, inevitably, in perinatal morbidity. But irrespective of this, the 'outreach' capacity of the Finnish system (following up all missed appointments, etc.) must be stressed. So too, in our view, must the importance of adapting the functioning of these health centres to the needs and the difficulties of those whose attendance must be secured.

It is worth noting, also, that the obligations upon women in France to attend ante-natal care in force since 1971, intended to increase coverage, form part of a broader attack on handicap of perinatal origin (Wynn and Wynn, 1976). Other measures include the improvement in equipment and staffing of major obstetric departments; the establishment of more ICUs for newborn infants; and the regulation of minimum standards of equipment, staffing, size etc. binding on all establishments with maternity units, whether public or private. This latter has led to the closure and amalgamation of many small units. Moreover, it now appears that concern in France is not with coverage of ante-natal care (which is adequate) but with the poor quality, and often perfunctory nature, of the examinations given. Also, the striking reduction in 'class' differential in post-neonatal mortality rates suggests some levelling in social, economic and environmental conditions. It is noteworthy that, between 1956–60 and 1970–72, this reduction has been much greater than the (negligible) reduction in the class differential in neonatal rate – implying a greater relative levelling of environmental conditions than in obstetric care.

Conclusions and summary

Comparison of the British experience with that of other industrialized Western countries, on the basis of commonly used overall mortality rates, shows that British perinatal and infant mortality rates are distinctly higher than those of the four Nordic countries and of the Netherlands, and comparable with those of Western Germany. The rate of improvement in perinatal mortality enjoyed by Britain over the period 1960–75 was as good as that of most other countries, though the rate of gain is *now* poor. Moreover in the case of infant mortality all comparable countries have done better, especially France. Adult mortality patterns, especially in the younger age groups, compare reasonably with other countries.*

Why, then, might it be that infant mortality in particular presents so dismal a picture? Analyses quoted earlier suggest that infant death rates are associated with a number of characteristics of socio-economic and health systems. Low infant death rate seems clearly to be associated with per capita GDP, and there is some evidence for an association with an egalitarian income distribution. (In other words distributional aspects of society – and the extent of income inequalities – may be related to national performance in the infant mortality rankings.) So far as health policy is concerned, it seems that extent of provision of nurses and midwives, and of hospital beds, are more important than provision of physicians. Not unrelated, it seems that a relative emphasis upon preventive, ante-natal and child health services within health policy is required. International comparison here may thus have implications for policy.

It is possible, of course, that the superior performance of Sweden, Netherlands etc. might be attributed to difference principally in the extent of internal inequalities. Thus, if the perinatal mortality rate for all England and Wales were equal to that of social classes I and II, or the infant death rate equal to that obtaining in Oxford RHA, there would be little difference between these countries and ours. The second question, then, is whether the inequalities in health between social classes and regions, found in Britain, also exist elsewhere.

---

* It has, however, recently been noted that whereas the death rates among men aged 45–54 from coronary heart disease in Australia, Canada, Finland and America are now *declining*, those in England and Wales have merely *stopped rising*. The reasons for decline remain to be explained (Morris, 1979).

Briefly, the evidence – although disparate and not permitting comprehensive comparison – suggests that they do. The evidence relating to France and Germany (in the first case on an occupational basis, in the second on a regional basis) indicates disparities broadly corresponding to those of Britain. Finland also seemed comparable. So too did the Netherlands, at least in terms of the total range of regional inequality noted. Only in the cases of Norway and Sweden did a significantly smaller inequality appear to obtain. Moreover, in both these cases the extent of regional inequality (at least on the index of adult male mortality rate) seems to have fallen consistently over the years. American evidence on changing inequalities suggests an improvement in the case of infants and access to medical services, but not in adult mortality or morbidity.

If the evidence for changes in the extent of inequalities is slight (and in the American case ambiguous), that for the success of specific policies designed to reduce inequalities is slighter still. Clearly, as the study by Rumeau-Rouquette *et al.* showed, various dimensions of comparison can produce discrepant results, and changes in extraneous variables may often interfere. Of course, this study also suggested that reductions in inequality of access to, or utilization of, pre-natal care can come about.

None of the results quoted enables us to deal with the question of the relative importance of inequalities in provision or utilization of health services on the one hand and other forms of inequality on the other in determining inequalities of outcome. (Although it is noteworthy that provision of physicians is more equal on a regional basis in England than even in the Netherlands.) An aspect of this question is that of the intervention of social class or related factors between morbidity and use of health services. Is it *commonly* the case that working-class or low-income individuals or families have less recourse to the health services when they are sick? There are relatively few studies to draw upon.

One important study was carried out by Purola *et al.* in Finland in 1964, just prior to the introduction of much expanded health insurance (Sickness Insurance Act), which for the first time covered primary medical care. Methodologically this study, like the General Household Survey, was based on a questionnaire administered to a representative sample of non-institutionalized families (not households). Questions covered self-reported morbidity, use of health services, income etc. The most important conclusion for our present purposes was that the number of consultations with a GP in a given period of time was proportional to income, when number of days of reported sickness was held constant. A similar relationship obtained in the case of the chronic sick. On the other hand, the number of days spent in hospital was not a function of income. Moreover, since it was known that incomes in rural areas were lower than in urban areas, and it had been established that distances to physicians were greater in rural areas and that consultation rates were inversely proportional to distance, the effects of income were examined holding both morbidity and distance constant. The effects of income on GP consultation rates and those of distance were independent of each other (Purola *et al*, 1968).

The Finnish Sickness Insurance Act was designed to reduce the financial disincentive to making use of physicians' services. It does not appear however that organizational or financial arrangements can wholly compensate for income inequalities in bringing about parity of usage.

An analysis by Salkever of data collected in five countries with very different health systems (Liverpool, Helsinki, Lodz, Baltimore and north-west Vermont, and an area of Saskatchewan) – in the context of a WHO study – throws some light on this (Salkever, 1975). Relating probability of contacting a physician to an index of ill-health (perceived seriousness of condition; days restricted activity; days in bed), according to income, Salkever found first that in all cases except Saskatchewan low-income children fared worse. That is, their reduced utilization was independent of the organization and costs of health care. Among adults, it appeared that the clearest association of low income with low utilization was found in Liverpool. If American and French experiences are any guide, this is one aspect of the cause of health inequality which can be corrected.

Chapter 6

Towards an Explanation of Health Inequalities

Death rates in present-day Europe have reached what appear to be their lowest points in the history of human society. The twentieth century has witnessed a dramatic decline in the rate of infectious disease, as well as the introduction of powerful therapies for its treatment. Common causes of death like TB and diphtheria, often linked with poverty and material deprivation, have greatly diminished, though they have been replaced by new diseases, some of which have been linked in particular studies with affluence and material abundance. On that account inequalities in health might have been expected to diminish. But the evidence which we have presented in earlier chapters suggests that this has not been the case. In this chapter we ask why occupational class continues to exert so significant an influence on health in Britain.

There are a number of approaches to an explanation, though none in our view provides a wholly satisfactory answer. Indeed, the variable of occupational class is in itself multifaceted, and its influence probably varies according to age or stage in the life-cycle and according to the natural history of disease.

Theoretical approaches

Theoretical explanations of the relationship between health and inequality might be roughly divided into four categories:

1. Artefact explanations.
2. Theories of natural or social selection.
3. Materialist or structuralist explanations.
4. Cultural/behavioural explanations.

In some respect each one of these approaches sheds light on the observed relationships between class and health in present-day Britain. We shall first describe and discuss in general terms the four approaches and then go on, by reference to the problems of different age groups, to show that any satisfactory explanation must build essentially on the ideas of the cumulative dispositions and experience of the lifetime, and of multiple causation.

The artefact explanation

This approach suggests that both health and class are artificial variables thrown up by attempts to measure social phenomena and that the relationship between them may itself be an artefact of little causal significance. Accordingly, the failure of health inequalities to diminish in recent decades is believed to be explained to a greater or lesser extent by the reduction in the proportion of the population in the poorest occupational classes. It is believed that the failure to reduce the gap *between* classes has been counterbalanced by the shrinkage in the relative size of the poorer classes themselves. The implication is that the upwardly mobile are found to have better health than those who remain, or that their health subsequently improves relative to the health of those they join. We would make two comments. One is that informed examination of successive census reports shows that the poorer occupational classes have contracted less sharply than often supposed (see Appendix, Tables 1 and 2). The other is that indicators of relatively poor progress in health apply to much larger sections of the manual occupational classes than just those who are 'unskilled' (see p. 60, for example).

Natural and social selection

Occupational class is here relegated to the state of dependent variable and health acquires the greater degree of causal significance. The occupational class structure is seen as a filter or sorter of human beings and one of the major bases of selection is health, that is, physical strength, vigour or agility. It is inferred that the Registrar General's class I has the lowest rate of premature mortality because it is made up of the strongest and most robust men and women in the population. Class V by contrast contains the weakest and most frail people. Put another way, this explanation suggests that physical weakness or poor health carries low social worth as well as low economic reward, but that these factors play no causal role in the event of high mortality. Their relationship is strictly reflective. Those men and women who by virtue of innate physical characteristics are destined to live the shortest lives also reap the most meagre rewards. This type of explanation has been invoked to explain the preponderance of individuals with severe mental disorders in social class V (a thesis which was reviewed critically in, for example, Goldberg and Morrison, 1963). It is postulated that affected people *drift* to the bottom rung of the Registrar General's occupational scale.

Similar selective processes are thought to occur with other forms of disease even though the extent of drift may not be so great and there is little actual evidence of it.

Materialist or structuralist explanations

The third type of explanation emphasizes the role of economic and associated socio-structural factors in the distribution of health and well-being, and, because it is frequently misunderstood, requires fuller exposition. There are several separate strands of reasoning within it which can be ordered more or less according to the extent to which the primary causal significance is assigned directly or indirectly to the role of economic deprivation. Amongst explanations which focus on the *direct* influence of poverty or economic deprivation in the production of variation in rates of mortality is the radical Marxian critique. With the benefit of a century's hind-sight the validity of much of this nineteenth-century theory of the relationship between health and material inequality has been accepted today, especially for the earlier phase of competitive industrial capitalism (Stedman-Jones, 1971; Thompson, 1976). Exploitation, poverty and disease have virtually become synonymous for describing conditions of life in the urban slums of Victorian and Edwardian cities, as they are today for the shanty towns of the under-developed world.

But can it be so readily applied to contemporary health experience? Can the premature mortality of the working class still be directly attributed to subsistence poverty and exploitation? It is true that a relationship between material deprivation and certain causes of disease and death is now well established, but then so is the capacity of the capitalist mode of production to expand the level of human productivity and to raise the living standards of working people. Economic growth of the kind most readily associated with the European style of industrialization has in itself been credited with the decline in mortality from infectious disease during the nineteenth and twentieth centuries (cf. McKeown, 1976; Powles, 1975). Today death rates for all age groups in Britain are a fraction of what they were a century ago and many of the virulent infectious diseases have largely disappeared (cf. Morris, 1975; OPCS, 1978), and the 'killer' diseases of modern society – accidents, cancer and heart disease – seem less obviously linked to poverty. Against this background, the language of economic exploitation no longer seems to provide the appropriate epithet for describing 'Life and Labour' in the last two decades of the twentieth century. Through trade-union organization and wages council machinery it is now argued that labour is paid its price and, since health tends to be conceptualized in optimum terms as a fixed condition of material welfare which, if anything, is put at risk by affluent living standards, it is assumed by many that economic class on its own is no longer the powerful determinant of health that it once was.

The flaw in this line of reasoning is the assumption that material subsistence needs can be uniquely and unambiguously defined in terms independent of the overall level of economic development in a society. People may still have too little for their basic *physiological* as well as social needs. Poverty is also a relative concept, and those who are unable to share the amenities or facilities provided within a rich society, or who are unable to fulfil the social and occupational obligations placed upon them by virtue of their limited resources, can properly be regarded as poor. They may also be relatively disadvantaged in relation to the risks of illness or accident or the factors positively promoting health.

It is worth illustrating how this can happen. New types of industrial process can introduce entirely new risks for the workforce or the population in the area. Certain forms of building or construction or town planning can introduce new hazards for adults as well as children. Changes in distances from work, type of participation in the local community and in leisure can alter the balance for many people in their access to health services as well as their knowledge about health. People living alone who have a fall, or people who have a heart attack, face different problems in different communities. Warnings about undesirable food and other products (inflammable clothing and furniture, for instance), as well as the latest information about the means of obtaining a healthy diet, may or may not be communicated, depending on the social circumstances. Many other examples of how new problems of health arise in a changing society might be given. The material deprivation of some sections of the population can paradoxically grow even when their income increases, relative to changing structures and amenities.

How far might differences in access to resources help to explain this? How unequal is the distribution of wealth in Britain? Historically the structure of living standards has been slow to change. Personal wealth is still concentrated in the hands of a small minority of the population, as reports of the Royal Commission on the Distribution of Income and Wealth have shown.

The question whether the richest men and women in Britain have maintained their economic position at the expense of less well-endowed citizens eludes a categorical answer. The Royal Commission has referred to the 'remarkable' stability of the unequal distribution of income over the past two decades (see also Appendix, Table 4). Moreover there is no doubt that the proportion as well as number of the population dependent on a subsistence or near-subsistence income from the state has grown. For some groups, and especially manual groups, relative lifetime resources will have been reduced. Earlier retirement, unemployment and redundancies, single-parent status and disablement, as well as the proportionate increase in the elderly population, all play some part in this development. For recent years Table 32 shows the tendency for those at the lowest relative income standards to increase in number and proportion.

Table 32: *Numbers of persons in poverty and on the margins of poverty* (*Family Expenditure Survey*)

Income relative to supplementary benefit	Britain (000s)			
	1960*	1975	1976	1977
Under supplementary benefit standard	1,260	1,840	2,280	2,020
Receiving supplementary benefit	2,670	3,710†	4,090†	4,160†
At or not more than 40 per cent above standard	3,510	6,990	8,500	7,840
Total	7,740	12,540	14,870	14,020
Per cent of population	14.2	23.7	28.1	26.6

*From B. Abel-Smith and P. Townsend, *The Poor and the Poorest*, Bell, 1965, pp. 40 and 44. The data are for the UK and are on a household rather than an income unit basis. It should be noted that this column is based on national assistance scales, not supplementary benefit scales.

†Drawn separately from a supplementary benefit sample inquiry with people drawing benefit for less than three months excluded. In the FES, such people are categorized according to their normal income and employment.

Sources: For 1960, Abel-Smith and Townsend, 1965, pp. 40 and 44. For 1975–7, DHSS (SR3), Analyses of the FES.

There is therefore a paradox: while we would not wish to assert that the evidence is consistent and complete, the proportion of the population with relatively low lifetime incomes (in the widest sense of 'income') seems to have increased in recent decades, just as the proportion assigned to classes IV and V seems to have decreased, though the latter continue to comprise more than a quarter of the population. While economic growth has improved the access of both groups to income and other resources, other groups have gained in proportion, and since neither facilities nor knowledge is a finite commodity, those with relatively low incomes (in increasing numbers) have remained relatively disadvantaged.

So it has been with health. Occupational classes IV and V may in time catch up with the contemporary levels achieved by I and II but by that time the latter groups will have forged even further ahead. There is nothing fixed about levels of physical well-being. They have improved in the past and there is every likelihood that they will improve in the future. But class inequalities persist in the distribution of health as in the distribution of income or wealth, and they persist as a form of relative deprivation.

Unfortunately the opportunity for examining the association between income and health is restricted by lack of information and the role played by material factors in creating the pattern of health and ill-health which can be found in the population is complex. Occupational class is multifaceted in 'advanced' societies, and apart from the variables most readily associated with socio-economic position – income, savings, property and housing – there are many other dimensions which can be expected to exert an active causal influence on health. People at work, for instance, encounter different material conditions and amenities, levels of danger and risk, degree of security and stability, association with other workers, levels of self-fulfilment and job satisfaction and physical or mental strain. These dimensions of material inequality are also closely articulated with another determinant of health – education.

Two other related theoretical approaches should be mentioned. Each is concerned with the effect of macro-economic variables – levels of production, unemployment etc. – on health. First an American social scientist, Harvey Brenner, making use of time-series data trends in the US economy and fluctuations in rates of mortality, purports to show that recessions and wide-scale economic distress have an impact on a number of health indicators, including foetal, infant and maternal mortality, the national mortality rate – especially of death ascribed to cardio-vascular disease, cirrhosis of the liver, suicide and homicide rates – and on rates of first admission to mental hospitals (Brenner, 1973, 1976 and 1977).*

In fitting the data on economic trends, essentially unemployment, to health indicators, Brenner suggests there is a delayed effect of between two and five years, choosing the lag to obtain the best fit. By doing this he purports to be able to estimate both the initial impact of recession on the dependent variable as well as the cumulative impact over the space of several years. He also posits time lags of varying numbers of years between economic changes and changes in various health indicators (on a purely empirical basis) and in doing so claims to establish the direction of causality in a temporal sequence as well as suggesting the length of time involved. A major

* Studies of this kind were actually carried out by Morris and Titmuss in the 1940s, in an attempt to examine the effects of the violent economic fluctuations of the 1920s and 1930s upon a variety of health and mortality indicators (see, for example, Morris and Titmuss, 1944a, 1944b).

problem with such research, even if validated, is, of course, the causal mechanism. *How* does unemployment increase mortality? Brenner makes use of the somewhat ill-defined concept of 'stress' to link the two.

The second approach, in opposition to Brenner's, is concerned to disprove the common assumption that economic growth leads to an increase in general levels of health. In advanced capitalist societies, it is argued, profit is realized through hazardous, punishing and physically stressful work. Time-series data on employment and death rates are here presented in such a way that high rates of mortality appear to follow on from low rates of unemployment and high levels of prosperity (Eyer, 1975, 1977a, 1977b). In periods of high unemployment this is supposed to be the combined result of weakened institutionalized pressures to consume, relief of workers from stressful work routines, an increase of social solidarity (unlikely as this may seem), the added stimulation of supportive relationships and networks, and in general a more varied and more elevated meaning for human existence.

Cultural/behavioural explanations

A fourth approach is that of cultural or behavioural explanations of the distribution of health in modern industrial society. These are recognizable by the independent and autonomous causal role which they assign to ideas and behaviour in the onset of disease and the event of death. Such explanations, when applied to modern industrial societies, often focus on the individual as a unit of analysis emphasizing unthinking, reckless or irresponsible behaviour or incautious life-style as the moving determinant of poor health status (cf. Fuchs, 1974). What is implied is that people harm themselves or their children by the excessive consumption of harmful commodities, refined foods, tobacco and alcohol, or by lack of exercise, or by their under-utilization of preventive health care, vaccination, ante-natal surveillance or contraception. Some would argue that such systematic behaviour within certain social groups is a consequence only of lack of education, or individual waywardness or thoughtlessness. Explanation takes an individual form. What is critical, it is implied, are the personal characteristics of individuals, whether innate or acquired – their basic intelligence, their skills obtained through education and training, their physical and mental qualities, and their personal styles and dispositions. Others see behaviour which is conducive to good or bad health as embedded more within social structures – as illustrative of socially distinguishable styles of life, associated with, and reinforced by, class.

Tables 33, 34 and 35 provide the kind of data sometimes used to illustrate a cultural/behavioural type of explanation. Certain styles of living, like a diet strong in carbohydrates, cigarette-smoking and lack of participation in sporting activities, are known to cut across class. It is implied that there are individual or, at most, sub-cultural life-styles, rooted in personal characteristics and level of education, which govern behaviour and which are therefore open to change through changes in personal activities or educational inputs. However, data of the kind illustrated in these tables are not easy to interpret. For one thing, the observations are themselves only indicators which are subject to qualification if their meaning is to be put into context.

Table 33: *Household food consumption by income group (oz./person/week)*
(*Great Britain, 1979*)

Income group	Food				
	white bread	brown, including wholemeal bread	sugar and preserves	potatoes	fresh fruit
A	17	5.3	11	39	25
B	22	4.5	12	40	20
C	26	4.3	13	48	16
D	29	4.3	15	48	15

Gross weekly income of head of household: A = £145+; D = less than £56 per week.

Source: Adapted from *Household Food Consumption and Expenditure*, HMSO (see Morris, 1979).

Table 34: *Cigarette-smoking by socio-economic group (males and females aged 16 +)*
(*1980*)

SEG	Current smokers %	
	Men	Women
Professional	21	21
Managerial	35	33
Intermediate non-manual	35	34
Intermediate manual	48	43
Semi-skilled manual	49	39
Unskilled manual	57	41
All	42	37

Source: *General Household Survey*: OPCS Monitor, 28 July 1981.

Table 35: *Active leisure pursuits by males: ratio of participation rates, non-manual to manual workers, by age (males aged 16 or over engaging in each activity in the four weeks before interview) (Great Britain, 1977)*

	Age group		
	16–29	*30–59*	*60+*
Squash/fives	4.4	6.9	*
Athletics (incl. jogging)	3.3	3.3	*
Rugby	2.9	*	*
Golf	2.8	3.2	4.9
Badminton	2.8	2.8	*
Cricket	2.4	1.7	*
Tennis	2.4	4.1	*
Table-tennis	1.7	3.1	*
Swimming outdoors	1.6	2.1	*
Walking (more than 2 miles)	1.6	1.8	1.7
Bowls (indoor)	1.4	1.3	1.1
Bowls (outdoor)	1.4	1.4	1.6
Playing football	1.1	1.6	*
Swimming (indoor)	1.1	2.2	*
Dancing	0.9	1.1	1.2
Gymnastics/yoga/keep fit	0.9	2.1	*

* Ten or fewer participants in either manual or non-manual group.

Source: *General Household Survey*, 1977.

Thus, a balanced diet, or balanced physical activity, to promote health is easy neither to define nor measure. People who eat one type of food to excess may make up for that disadvantage in some other respect. And manual workers who are spectators rather than active sportsmen include those who have to exert physical strength and agility in their everyday jobs.

Again, the data can be interpreted in other ways than in relation to level of knowledge or education, or personal responsibility. Commercial advertisements are planned to 'educate' tastes, and the education provided in schools is not always calculated to prepare young people to ward off influences upon their consumption and behaviour which may be undesirable for health. Moreover, access to good food and sports facilities depends also on the area in which people live and the resources they can command, and not only their personal characteristics or behaviour, or education. But, in emphasizing these reservations we must also call attention to the *cumulative* importance of those contributions to personal behaviour made by genetic endowment of attributes, the influence of family upbringing and practices and the evolution of modes of self-management which contribute to wide differences in health achieved by different members of the same occupational or socio-economic class.

The interpretation of level of personal knowledge or education as a causal factor in health illustrates our theoretical problem. It is on the basis of success or the lack of it at school that children are selected for manual and non-manual work and, as we have seen, this occupational distinction plays an important part in measured health status differentials. But we can go further. Bernstein has argued that distinctive patterns of child rearing and socialization, such as those which tended to differentiate between working-class and middle-class families, produce quite different linguistic capacities which are in turn correlated with quite different intellectual approaches to the social world (Bernstein, 1971). The working-class child is rendered at a particular disadvantage on account of these differences because of the *fit* which exists between middle-class norms of socialization and the dominant structure of the educational system. The outcome of this is that children from middle-class homes enter the school system already equipped with the appropriate mode of communication and, as a result, they have more successful educational careers and leave school with a greater facility to manipulate their social and economic environment (which of course includes health services) to personal advantage. These ideas carry the variable of education far beyond the simple idea of the transmission of knowledge and skills. They imply that the educational system tends to be substantially developed and maintained in conformity with the class system or with that pattern of differential material advantages or disadvantages, and social opportunities or obstacles, which govern both the place taken in the system by the individual child and the chances of that child having a successful career within the system. On this reasoning, level of education becomes difficult to treat as intrinsically independent of class.

More theoretically developed as the basis for cultural/behavioural explanations is the 'culture of poverty' thesis – which has much in common with the idea of 'transmitted deprivation'. As originally proposed by Oscar Lewis, an anthropologist who studied poor communities in Central America and, later, migrant groups in New York, the 'culture of poverty' was intended to apply only to market-organized social structures with poorly developed public systems of health, welfare and income maintenance (cf. Lewis, 1967). Starting from a distinct cultural anthropological perspective, Lewis argued that human existence in any given environment involves a process of biological and social adaptation which gives rise to the elaboration of a structure of norms, ideas and behaviours. This culture over time acquires an integrity and a stability because of the supportive role it plays in helping individuals to understand and cope with their environment but, through its influence on socialization practices and the like, it also comes to have an important autonomous influence in the social consciousness of individuals. The integrity of the culture ensures its autonomous survival even when the material base from which it emerged has changed or been modified. It is for this reason that people cling on to outmoded ideas or old-fashioned practices which do not seem to accord with the changed material realities of modern existence. The 'culture of poverty' thesis has been widely criticized by British social scientists (Holman, 1978, Chapter 3; Rutter and Madge, 1976; Townsend, 1979, pp. 65–71).

Consider, for example, the diffusion of the acceptance of the idea of family planning, which is generally agreed to have been first adopted by the professional classes (Banks and Banks, 1964), from whence it diffused to poorer classes. On the basis of the 'culture of poverty' thesis this should not have happened or, at least, there should have been more evidence of stiff resistance to the adoption of the practice. However, the fact that family planning has spread rapidly to all classes is one strand of historical evidence which is felt to cast doubt on the 'culture of poverty' thesis. The implication of that example is that the beliefs and values of poorer sections of the population are less autonomous, and more dependent upon conventional or orthodox beliefs and values, than has been assumed by proponents of the thesis. Instead social scientists have felt it right to place emphasis on the material circumstances of families and their access to the means of contraception in explaining class variations in the readiness or otherwise to adopt new methods of family planning. While recognizing the force of many of their criticisms we believe it is difficult to settle questions of interpretation like that of family planning one way or the other. We are aware that even if it is difficult to make a case for separately identifiable sub-cultures that does not dispose of the possible role of cultural variations in contributing to any overall explanation of variations in health.

Choosing between such complex and sometimes competing approaches, when applied to evidence as complex as that which we have assembled, is a daunting task. We must make clear our belief that it is in some form or forms of the 'materialist' approach that the best answer lies. But there can be little doubt that amongst all the evidence there is much that is convincingly explained in alternative terms: cultural, social selection and so on. Moreover, it may well be that different kinds of factors, or forms of explanation, apply more strongly, or more appropriately, to different stages of the life-cycle. This possibility has guided the presentation of our data.

Birth and infancy

Today the greatest risk at child-birth is among mothers who are older and who have already had several children. Such cases, of course, were more prevalent in Victorian society, where knowledge about birth control was scanty and where rather different ideologies about family size existed. In recent years the percentage of mothers in classes IV and V having a fourth or fifth child has decreased, but remains higher than in classes II and III. It could therefore be that higher rates of still-birth or perinatal death are a consequence of differences in maternal age and 'parity' (family size) between the classes. But class inequalities in rates of death at birth and throughout the first year of life are found even when parity and maternal age are held constant (Morris and Heady, 1955; Morris, 1975). While age and parity exert an important influence on the risk of all still-births, the significance of these variables is much more evident among the wives of semi-skilled and unskilled manual workers. The risk of still-birth for the wives in professional and managerial households is lower no matter what their age or their previous record of pregnancies. (Similarly for perinatal death rates: at all ages and parities, the class differential remains.)

Rates of post-neonatal mortality differ somewhat – class differences are generally greater among young mothers under the age of 25 – but overall the broad pattern remains the same. The inescapable conclusion is that occupational class differences are *real* sources of difference in the risk of infant mortality.

Equally importantly, there are similar differences in the class incidence of low birth-weight which, as we shall see, can have, except under the most advantageous conditions, long-term implications for the health and development of the young child.

There are a number of explanations for this situation. Several studies have pointed to the importance of the mother's health, and the quality of obstetric care received, and there can be no doubt, on the basis of the evidence we have presented so far, that these are class-related (Hellier, 1977; Doll, Hill and Sakula, 1960).

Other explanations tend to be more complex. Studies over the last twenty years suggest that genetic factors play a 'predisposing' role in giving rise to congenital defects, with adverse environmental factors acting as a trigger (Lawrence, Carter and David, 1968; Janerich, 1972).

Work in the 1950s ascribed class differences in infant mortality to selective processes in mating and marriage (Illsley, 1955). Tall women married above their father's occupational class, short women below it, and these physical characteristics of women were then associated with different rates of infant mortality, the taller mothers having lower rates of infant death. The study concluded that higher-class men appeared to be recruiting as wives the most effective child-bearing women.

'Transmitted nutritional deprivation' offers another variant on the theme of selection (Baird, 1974). It suggests the existence of a vicious cycle of nutritional deprivation which leads to low birth-weight and congenital mal-formation. This cycle is difficult to break because, the evidence suggests, it originates in the nutritional deprivation of the mother not at the time of giving birth but *at the time of her own birth.* By this account, perinatal death and low birth-weight are seen as caused, in part, by the effects of nutritional deprivation upon the reproductive capacity of the mothers of the infants. These explanations are based upon data accumulated on the childbearing population of Aberdeen over many years, and they offer valuable insights into the mechanisms and processes whereby social class differences in mortality are produced and perpetuated.

If the relative importance of factors such as these in determining rates of perinatal death, and of handicap among survivors, is controversial, the situation is somewhat clearer in the *post-neonatal period.* When we look at causes of death in infancy which exhibit the steepest class gradients, there is much evidence to suggest that the important causal variables are contained within the socio-economic environment. The causes of death which are most likely to be associated with the nutritional status of the mother have the shallowest of gradients, while respiratory disease and accidents show steep class gradients. These observations lead us directly to consider the role of material deprivation on the life chances of the infants, and to the hypothesis that any factors which increase the parental capacity to provide adequate care for an infant will, when present, increase the chance of survival, while their absence will increase the risk of premature death. The most obvious of such factors fall within the sphere of material resources: sufficient house-hold income, a safe, uncrowded and unpolluted home, warmth and hygiene, a means of rapid communication with the outside world, for example a tele-phone or car, and an adequate level of manpower – or womanpower (two parents would normally provide more continuous care and protection than one). In addition to these basic material needs must be added other cognitive and motivational factors which are not independent of the distribution of material advantage. Those factors would include knowledge, certain skills and resources in verbal communication and a high level of motivation to provide continuous and loving care. When all these factors are present the infant's chance of survival is very good indeed. When some or even many of these are absent, the outlook is less propitious. Moreover, it should not be forgotten that these very same factors play a part in determining the development of the infant's own cognitive/linguistic and other skills. Competences acquired at this stage of life can profoundly influence later intellectual (and hence educational) achievement.

Table 36: *Causes of death from accidents of children aged 1–14 years (1968–74)*

Type of accident (or violence)	Total age 1–14 years	
	Number	%
Total accidents and violence	10,877	100.0
All accidents	10,204	93.8
Motor vehicle collision with pedestrian	3,656	33.6
Other motor vehicle collisions	1,199	11.0
Other transport accidents	619	5.7
Accidental poisoning	276	2.5
Falls	625	5.7
Fires	904	8.3
Drowning	1,401	12.9
Inhalation of food or other object	343	3.2
Accidental suffocation	375	3.4
Blows, cuts, explosions etc.	460	4.2
Accidents caused by electric current	150	1.4
Other accidents	196	1.7
Total violence	673	6.2
Suicide	33	0.3
Homicide	417	3.8
Injury undetermined whether accidentally or purposely inflicted	223	2.1

Source: OPCS.

Childhood: 1–14 years

The most important causes of death amongst all children aged 1 to 14 are, in descending order, accidents (with a small number of deaths also due to poisoning and violence – see Table 36), respiratory disease, neoplasms, congenital abnormalities and infections. Among 1- to 14-year-olds, and this we wish to stress, *almost all* the differences in mortality between occupational classes I and V are due to accidents, respiratory disease (bronchitis and pneumonia) and to a much lesser extent congenital abnormality. Among older children, deaths from accidents remain highly class-related, though deaths from respiratory disease become less so.

It follows that one approach to explaining this situation is to unravel those aspects of the social situations responsible for respiratory disease and for accidents. There are a number of epidemiological studies which help us to do this.

A study in 1966, for instance, found that the principal correlate of respiratory symptoms was the extent of air pollution in the child's area of residence (Douglas and Waller, 1966). But there was no tendency for working-class children to be more concentrated in high-pollution areas and social class had a small independent effect.

A more recent study in the mid-seventies took 2,000 children living in Harrow (which consequently did not permit consideration of a range of air pollution levels) and concluded: 'Illnesses occurred much more commonly in infants born to families which had several other children already, and in those families where the parents had respiratory disability or were smokers' (Leeder, Corkhill, Irwig, Holland and Colley, 1976). When all variables were taken together the most important proved to be: (i) bronchitis/pneumonia in siblings; (ii) parent smoking (affecting air inhaled by children); (iii) number of siblings (and likelihood of infection); (iv) parental history of asthma/wheeze. Class had no effect independently of these factors; but both smoking and family size are clearly related to class.

A third study of over 11,000 children aged 6 to 10 in a number of urban environments looked more directly at the interplay of social class and physical environment (Colley and Reid, 1970). It concluded that at the equivalent levels of air pollution children of occupational classes IV and V were much more likely to suffer from respiratory diseases than their counterparts in occupational classes I, II and III. Air pollution in short was an exacerbating factor. More directly, it reaffirmed that a past family history of respiratory disease is closely associated with a chronic cough in the 6- to 10-year-olds. It also once more found a clear class gradient in respiratory disease.

The general implication seems to be that the class gradient in bronchitis is largely a consequence of parental smoking, family size (and the increasing likelihood of infection by siblings), and a parental history of lung disease (which may also to some degree genetically place the child at risk). Parental history of lung disease is, of course, as shown independently, a function of type and severity of occupation. Environmental pollution is also implicated, and may be a particular danger for those children made vulnerable through other factors.

The second condition responsible for much of the gradient in child mortality is accidents. Among child pedestrians, for example, the risk of death from being hit by a motor vehicle is multiplied by five to seven times in passing from class I to class IV; for accidental death caused by fires, falls and drowning, the gap between the classes is even greater. These substantial differences demonstrate the non-random nature of these events. While the death of an individual child may appear as a random misfortune, the overall distribution clearly indicates the *social* nature of the phenomena. How is it to be explained?

Accidents have two primary causes: either environmental hazard, or dangerous behaviour reflecting carelessness, adventure or irresponsibility. These primary causes involve both material and cultural factors and indeed a full explanation of inequalities in the risk of death in childhood implicates each of them.

To begin with, the class pattern of accidents has to be seen in the light of the great differences in the material resources of parents, which may place significant constraints on the routine level of care and protection that they are able to provide for their children. Children of parents in occupational classes IV and V are amongst the poorest members of their age group in the population. Their opportunities to play safely within sight or earshot of their parents are less than those of their better endowed peers higher up the social scale. Furnishings, including forms of heating in the home, are likely to be less safe, as are the other domestic appliances which they encounter.

Differences in the material resources of the household also mean that the children of semi-skilled and unskilled workers are more likely to be thrown on to their own devices during holidays and out of school hours, which alone would be sufficient to increase the probability of their being involved in an accident.

It is impossible to escape the conclusion that in the context of childhood the most straightforward of material explanations is capable of providing a simple chain of causation by which the pattern of health inequality is illuminated. Households in occupational classes IV and V simply lack the means to provide their children with as high a level of protection as that which is found in the average middle-class home. This can mean both material and non-material resources. A study in Camberwell in south London, for example, concluded that one of the reasons for the greater prevalence of accidents in working-class homes is the higher incidence of stressful life events experienced by mothers. Such women lack the means to resolve the recurrent setbacks which dominate their domestic lives and are less well equipped to provide continuous and vigilant protection: 'The mother's psychiatric state and the presence of a serious long-term difficulty or a threatening life event were related to increased accident risk to children under 16. These factors were more common among working-class children, and in so far as they are causal, they go a long way to explain the much greater risk of accidents to working-class children' (Brown and Harris, 1978).

One recent study, valuable because it reports a field survey, focused on a sample of boys of 6 to 7 and 10 to 11 years old from severely deprived large families in Birmingham known to the social services department. Children were compared with a control group of similarly aged children, living in the same area but not under social service department supervision. The study was published in two parts.

In the first Brennan (1973) focused on medical characteristics. She found that both groups of children were below national age norms in height but that the sample children were more so. There was a high degree of visual impairment among both groups but again it was more marked among the sample children. (Moreover of the forty-six sample children who suffered visual impairment only one wore spectacles.) There was a higher degree of hearing loss among the sample children. Finally 78.2 per cent of sample children as against 58.9 per cent of control children were diagnosed as having some illness on clinical examination, far higher than indicated for the city as a whole from school health records, the most important being respiratory disorders, orthopaedic defects, speech defects, skin disorders and chest complaints.

The second study, with a cultural approach (Wilson and Herbert, 1978), also considered the 3–4-year-old siblings of those older brothers, and made extensive use of interviews, observation over a long period and psychological test data. This study vividly illustrates the nature and the effects of severe poverty on family life and on child development. It suggests that ill-health, inhibited cognitive development and behaviour problems are associated in a general 'poverty syndrome'.

Accidents to the children were common: thirty-four out of fifty-six families had experienced severe accidents (one child had lost an eye, sixteen suffered burns or scalding needing skin grafts).

Particularly striking was the extent to which ill-health was found to cluster in families. Of the fifty-six families studied: 'In forty families all, or most, members of the family were reported as having had much illness, or as suffering from defects or conditions which affected their activities. Respiratory diseases were most frequently mentioned, followed by gastric conditions and skin conditions.' Moreover, 'only four among the sixteen fitter families can be truly said to be healthy and obstetric problems were frequently mentioned'.

The authors concluded:

The children, in the process of growing up, have many shared experiences. They live in overcrowded conditions, being members of large families; their homes are inadequate by current standards; the neighbourhoods are rough and disliked by most who have to live in them. They experience poverty, by which we mean that they go short of things considered essential or normal by others around them. Most, if not all, the children have first-hand knowledge of illness, disability, accidents and mental stress expressed in a variety of symptoms. (p. 104)

The objective is survival, the operative unit is the family. The needs of individuals must take second place. Decisions were made at family level and related to the main wage earner or recipient of benefit rather than to the needs of individual children. (p. 186)

Finally there is considerable evidence that material deprivation affects physical development in young children and that ill-health contracted in childhood can dog an individual for life. Several studies, for example, have pointed to the effect of nutritional deprivation not only on physical growth, but also on the brain and nervous system. Some of the evidence is circumstantial, but laboratory experiments on animals suggest that malnutrition during the period of rapid brain growth – the first six months after birth – can affect the size and number of brain cells in several ways that can never later be compensated for (Birch and Gussow, 1970; Eichenwald and Fry, 1969). The implications for children from poor families in modern Britain who have a meagre diet are unclear, but few would disagree with the view expressed in an official publication that 'a hungry child is unlikely to be alert during lessons' (DHSS, *Eating for Health*, 1978).

Poor physical development also renders children susceptible to illness, and several reports have suggested that this may then persist. A study of 1,000 Newcastle families illustrates how repeated respiratory infections in the first five years, if inadequately treated, can lead to some degree of disability at the age of 15 (Miller, Court, Knox and Brandon, 1974).

Studies such as this – there are many more – suggest, as one government inquiry put it, that inadequately treated bouts of childhood illness 'cast long shadows forward' (the Court Report). Working-class children are more likely to suffer from them and less likely to be adequately treated for them.

Adult life

Among adults, as we have already seen, health differences between occupational classes have remained or have even widened. The phenomenon is principally one of relative deprivation – the maintenance of big differences in life chances against the dynamic background of a growing economy.

Explanations for this continued inequality have taken a number of forms. The twentieth century has witnessed and will continue to witness a series of revolutionary changes in the structure of occupations. To date these changes have resulted in some contraction of the size of the semi- and unskilled manual labour force and an expansion in non-manual occupations (see Appendix, Table 1). These changes have given rise to alterations in the age composition of each occupational class, older workers tending to be found in the contracting areas – though not as emphatically as some people suppose – and younger and more recent recruits to the workforce in the expanding area. Besides making comparisons between the occupational classes over time somewhat difficult, these shifts in the occupational structure in themselves offer an analytical solution to the continuing pattern of health inequality, for it is argued that the higher death rates of social class IV and V are, at least in part, a reflection of the older age structure of these occupational groups. The same argument has been used conversely to explain, to a small extent, the relatively low death rates of social class I.

In any event, Fig. 8, on the relationship between age and occupation for some of the major causes of death, shows that for all causes except malignant neoplasms class gradients are steepest in early adulthood and most shallow in the decade before retirement. The artefact explanation does not throw light on these observed patterns of fatal disease incidence amongst younger men.

These same distinctive trends also highlight the limitations of the thesis that the health gap is caused by age-related processes of social mobility. Occupational drift throughout the span of working life may help to contribute to class differences among the over-fifties but it cannot be said to be the cause of class inequalities between the ages of 15 and 45 years.

The limitations of these explanations especially among the male workforce of 45 years and under leads to a consideration of the direct role of material life on the production of health differentials. The most obvious starting point is the division between manual and non-manual occupations. Men engaged in manual occupations routinely confront a much higher degree of risk to

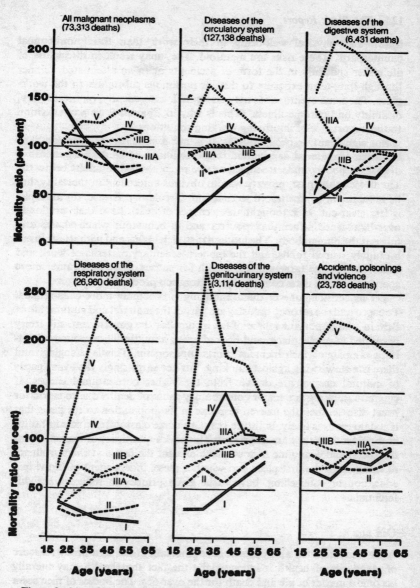

Figure 8. *Mortality ratios by occupational class, age and cause of death (men 15–64, England and Wales). (Source: Occupational Mortality 1970–72, H M S O, 1978, pp. 44–5.)*

health and physical well-being in their work than their non-manual counterparts. These risks are manifold. They may result in direct loss of life either suddenly in the form of accidents or in an attenuated manner through long-term exposure to dust or poisonous substances in the work-place. The same eventualities may also entail, antecedently, physical injury, disability and chronic illness. (This is why in Chapter 9 we pay attention to the importance of improving working conditions.)

But significant as occupation is, it is not a sufficient explanation. The influence of material deprivation in the aetiology of modern degenerative diseases is poorly understood, especially when applied to adults below the age of 45. In the past, poverty was an obvious antecedent in mortality, but its influence in deaths traced to cancer or circulatory disease, for example, is less clear-cut. It is thought these causes of death have their origins in over-indulgence rather than poverty and in behaviour which abuses and misuses the human body. The modern diet, rich in fats and with its emphasis on highly refined foods, and the modern sedentary patterns of work and leisure, are prime targets in the search for causes, as is, at a rather more specific level, the mass consumption of tobacco products.

Let us consider one of these. Smoking is becoming more class-related. Tobacco and the tobacco industry are part of the material and cultural life of Britain – an important source of tax income for the government, still freely permitted in public places and backed up by a multi-million pound advert-ising campaign which includes sports sponsorship. This is changing, and there is a slow swing against smoking, but not surprisingly the avant garde of cultural change are drawn from the higher occupational classes. If cigarette smoking is a major contributory cause of deaths due to cancer or heart disease, then the uneven response in the population to the news that it is dangerous is likely, in future years, to make class differentials in health even wider than they are at present. This raises questions, of course, about the social and economic factors which explain the fact and the prevalence of smoking in the first place and whether these, independent of individual education or counselling, have to be given priority in reducing the dif-ferentials.

Old age

After retirement the appropriateness of mortality rates as a proxy measure of standards of health is increased by the fact that health may literally become a matter of life and death for the over-65s. The bodies of men seem to exhibit the effects of wear and tear sooner than those of women and those of manual workers sooner than those of non-manual, and the manifestations of degeneration in disease become more frequent. What has to be remembered is that these outcomes are the end product of inequalities in the use made of, and the demands upon, the human body earlier in the lifetime and the kind of environment in which human beings have been placed.

This interpretation suggests that inequalities in health are the direct reflection of inequalities in the social division of labour. In the collective effort of social production, some workers' bodies wear out first. But inequalities in health at the end of the lifetime also emanate from the distribution of rewards associated with the social division of labour. Old age is a time of poverty, albeit poverty expressed in the form of relative deprivation, which among Britain's aged can mean material scarcity in very real terms, as deaths from hypothermia among the old reveal in severe winters. A recent DHSS report estimated malnutrition at 7 per cent among a sample of the elderly who were studied (DHSS, 1980, p. 3). In old age the relationship between income and the capacity to protect personal health is stronger perhaps than at any other time in the life-cycle, and in general it is likely that individuals who are well endowed through generous or index-linked pension schemes will lead the healthiest, the most comfortable and the longest lives after retirement. These material fortunes or misfortunes of old age are closely linked with occupational class during the working life. To have secure employment and an above-average income when one is at work is to be better able to provide for one's retirement. It is in this way that continuity in the distribution of material welfare is sustained, and inequalities in health perpetuated, from the cradle to the grave.

Conclusions

Several conclusions can be drawn from this look at different stages in the human life-cycle. First, while cultural and genetic explanations have some relevance – the latter is particularly important in early childhood – more of the evidence is explained by what we call 'materialist' or 'structural' explanations than by any other.

Secondly, some of the evidence on class inequalities in health can be understood in terms of specific features of the socio-economic environment: features such as accidents at work, overcrowding and smoking, which are strongly class-related in Britain. Since such features are recognized objectives of various areas of social policy we feel it sensible to offer them as contributory factors, to be dealt with in their own right, and not to discuss their incidence further in social-structural terms. The same is true of other aspects of the evidence which we feel show the importance of health services

themselves. Ante-natal care, for example, is important in preventing perinatal death, and the international evidence presented in Chapter 5 suggests
that much can be done through improvement of ante-natal care and of its
uptake. The international evidence also suggests the importance of preventive health within health policy, despite studies, to which we alluded earlier,
which suggest that few of the differences in mortality either between nations,
or between British regions, can be explained in terms of health care provision.
But beyond this there is undoubtedly much which cannot be understood
in terms of the impact of such specific factors. Much, we feel, can only be
understood in terms of the more diffuse consequences of the class structure:
poverty, work conditions (and what we termed the social division of labour)
and deprivation in its various forms in the home and immediate environment, at work, in education and the upbringing of children and more
generally in family and social life.

It is this acknowledgement of the complex nature of the explanation of
health inequalities – involving access to and use of the health services;
specific issues in other areas of social policy; and more general features of
class, material inequality and deprivation – which informs and structures
the recommendations we make in Chapters 8 and 9.

Chapter 7

The Need for More Information and Research

The scope and quality of national statistics relating to health and mortality in Britain are exceptionally good. Our task in compiling this report would have been much more difficult in most, if not all, other European countries. We have drawn on routine birth and death statistics, statistical returns collected for administrative and management purposes such as the hospital in-patient enquiry (HIPE), annual surveys like the GHS and the National Food Survey, the three national birth cohort studies and specific research projects.

Nevertheless there are gaps and imperfections which we feel necessitate either the initiation of further research or modification of the regular instruments of data collection.

There is a real need for continuing assessment of the development of children from birth to at least through primary school. It needs to be undertaken in relation to occupational class and must include surveillance of the nutrition of children. Studies of the kind we have in mind were in fact initiated in 1971, when the availability of school milk was reduced and the price of school meals raised, under the auspices of the Committee on Medical Aspects of Food Policy (COMA), and are still being carried out. Some of the findings of this work are discussed in Chapter 9, where we present our recommendations for policy relating to school meals and milk. The feasibility of surveillance of this kind has now been demonstrated, and the assessment of children's growth in relation to class and nutrition should become a matter of routine.

We recommend that school health statistics should routinely provide the results of tests of hearing, vision, and measures of height and weight, in relation to occupational class. Authorities might also be requested to report separately on schools in inner city areas, or to differentiate between a wide range of urban/rural locations. *As a first step we recommend that local health authorities, in consultation with education authorities, select a representative sample of schools in which assessments on a routine basis be initiated.* We should also like to see progress towards routine collection and reporting of accidents to children. Such reporting should ultimately distinguish not only between occupational classes and age groups, but also locations of accident

– on the road, at home, in school or elsewhere – and when appropriate the articles or building design features involved in accidents. At present the only national source of information is the HIPE. However, not only does HIPE fail to record occupational class, it also omits the vast bulk of accidents not requiring in-patient admission.

We recognize there are difficulties in working towards a national system of child-accident reporting, which may require the co-operation not only of hospital accident and emergency departments, and the police in the case of traffic accidents, but conceivably of health visitors also. In view of the importance of the topic, *we recommend that representatives of appropriate government departments* (*Health and Social Security, Education and Science, Environment, Trade, Transport, and the Home Office*), *as well as of the NHS and of the police, should consider how progress might rapidly be made in improving the information on accidents to children, nationally and locally.*

A further area where a concept of health broader than acute sickness has to be employed is in relation to the distribution of impairment and disability. We would like to see local authorities reporting systematically on numbers of disabled as well as, however crudely, on assessments of the severity of disablement. In the late 1970s local authorities began to classify handicapped people by the self-care criteria (whether they could wash and dress, and look after themselves in an elemental way), but that classification is not yet comprehensive, even for the physically handicapped, and needs to be extended, above all to the mentally handicapped. Social service departments and local officers of the Department of Employment should seek to introduce categorizations of severity, preferably on the basis of limitation of activity. This would permit comparison of priorities between services, as well as between authorities.

We would also like to draw attention to the importance of the National Food Survey, for which the Ministry of Agriculture, Fisheries and Food has responsibility. This annual survey is the principal source of information on the food purchased and consumed and hence the diet of the population, and is therefore of great importance. There are, however, problems relating to the low response rate of the survey. We feel that much could be done, through greater recourse to epidemiological expertise, to transform the survey into a more effective instrument of nutritional surveillance in relation to health.

We recommend that consideration be given to the development of the National Food Survey into a more effective instrument of nutritional surveillance in relation to health, through which various 'at risk' groups could also be identified and studied. We fully recognize that such a development may raise questions about proper responsibility for the survey.

Finally, *the importance of the problem of inequalities in health and their causes, as an area for further research needs to be emphatically stated. We recommend that it be adopted as a research priority by the DHSS and steps taken to enlist the expertise of the Medical Research Council (MRC), as well as the Social Science Research Council (SSRC), in the initiation of a programme of research. Such research represents a particularly appropriate area for departmental commissioning of research from the MRC.*

A strategy for advance

In our view, the six areas in which further research – leading, it should be said, in some instances to improved or augmented administrative statistics – is essential are:

   a. surveillance of the development of children, especially in relation to nutrition and accidents;

   b. better understanding of the health effects of such aspects of what can be regarded as individual behaviour as smoking, diet, alcohol consumption and exercise;

   c. the development of area social condition and health indicators for use in resource allocation;

   d. health hazards in relation to occupational conditions and work;

   e. better measures of the prevalence and course of disability, and the degree of its severity.

   f. study of the interaction of the social factors implicated in ill-health over time, and within small areas.

The importance of each of these derives from its relevance to our overall strategy of developing new policy.

In order to study the dynamics of child health – the process by which ill-health and educational under-achievement (whether a consequence of handicapping conditions, absence from school or cultural factors) develop together and so perpetuate the link between health and social class – it is necessary to turn to longitudinal studies.

In our view three issues upon which research needs to be brought to bear are:

   i. the *interaction* of processes leading to physical and mental disadvantage, handicap and ill-health;

   ii. the role which services related to child health play, and might play, in inhibiting the cumulation of disadvantage;

   iii. the routes by which some children escape what is for most born into similar conditions an unenviable fate.

Conclusions and recommendations

We have made various recommendations which will improve and extend the quality of class-related health and health service utilization data on a regular basis and enhance knowledge of their interrelationships.

It is argued, in relation to health, that the monitoring of ill-health (itself still so imperfect) should evolve into a system also of monitoring health in relation to social and environmental conditions. Two areas where progress could be made are (i) in relation to the development of children, and (ii) in relation to disability. Certain modifications to community health statistics are proposed:

We recommend that school health statistics routinely provide locally and nationally, in relation to occupational class, the results of tests of hearing, vision, and measures of height and weight. As a first step we recommend that local health authorities, in consultation with education authorities, each select a representative sample of schools in which assessments on a routine basis be initiated.

We should also like to see progress towards the routine collection and reporting of accidents to children, ultimately distinguishing the age and occupational class of the parents as well as the location and circumstances of accidents. In relation to traffic accidents there should be better liaison between the NHS and the police, both centrally and locally.

We recommend that representatives of appropriate government departments (Health and Social Security, Education and Science, Environment, Trade, Transport and the Home Office), as well as the NHS and the police, should consider how progress might rapidly be made. The Child Accident Prevention Committee, if suitably constituted and supported, might be a suitable forum for such discussions, to be followed by appropriate action by government departments.

In relation to the disabled, we should like to see local authorities reporting systematically on numbers of disabled as well as (however crudely) on assessments of severity of disablement applying to mentally handicapped people, elderly people in residential homes and other groups of handicapped people, as well as the general classes of the handicapped, as at present.

In our view it is the extent to which need is unmet, rather than pressure upon existing services, which should form the basis for planning, and it is this view which has underpinned our recommendations. Turning, then, to the health services themselves, it is clear that systematic knowledge of the use made of the various services by different social groups is extremely scanty. We recognize that the collection and central reporting of occupational data within the context of the various administrative returns pose problems of feasibility and accuracy. Nevertheless we feel that the desirability of such information is such that further thought should be given to how these problems might be overcome, within the context of the current review of health service statistics.

Further, we draw attention to the importance of the National Food Survey as the major source of regular information on the food purchase (and hence nutrition) of the population. *We recommend however, that consideration be given (drawing upon epidemiological expertise within the OPCS and elsewhere) to development of the National Food Survey into a more effective instrument of nutritional surveillance in relation to health, through which various 'at risk' groups could also be identified and studied.*

Beyond this, we feel that the six areas in which further research is needed are:

- surveillance of the development of children, especially in relation to nutrition and accidents;
- better understanding of the health effects of such aspects of behaviour as smoking, diet, alcohol consumption and exercise;
- the development of area social conditions and health indicators for use in resource allocation;
- health hazards in relation to occupational conditions and work;
- better measures of the prevalence and course of disability, and the degree of its severity;
- study of the interaction of social factors implicated in ill-health over time, and within small areas.

Though these issues are in an obvious sense quite distinct, yet they can also be seen as aspects of an overall strategy, and it is this strategy which we particularly wish to commend. Our concern is with the interaction of variables traditionally seen as directly implicated in ill-health (such as smoking behaviour and work conditions) with social variables. It will be necessary to examine the effects upon the health of social groups of a wide range of social and behavioural variables, implying further work both on the development of health indicators and upon the way in which disadvantageous social and environmental conditions may give rise to or exacerbate the effects of patterns of dietary behaviour, leisure behaviour etc.

The importance of the problem of social inequalities in health and their causes, as an area for further research, needs to be emphatically stated. *We recommend that it be adopted as a research priority by the DHSS, and steps taken to enlist the expertise of the Medical Research Council, as well as the*

Social Science Research Council, in the initiation of a programme of research.
Such research represents a particularly appropriate area for departmental
commissioning of research from the MRC.

While we ourselves have not attempted to develop a research strategy in
detail within this report, it is our view that two types of study are needed.
First, a study of the interaction of social and environmental variables over
time, and their relationship to the (healthy) development of children. The
longitudinal approach, as in the existing cohort studies, is appropriate here.
Second, a study carried out in a small number of carefully selected places.
Such a study would concern itself with the whole range of social conditions
relevant for health, as well as patterns of behaviour which may in some senses
be damaging to health. Crucial for further progress in the elimination of
health inequalities is greater understanding of the interactions of this complex set of variables: social and individual. Such interactions will necessarily
have both diachronic and locational dimensions, and the studies we have in
mind will be sensitive to, and permit elucidation of, both.

Chapter 8

Planning the Health and Personal Social Services

Any strategy for improving health inevitably involves both the health care system and a range of social policies not immediately related to that system. In this chapter we look at those services which fall under the general administration of the Department of Health and Social Security, while in the next we outline some of the major changes which need to be made in other areas of social policy.

Objectives and principles

We believe the health and social services should adopt a three-fold scheme of priorities:
* Priority for children to have a better start in life.
* Priority for disabled people bearing the brunt of cumulative ill-health and deprivation to improve their quality of life and reduce the need for institutional care.
* Priority for preventive and educational action to encourage good health.
   We shall look at each of these in turn.

1. Priority for children at the start of life

The wide gap in life prospects between babies born of members of different occupational classes – amongst the widest we have found in society – together with the likelihood that the beneficial effects of any reduction in that gap will be carried over into adult life and may lead to savings in health expenditure, demands that action be taken at this stage.

It would be wrong to suppose that improvements in infant and child care could be fully effective without paying heed to the need for improvements in the living standards of their families and the physical constitution and access to health services of their parents. Nevertheless some specific action aimed at this age group is possible. The great majority of 'excess' infant deaths in classes I V and V are attributable to congenital abnormalities and other complications of birth and the period immediately afterwards, and in later infancy and childhood to accidents, respiratory diseases and gastro-intestinal infections. As we shall go on later to show, this means that special measures need to be taken to improve the quality of community health services, especially those devoting resources predominantly to children and those which reduce risks of ill-health, injury and accidents.

2. Priority for disabled people bearing the brunt of cumulative ill-health and deprivation

It cannot be sufficient to plan only for the next generation or to take steps to prevent certain health problems arising in the future. The cumulative deprivations of a lifetime are a potent source of class inequality in health. Those who are the worst victims of past and current industrial and social practices, who have been exposed for prolonged periods to bad housing, poor working and environmental conditions and low incomes, also deserve services to improve their health and to enable them to cope with disabilities. As with our first priority area, a marked shift of resources to community health and welfare services is called for.

3. Priority for the preventive services

Greater equality in health depends upon a high national standard of knowledge about self-care, the care of children and other dependants, and the pursuit of activities conducive to health which themselves depend on such factors as high standards of home-keeping, good education and widely diffused recreational and sporting activities. This suggests a coherent national programme of enormous scope and we can only hope to give illustrations in this and the next chapter of some of the most important parts of such a programme. They will include an expansion of health education, selective screening and strong anti-smoking measures. It is important, however, to convey at once the relative inexpensiveness of such measures. At the same time we are deeply conscious not only of the preposterously small part of NHS resources committed to 'preventive health', but also the lack of understanding by health authorities (and education authorities) of what is good health practice and how they might contribute to strengthening and supplementing such practice.

Planning

We know these concerns are not new, and indeed they are very much within the spirit of much recent government thinking. At least in theory, the whole period of the middle and late 1970s saw an emphasis on greater care in the community, as well as a higher priority for children, families with children, for the elderly and for preventive health measures.

Nevertheless at least two disconcerting observations need to be made about government priorities. First, objectives are not clearly defined. A good example is that of 'community care'. The DHSS itself seems to mean different things by this concept at different times. In one overall review of planning the department defined a primary objective for the elderly to be to develop domiciliary provision and encourage 'measures designed to prevent or postpone the need for long-term care in hospital and residential homes' (DHSS, *Social Care Research*, 1978, p. 13). But in the planning document *The Way Forward* in 1977 community care was defined as covering a whole range of provision, including community hospitals, hostels, day hospitals, residential homes, day centres and domiciliary support. Again the 1976 Priorities Document which represented new directions in government policy called for relatively higher growth rates for some services but gave no rationale for the percentage growth rates chosen. This laid them open to charges of arbitrariness.

We believe that a clear statement of what is planned and intended produces a better educated and more understanding public, a more democratic and accountable public service, and above all offers an opportunity to question and clarify any shortcomings there may be in the initial thinking.

There is certainly no mathematically precise or exact way of determining the relative priority of different services, but there is room for the development of more precise analytical tools. Although, for instance, there are problems in conceptualizing and measuring 'need' (Lind and Wiseman, 1978; Smith, 1980) *we consider there is no better alternative conceptual basis for developing a coherent rationale for the allocation of health care resources, and we recommend accordingly*. We shall return later to a discussion of 'need'.

Secondly, some of the changes recommended in the various priority documents are simply not materializing or are materializing so slowly as to be difficult to discern. The latest trends in spending on the personal social services, for instance, give little or no sign of the planned decline in spending on *residential* care, with the corresponding expected increase in *community* care. A summary of local authority planning returns does not bear out the change in emphasis recommended by the DHSS (*Local Authority Personal Social Services Summary of Planning Returns 1976–77 to 1979–80*, 1978).*
Even though the planned changes in the emphasis of spending were modest

* Later information shows that this statement still applies.

(extremely modest in some cases) the inability to fulfil even these limited objectives is disturbing.

We recommend a shift of resources within the national health service and the personal social services on a larger and more determined scale than so far accomplished towards community care and particularly towards the increased availability of care for young children. We see this as an important part of a strategy to break the links between social class or poverty and health.

What does this mean in practice? Table 37 illustrates what we have in mind. Column one shows actual expenditure on the various components of the health and social services in 1976/7. Column two is a projection of expenditure to 1981/2 and shows how modest the shift in resources sought by the last Labour government was. Column three (alternative 1) illustrates our idea of a more determined shift in emphasis assuming current planned levels of expenditure. This shows savings of £200 million in 1981/2 set against additional expenditure of £200 million (plus £30 million for an experimental action programme we shall explain further on). It doesn't imply a reduction in current levels of expenditure for any services but rather cuts in the anticipated growth (admittedly very small) in some areas. In our view the largest scope for reductions in rates of growth, if not in absolute costs, is in the pharmaceutical services.

Column four (alternative 2) is based on the belief that in fact current planned levels of expenditure, taking into account inflation and demographic changes, are inadequate and will do no more than permit an overall maintenance of existing levels. It follows that any reduction, even in anticipated growth, could end up as a real cut. Column four illustrates therefore how the shift in resources should be brought about on the more optimistic assumption that no service should be financed at a level below that previously forecast for 1981/2 and that additional resources could be made available. On this basis our proposals would require an additional £287 million, plus the £30 million mentioned before.

The setting-out of alternatives in Table 37 reflects a clear division of opinion within the Working Group. While we were completely in agreement on the importance of strengthening community and preventive services, two of us (DB and JNM) were opposed to obtaining the necessary resources by reducing expenditure on the hospital services, believing that these are already straitened by inflation and cash-limits; the others, on what may well be a sound appreciation of the financial outlook, were not so opposed to this. Naturally, all of us would wish to see additional resources.

These recommendations should, however, be thought of as money-saving in two senses. First, by reducing inequality and laying a better basis for the maintenance of health, the incidence of ill-health (and hence the need for

Table 37: *Planned and recommended revenue expenditure on selected services (£m.; November 1976 prices)*

Services to be given higher priority than at present	1976–7 actual	1981–2 DHSS projection (1978)	1981–2 Alternative 1	1981–2 Alternative 2
1. *Health and Welfare of mothers and pre-school and school children*				
Midwives	24	24	26	28
Family planning	12	15	20	21
Health visiting	47	63	66	70
Day nurseries	33	37	60	63
School health	51	51	60	65
Welfare food	18	19	40	43
Boarding out	20	26	28	30
Sub-total	205	235	300	320
2. *Family practitioner (other than pharmaceutical)*	440	494	514	547
3. *Care of disabled in their own homes*				
Home nursing	81	108	116	124
Chiropody	11	13	13	14
Home help	105	131	160	170
Meals	12	15	20	21
Day care	57	76	90	96
Aids, adaptations	13	14	30	32
Services for disabled	42	40	50	53
Sub-total	321	397	479	510
4. *Other specific preventive measures*	14	17	50	53
Total selected 'higher priority' services	980	1143	1343	1430
Recommended increases (Total 1, 2, 3 and 4)	—	—	+200	+287

Table 37: *Cont.*

Services to be given smaller priority than at present	1976–7 actual	1981–2 DHSS projection (1978)	1981–2 Alternative 1	1981–2 Alternative 2
5. *Acute in-patients and out-patients*				
6. *Mental handicap in-patients and out-patients*				
Mental illness in-patients and out-patients				
Residential care for elderly				
7. *Pharmaceutical services*				
Total selected 'lesser priority' services (5 + 6 + 7)	2992	3295	3095	3295
Recommended decrease 'lesser priority' services (5 + 6 + 7)	—	—	−200	0
Experimental ten-area programme			(30)	30

health care treatment) could be diminished. Second, by precautionary and supportive action the need for more expensive types of treatment will be reduced. While it may be true that many of those in hospital require additional resources, yet if fewer patients need be admitted or if the duration of stay can be safely reduced, there can still be scope for savings.

Resource allocation

The mid-seventies also saw a commitment to redistributing resources geographically across the country in a more appropriate fashion. There is abundant evidence that some parts of the country have historically had much higher health budgets and consequently more adequate facilities. Since these tend to be the better-off regions, health inequalities are reinforced.

In 1975 the government commissioned a DHSS Resource Allocation Working Party to investigate ways of establishing a formula for distributing resources that corresponded more closely to 'need' rather than historical practice. The working party interpreted its objectives as being to secure through resource allocation equal opportunities of access to health care for people at equal risk. We wish to endorse this objective.

Unlike the parallel priority document (1976) it did seek to establish a mathematically quantifiable definition of need as a basis for determining future resource distribution. This rested primarily on mortality rates, which were taken as a proxy for morbidity rates. The procedure was, essentially, to take the age and sex structure of a population together with the average death rates for people of different sexes at different ages and then to 'weight' a region's population according to its need for various services – hospital, GP, ambulance etc. These services were costed and target revenues set accordingly. The RAWP proposal was that those regions furthest from their targets should have relatively larger growth budgets than those nearer, or, in the case of regions in the south-east of England (the so-called rich regions), already well past it. The more difficult questions of exactly how to redistribute resources more fairly at area and district level were largely ignored.

The RAWP formula was complicated and we were unable to get a complete picture of how its method was being applied around the country. Between 1976 and 1979 at least nine of the fourteen health regions had only partially implemented it. Four had not yet analysed their populations according to average death rates and five had not done this in relation to the particular need for general hospital care. Even among the remaining five, progress appeared to be cautious in moving towards targets for particular services.

We believe there are several points which deserve further attention. First, neither RAWP principles nor RAWP methodology has been consistently applied at area or district level and some of the misunderstandings about it have arisen because of the lack of precise illustrations at health district level of the actual and desirable operation of different services. This leads us to recommend that health authorities should consider increasing the volume of information collected and published regularly for each health district about: (a) health experience (indicators of morbidity, mortality and positive health); (b) rates of usage of health and health-related services (including GP consultations, out-patient attendance, home nursing and health visits and in-patient and residential care); and (c) social and environmental conditions.

Secondly, there has been insufficient thought given to how the concept of need could be enhanced by additional indicators. Are there, for instance, indicators of social deprivation which might be used independently or to supplement death rates in developing a formula for resource allocation?

There is in Britain a long tradition of study of the relationship between social conditions and death rates. While surveys like the General Household Survey do not break down information into sufficiently small areas, census data, although biased towards housing information and quickly out of date, does offer material on a range of deprivation-related factors at local authority and ward level.

One study in 1961 used a variety of census indicators, plus climatic and air pollution indicators, in the attempt to explain differences in adult mortality rates between the larger county boroughs of England and Wales. Multiple regression techniques allowed these authors to show, for example, that 'social conditions' (an indicator combining amount of overcrowding, social class, average educational level etc. was used), air pollution levels and inclement climate were independently associated with mortality rates from bronchitis (Gardner, Crawford and Morris, 1969).

More recently a second study, using 1971 census data together with 1971 mortality rates for children aged 0 to 4 and 5 to 14, sought to relate the death rates for children to social need variables, also at county or metropolitan borough level (Brennan and Lancashire, 1978). It found significant correlations between mortality rates, especially for the younger children, and extent of overcrowding, lack of basic amenities, extent of unemployment among male working population and extent of council house occupancy.

A significant correlation was also obtained with the proportion of unskilled workers, and the authors then examined whether or not social class composition (understood in the restricted sense of the percentage of population in class V), housing variables (density, possession of amenities) and unemployment rate are *independently* related to mortality rates. Calculation of partial correlations (housing variables and unemployment rate held constant) showed that the effects were independent of each other in the case of the under-5s.

Although this kind of analysis cannot be extrapolated to causes of mortality at the individual level, it is important here in suggesting that areas having high unemployment rates, *or* bad housing, *or* a high proportion of unskilled workers, or worse, all three, are likely to have high rates of child mortality especially in the first five years of life. The authors also conclude that the percentage of population in social class V *alone* will inadequately

Table 38: Highest-ranking local authority areas on each of eight 1971 census and mortality indicators (England)

1 Households with more than one person per room (per 1,000 households)	2 No. unemployed per 1,000 persons	3 No. unskilled workers per 1,000 economically active	4 Married couples with four or more children per 1,000 families	5 Perinatal mortality rate (average 1974–6)	6 Infant mortality rate (average 1974–6)	7 Adjusted mortality ratio (1976)
Knowsley	Knowsley	Tower Hamlets*	Knowsley	Wolverhampton	Rochdale	Salford*
Islington*	Liverpool*	Southwark*	Liverpool*	Sandwell	Oldham	Tameside
Hackney*	S. Tyneside	Newham*	Manchester*	Liverpool*	Salford*	Gateshead*
Tower Hamlets*	Sunderland	Knowsley	Birmingham*	Gateshead*	Wolverhampton	Liverpool
Lambeth*	Manchester*	Liverpool*	Cleveland	Salford*	Manchester*	S. Tyneside
Kensington/Chelsea	Newcastle	Cleveland	Sefton	Rochdale	Bradford	Tower Hamlets*
Hammersmith	Cleveland	Humberside	Hackney*	Bolton	Calderdale	Durham
Southwark*	Gateshead*	Salford*	Lambeth*	Manchester*	Kirklees	Bolton
Brent	Hammersmith	Newcastle*	Newham*	Walsall	Walsall	Wirral
Camden*	Tower Hamlets*	Islington*	Salford*	Knowsley		N. Tyneside
			Wirral			
			S. Tyneside			
			Sunderland			
			Lewisham*			

*indicates Inner City Partnership Scheme area

Note: Adjusted Mortality Ratio (AMR) is the local death rate standardized for population age/sex structure and divided by the national rate.

Sources: Columns 1–4 Imber, 1977; 5–6 DHSS/OPCS (unpublished); 7 OPCS *Local Authority Vital Statistics 1976*.

reflect the extent to which social factors pre-disposing to high infant mortality are present in an area. Of course more 'inclusive' measures of class composition remain to be examined in relation to mortality. Table 38 shows which metropolitan districts and non-metropolitan counties show up worst on each of four census social indicators, and three indicators of mortality (using recent mortality data). The frequent appearance of certain areas notably in the north-west and the north-east is apparent. Further work on relationships between indicators of social disadvantage and of mortality is needed.

Third, we do not believe that a more equitable distribution of resources alone, without parallel attention to *how* these resources are to be used, will greatly serve to reduce inequalities in health care, still less in health. In the debate on the RAWP recommendations too much attention has been concentrated on criteria of the need for health care and too little on the effects upon health of allocating resources to one type of service rather than another. We believe that 'need' for health care must govern the definition of priorities and that at the present time the definition of such need shows the case for making a more pronounced shift of resources towards community and preventive health care. This leads us to suggest a possible modification to the implementation of the RAWP philosophy.

At present, the proposal is that weighted populations for each kind of health service are combined on the basis of the share of total revenue which each of these services currently represents, that is 8.8 per cent for community health, 55.9 per cent for non-psychiatric in-patients etc. We believe that this process should reflect not *current* distribution of expenditure but that which is *aimed* at in the planning of services. That is, if community health is a *priority* (and is intended to absorb, say, 10 per cent of total resources, excluding those for family practitioner services, within 5 years' time) then it is this figure which should be used in the combining of weighted populations. *We therefore recommend that the resources to be allocated should be based on the future planned share for different services, including a higher share for community health.*

In saying this we reiterate the Royal Commission's endorsement of the Expenditure Committee's view that: 'the expenditure planning and priority setting of DHSS should be synchronized so as to enable Parliament to examine the relationship between the two' (*Ninth Report from the Expenditure Committee.* Session 1976–7, 1977, p. lvi; and see also *Report of the Royal Commission on the NHS*, 1979, p. 56).

A district action programme

To ensure the vigorous implementation of the three-fold priority programme we outlined at the beginning (p. 133) we also propose the establishment of what we have called a *district action programme*. It would be adopted nation-wide and would involve additional modifications to the present structure of care not so far seriously pursued by government policies. It is a four-point programme.

1. The health and welfare of mothers, pre-school and school children

The under-utilization of the community and preventive health services by poorer groups is well documented. While we cannot assess the *extent* to which this is a consequence of the inequitable provision of services – so that, for example, working-class women might have longer journey times and waiting times in visiting child health clinics – we have known for a long time that under-utilization is associated with organizational and cultural aspects of services. One authority puts the problem as follows:

Under-utilization of ante-natal and child-health services results from inadequacies in the services themselves and particularly from their insensitivity to the uncertainty and conflict of responsibility mothers feel regarding the question of their baby's health. Two particular areas of inadequacy are highlighted by recent research: firstly, inadequacies as regards the organization of ante-natal clinics (timing of clinics and length of waiting, location of clinics, facilities for children and other relatives, etc.) and secondly, inadequacies as regards the actual content of the check-up (lack of individual attention and advice tailored to the individual's needs, lack of privacy, etc.). (Graham, 1978)

We recommend that areas and districts should review the accessibility and facilities of all the ante-natal and child-health clinics in their areas, and develop plans to increase utilization by mothers. On the basis of our own experience this must include such reforms as experimenting with evening and weekend opening, the dispersion of ante-natal sessions from hospitals covering large catchment areas to new centres in small areas, and the humanization of ante-natal procedures and settings, especially in clinics in hospitals. One clinic which we visited was described, not unfairly it seemed, as a 'cattle market'.

The DHSS should furthermore publicize factors which explain high utilization in some areas, like Liverpool, and low utilization in others, like Salford. Wherever possible clinics should be established in conjunction with group practice and health centres, in partial fulfilment of the recommendations of the Court Committee. As some commentators have pointed out, relatively few general practitioners are keen to devote more time to practising preventive medicine, and a change in outlook will take a long time to bring about (Alberman, Morris and Pharaoh, 1977, p. 394), but it might be encouraged if more health visiting staff were seconded full-time or part-time to group practice. There is room for experiment, and it is possible for some health visitors to combine territorial and team responsibilities. There is an even more powerful case to be made out for the secondment of social work staff, but in this case knowledge of welfare rights would be a very necessary part of their skills. Ease of access, good facilities, respect for the individual and availability of care and advice throughout infancy and childhood might be the watch-words of any planned development of services.

We should perhaps, at this point, mention the experiments in France and Finland (see Chapter 5), where ante-natal care is supported by financial inducements. We have examined these but we are not convinced that reluctance on the part of mothers to attend clinics is the real key to their under-utilization in Britain. In Finland the establishment of a national network of clinics in 1945 preceded the introduction of payments and may have been the key factor in encouraging high rates of attendance. In France ante-natal payments were introduced many years before the dramatic improvements in the French perinatal mortality rate.

One of the problems we face in Britain is that with the huge proportion of hospital births it can be difficult securing the involvement of GPs at an early stage in the life of a child. There are a number of possible solutions to this. One, already mentioned, is the association of more ancillary staff with primary care teams. We would then urge that the teams should generally be constructed on the basis of two and at most three general practitioners so that some contribution might be made to the vitality and integration of the local community. Another is immunization, where GPs have a much better knowledge of family history and the health and development of a child and are in a much stronger position to know about untoward reactions. In principle we advocate such a policy, though we recognize that for some time to come there will have to be back-up provisions in the community where the medical service is inadequate.

Unfortunately this inadequacy is disturbingly widespread and we were very concerned about the standard of GP service in some poor areas with high mortality. There are single-handed general practitioners who live at a considerable distance from the areas in which their patients reside, have little knowledge of or interest in local culture – which leads them to prescribe or otherwise treat patients inappropriately – who rely for a disproportionately large part of the year, the week or the day on the deputizing services, and take little or no interest in the possibilities of new health centres, group practice or other forms of collaboration among and between health service and social service professional personnel.

Some are considerably older than 65 and others are new to practice in this country and include those who are virtually in transit to other career destinations. There are some who have resorted to work in these areas because they have been unsuccessful elsewhere and are exposed here to less criticism. As the Royal Commission said of declining urban areas, 'Many health professionals are coping courageously and effectively in these areas, but there is evidence in some places that services are inadequate. The GPs tend to be older and to have large lists. The accepted view today is that a GP will work most efficiently in a group practice or partnership with several other GPs and there may be some connection between the extent of single-handed practice and low quality of care, although there are many excellent single-handed GPs. More single-handed practices are found in the inner city areas' (*Report*, 1979, p. 88). For the inner London area, these problems have been well documented in the Acheson Report (London Health Planning Consortium, 1981).

We are aware that some of the best and most dedicated members of the medical profession also work in these areas and that the problems of quantifying the problem are immense. Nevertheless we are in no doubt that the problem is sufficiently serious to demand action. The Royal Commission took a similar view and recommended, among other things, close supervision of deputizing services, a review of controls on the appointment of GPs, the offer of an assisted voluntary retirement scheme to GPs, a study of the feasibility of introducing a compulsory retirement age, the introduction of audit or peer review of standards of care and treatment and the development of health centres as a priority in inner city areas.

We accept this, but we would want to go further. *We recommend that the professional associations as well as the Secretary of State and the health authorities should accept responsibility for making improvements in the quality and geographical coverage of general practice, especially in areas of high prevalence of ill-health and poor social conditions. Where the number or scope of work of general practitioners is inadequate in such areas we recommend health authorities to deploy or redeploy an above-average number of community nurses attached where possible to family practices.* The review of coverage must include definitions of desirable standards of practice and keeping abreast of modern methods of practice as well as advancement in medical knowledge, and not only questions of remuneration and inducement. *We further recommend that the distribution of general practitioners should be related not only to population but to medical need, as indicated by SMRs,*

supplemented by other indicators, and that the per capita basis of remuneration
be modified accordingly.

One possibility deserving careful consideration is the attachment of additional, newly qualified G Ps to existing group practices and health centres for periods of, say, two to five years. Every effort should be made to provide housing temporarily or permanently within the areas. One problem of the poor areas is that health centres are not yet the main form of medical organization. In Gateshead only a fifth and in Tower Hamlets fewer than a tenth of G Ps are in health centres. Previous studies have demonstrated that a more effective policy deserves to be adopted. 'The NHS has not brought about any dramatic shift in the location of GPs ... Areas which are currently facing the most serious shortages seem to have a fairly long history of man-power difficulties, while those which are today relatively well supplied with family doctors have generally had no difficulty in past years in attracting and keeping an adequate number of practitioners...' (Butler, Bevan and Taylor, 1973). A separate study of mortality and GP statistics in 1972 and 1973 found a significant lack of correlation between measures of illness and death and the number of GPs, suggesting that the supply of GPs is not matched to health care need (Forster, Frost, Francis and Heath).

We believe the evidence suggests that it is precisely those areas most in need of good medical facilities – judged on the basis of rates of mortality and morbidity – which are often least likely to have them.

Education facilities are another area that causes us concern. With the relative increase in number of one-parent families and increased employment of young mothers with children, the problem of facilities for those without relatives living nearby is considerable. Present plans for the expansion of day nurseries are meagre, and the rate of expansion needs to be larger. Within the proposed Health Development Programme at national level *we recommend the financing of new services for children under 5 from the savings that are being made as a result of the decline in the school population.* This proposal is further elaborated below (Chapter 9, pp. 172–5).

School health services are another neglected but valuable resource. They make it possible, for instance, to monitor the health of children in certain types of family more frequently, and there are possibilities of relating health surveillance to teaching about health and the health service. At the same time there have been a number of suggestions that all health services for children should be more tightly integrated. A Scottish working party expected that 'in the course of time much routine school health work will be carried out by primary care teams but the more specialized aspects such as the assessment of handicapped children will be the responsibility of paediatricians working closely with other professional colleagues' (*Towards an Integrated Child*

Health Service, 1973, p. 101). Like the working party, we recognize that there will have to be different systems of provision of school health care for some time to come, but *recommend that every opportunity should be taken to link revitalized school health care with general practice, and to intensify surveillance and follow-up both in areas of special need and for certain types of family.* For this purpose we take the view that certain assessments can be undertaken by health visitors and social workers, especially where they are already working in association with group practice. Much of this has already been accepted, at least in principle, by Ministers.

One area of school health which requires separate attention is the child guidance system. This has traditionally provided psychiatric care for a relatively small number of maladjusted children on an intensive basis. There is evidence of long waiting lists, misunderstood systems of queueing, and a negative image of the work among parents (Fitzherbert, 1977, pp. 85–96). At the same time there is evidence from surveys in the Isle of Wight and in London (Rutter *et al.*, 1970, 1975) of a very much higher prevalence of maladjustment among children than had been thought, or than could be helped by traditional psychiatric methods. Consequently there is a growing view, which we share, that the emphasis must increasingly be upon preventive methods and upon increasing co-operation between psychiatrists, educational psychologists and teachers. For example, the so-called 'nurture group' pioneered by Marjorie Boxall provides a special therapeutic environment to compensate for inadequate early experience *within* the school from which children are gradually returned to normal classes. Such experiments should be encouraged and evaluated.

For handicapped children Ministers have already accepted in principle the establishment of District Handicap Teams. The teams can help to provide careful diagnosis and continuing help and advice and support to handicapped children and their parents. *We recommend that an assessment which determines severity of disablement should be adopted as a guide to health service priorities, and that this should be related to the limitation of activities rather than loss of faculty or type of handicap.* This procedure would help to equate the provision of services for mentally handicapped as well as physically handicapped children.

2. The care of disabled and elderly people in their own homes

When disablement is understood in terms of functional limitation it becomes possible to rank severity and provide a better guide to the selection of priorities. For example, conventions about the division of clients according to type of handicap, or the conventional categorization of patients as requiring hospitalization, residential care, sheltered housing or domiciliary support, may need to be re-examined. Many people seem to find themselves in a particular category more by chance than for any specific medical reason. Moreover the quality of care provided by the different types of institution, judged by costs, manpower, amenities etc., may bear little relation to need.

We believe disabled people suffer two distinct forms of inequality. One is inequality of opportunity for treatment for those in different types of hospital. *We recommend a review of the distribution of facilities and services between acute and long-stay units and also of the distribution of elderly patients in geriatric, psychiatric and general hospitals.*

The second form of inequality is in opportunities for care, rehabilitation, occupation, privacy and social relations between hospital patients and residents of local authority, voluntary and private homes on the one hand and disabled people living in their own homes on the other. These inequalities have attracted rather less attention than inequalities in services for people in different areas.

Both these forms of inequality require attention. However, we believe the first step in doing this is to clarify the meaning of community care and give much greater emphasis to the tendencies towards that objective favoured in government planning documents.

For instance the Jay Committee, which reported on mental handicap nursing and care in 1979, identified three broad sets of principles which should govern community care: (i) Mentally handicapped people have a right to enjoy normal patterns of life within the community; (ii) Mentally handicapped people have a right to be treated as individuals; (iii) Mentally handicapped people will require additional help from the communities in which they live and from professional services if they are to develop to their maximum potential as individuals.

The Committee concluded:

The mentally handicapped person should have access to the full range of services and facilities available to the general public and specialist services should be provided only where the general services cannot cope with a special need. But where special provisions are required they should offer a wide range of options in the three spheres of day, domiciliary and residential services. Mentally handicapped people in residential care should not be isolated from their neighbourhood or, more importantly, from their families. The staff who care for mentally handicapped residents should be compassionate and caring, but also professionally trained; their role should be to help each mentally handicapped person to develop mentally, physically and emotionally. Residents should live in small family-type groups sharing experiences informally with the staff, making their own decisions and taking necessary risks. (DHSS, Jay Committee, March 1979, p. 140)

In realizing such aims one obstacle in the development of services for mentally handicapped people, as for other groups of disabled people, is that responsibility for sheltered housing, as distinct from residential accommodation, is not the responsibility of the personal social services. As a result residential care is sometimes offered when sheltered housing would be the more rational choice. *We recommend that a Working Group, to include representatives of voluntary organizations concerned with relevant client groups, should be set up to review whether sheltered housing should be a responsibility of social service or housing departments and make recommendations.*

The elderly have also continued to have a poor deal from 'community care'. It has certainly not developed as rapidly as the general policy aims would suggest. The 1976 Priority Document argued:

> The general aim of policy is to help the elderly maintain independent lives in their own homes for as long as possible. The main emphasis is thus on the development of the domiciliary services and on the promotion of a more active approach towards the treatment of the elderly in hospital. But old people who can no longer continue to live independently in the community even with the support of all available health and social services will need long-term residential or hospital care. (DHSS, 1976, p. 38)

In practice, evidence of capacities among residents and their subjective preferences is not always given the attention it deserves. *We recommend that clear criteria for admission to, and for continuing residence in, residential care should be agreed between the DHSS and the local authority associations, and steps taken to encourage rehabilitation, and in particular to prevent homeless elderly people from being offered accommodation only in residential homes. Priority should be given to expansion of domiciliary care for those who are severely disabled in their own homes.*

It may even be that, in the light of evidence which emerges, numbers in residential care could be frozen and even reduced, thus freeing additional resources. At times the DHSS has seemed to favour such a policy (for example, DHSS, *Social Care Research*, 1978, p. 13). It is true that in the 1970s the population of residential homes became older. This does of course suggest a rising number who are likely to be substantially incapacitated – though that correspondence needs to be demonstrated – but there still remains considerable evidence that a large fraction of residents, perhaps two fifths or even more, do not require continuous or even substantial 'care and attention' in a residential setting (Table 39). This may not mean that it would be right or practicable to attempt to find alternative accommodation for many present residents, but it does suggest that alternative accommodation must be found in future for those who would otherwise be admitted unnecessarily.

Table 39: *Evidence of capacity of elderly residents in homes for self-care*

Date of study	Scope of study	Percent of residents with capacity for self-care (local authority residents only unless otherwise specified)
(i) 1958–9	National sample survey of homes in England & Wales	72% neither bedfast nor requiring help dressing 59% mobile outside home without assistance 52% (new residents only) with 'little or no incapacity for self-care'
(ii) 1963	National sample survey of homes in Britain	37% little or no incapacity for self-care 21% little or no incapacity for self-care *and* household management
(iii) 1969	National survey of homes in Scotland	67% complete capacity for self-care (i.e. able to wash, dress and use toilet) 48% 'fit', i.e. having complete capacity for self-care plus no impairment or only mild impairment of mobility, mental state and continence
(iv) 1970	National census of homes in England	45% minimally dependent (i.e. continent, mobile without assistance, able to eat and drink without assistance, *and* mentally alert)
(v) 1972	Survey of council homes in eight London boroughs	55% high or very high capacity for self-care
(vi) 1973	64 homes in Cheshire	63% able to wash, dress, feed and go to toilet unaided 42% no mobility problems, no assistance of any kind required *and* no behavioural problems

Sources: (i) and (ii) Townsend, 1962 and 1973; (iii) Carstairs and Morrison, 1972; (iv) DHSS, 1975; (v) Plank, 1977; (vi) Kimbell and Townsend, 1975.

Moreover we believe the tendency of the residential population to grow and become older reflects in part the social difficulties of elderly people, not just the fact that more of them are 75 and over. Factors such as lagging real incomes, displacement at younger ages from occupations and housing and especially the tendency for women increasingly to outlive men and to live alone all make life more difficult, and services have not developed fast enough to compensate.

Ironically another explanation is to be found in the reduction of the percentage of elderly cared for within the hospital system. For reasons of cost or professional definitions of medical or nursing need fewer elderly are to be found in hospital at any particular date, and the elderly residential population has grown at the same time as the hospital population has diminished. We are not sure this change-over has been entirely beneficial. The most severely disabled sector of the elderly population may now have *less* access to medical and nursing expertise than they used to and there may be less effort put into their rehabilitation.

Residential care is by far the most costly element in the personal social services and deserves a thorough review. In planning an efficient system of care for the elderly we may need to ensure that the minority of people in residential accommodation who are very frail and require close and continuous medical and nursing supervision and treatment for long-term conditions receive it in very small residential nursing hospitals, annexes and even day centres under local geriatricians. On the other hand, sheltered housing may be the best environment for that large fraction of people in residential accommodation whose disabilities are slight or at least not substantial, and perhaps in some instances also of residents whose disabilities are severe. *We therefore recommend that the present functions and structure of hospital, residential and domiciliary care for the disabled elderly should be reviewed in relation to their needs, in order to determine the best and most economical balance of future services.* We believe that such a review is likely to demonstrate the accelerated relative priority that deserves to be accorded to the development of domiciliary services. Strictly, the responses to the consultative document *A Happier Old Age* (DHSS, 1978) provide in some respects the material for just such a review. However, the issue deserves more sustained expert examination and research, especially into the subjective attitudes of elderly patients and consumers of residential and community services, than it appears to have attracted.

Overall, the care of disabled people, many of whom are *elderly* disabled people, requires more co-ordinated action by health and social service authorities than currently exists. The introduction of joint funding has encouraged more collaborative planning. *We recommend that this initiative should be developed and that there should be further central government funding of a more specific kind to encourage joint care programmes.* Within the general category of severely disabled people, sub-categories should be more clearly defined so that both types of authority can comprehend their individual but also joint responsibilities at different stages of chronic illness or disablement. *We further recommend that sums within the joint finance allocation should be reserved for payment to authorities putting forward joint programmes to give continuing care to disabled people – for example, post-hospital follow-up schemes, pre-hospital support programmes for families, and support programmes for the severely incapacitated and terminally ill.* Funding might be based on a percentage or per capita grant. Health and local authorities may be involved in broader types of in-service training and acknowledgement of the need to interchange staff between hospital and day centre, or hospital and home.

Like many policies, a more vigorous community care policy on behalf of disabled people in their own homes will encounter difficulties. Risks are involved in encouraging some people to continue living alone when disabled. Attempts to increase the pattern of social contacts in supplementation of support services for some elderly people living alone have not always met with success, and traditions of individual privacy, quite apart from the constraints of poverty and bad housing, do not make any easier the patterns of supportive social interaction which would better suit disablement in old age. In the long run a choice has to be made between the encouragement of further dependency on the part of disabled people in the hands of different professionals, and the ready availability in the community of support, including greater diffusion of information and expertise, reciprocation of services within the community, self-help, and all the risks of depending on spontaneous and other expressions of good-will among neighbours and generally in the community. This latter option is, of course, a form of 'prevention', for it would help people to deal with their own problems in their own homes and preserve for them the dignity of the status of responsible actors.

Finally, there has been a rapid expansion of the home help service. *In practice many home helps undertake a wide range of responsibilities on behalf of disabled people and we recommend that this should be formally encouraged, with short courses of training, specialization of some functions and with access to mini-bus transport, especially to day centres.*

3. Prevention: the role of government

A consultative document on prevention and health was published in 1976 and reprinted three times within the space of a year. This suggests widespread public interest. As Ministers stated in a foreword to the document, 'the preventive approach should permeate and inform all aspects of the health services'.

This will involve a change of outlook in the DHSS and more determined changes in organization and the allocation of resources. For the attainment of national objectives the distribution of information and knowledge about health and management of illness needs to be less hierarchical and more widely shared. In part this means taking a new view of health education. We have already called for the resurgence of the school health service and the introduction of special forms of teaching in the schools. But the issue is not simply the better instruction of individuals at key periods of their lives. As those concerned with health education are aware, there are at least three distinguishable sets of reasons for health education: (1) 'to produce changes in beliefs and behaviour in order to reduce mortality and morbidity; (2) to influence norms and values governing the use of health services; (3) to produce a general understanding of certain more diffuse "health" issues in order to obtain a population who have a general understanding of health issues and to avoid certain forms of "undesirable" or not directly definable "unhealthy" behaviour' (Tuckett, 1979, p. 4). A balance has to be struck between creating better and safer conditions of work, safer travel, well-regulated manufacture of food products and other goods and the creation of social and occupational conditions minimizing stress, as well as the conventional individual 'do-it-yourself' approach to health education.

While laying stress on the importance of designing and regulating appropriate occupational environmental and social structures, *we recommend that a greatly enlarged programme of health education, with a particular focus on schools, should be sponsored by the government. The DHSS and the DES, as well as other departments, would be involved, and at the local level health education in schools should be the joint responsibility of AHAs and LEAs.* Such a programme of health education would include new initiatives to use the media for publicity, a drive to involve young parents in a programme of health education arranged in conjunction with local clinics, and corresponding programmes for those caring for disabled people at home.

However, as we have seen, it is not sufficient to regard preventive medicine as a question of individual initiative and responsibility based upon more information, important though this is. We explained in Chapter 6 (pp. 110–125) how the very possibilities for such initiative and responsibility are themselves a function of social circumstances. We accept, for example, the importance of publicity for, and advice on, the importance of adequate diet and of exercise, for health. Yet, it is not always possible for people to act in what they know to be their own best interest, and there are strong occupational class trends of the familiar kind in recreation and exercise (Morris, 1979, 1980). While the value of exercise must be made clear through the media, *facilities* for exercise are also required. We therefore endorse the view of the House of Commons Expenditure Committee in 1977 (HC 169–i,

1977) that 'The Department of the Environment and local authorities [should] be required to make more adequate provision for physical recreation in any future major developments or redevelopments both public and private, particularly in inner city areas.' We consider also that additional grants for the establishment of facilities for physical recreation should be made available.

Vaccination and immunization are not used as much as they should be and in some cases, polio for instance, the rate of immunization has actually declined. Doctors and others in the NHS must convince members of the public of the importance of these preventive measures. Tougher measures against both smoking and alcoholism are also required. In general we would note that the government's response to the Expenditure Committee report (*Preventive Medicine*) contained in the White Paper *Prevention and Health* (Cmnd 7047, 1977) failed to provide the positive measures we believe necessary. *We recommend that national health goals should be established and stated by government after wide consultation and debate. Measures that might encourage the desirable changes in people's diet, exercise and smoking and drinking behaviour should be agreed among relevant agencies.*

In the case of smoking these measures are clear, and cannot rest upon exhortation alone. An anti-smoking policy must involve new forms of education and counselling but also preventive and stringent control measures. During recent years there has been disturbing evidence of a growing inequality in cigarette-smoking between rich and poor sections of the population. Between 1961 and 1980 men in professional occupations reduced their smoking by well over half, whereas unskilled workers reduced their consumption by much less. We take the view that unequal access to information about the effects of smoking has contributed powerfully to this trend. We recommend the adoption of the following measures, which should be seen not only as priorities in themselves, but as illustrative of the determined action which needs to be taken by government in relation to all necessary elements of a strategy for prevention:

i. *Legislation should be rapidly implemented to phase out all advertising of tobacco and sales promotion of tobacco products (except at place of purchase).*

ii. *Sponsorship of sporting and artistic activities by tobacco companies should be banned over a period of a few years, and meanwhile there should be stricter control of advertisement through sponsorship.*

iii. *Regular annual increases in duty on cigarettes in line with rises in income should be imposed, to ensure lower consumption.*

iv. *Tobacco companies should be required, in consultation with the trades* unions, to submit plans for the diversification of their products over a period of ten years with a view to the eventual phasing out of sales of harmful tobacco products at home and abroad.

v. *The provision of non-smoking areas in public places should steadily be extended.*

vi. *A counselling service should be made available in all health districts, and experiments in methods to help people reduce smoking should be encouraged.*

vii. *A stronger, well-presented health warning should appear on all cigarette packets and such advertisements as remain, together with information on the harmful constituents of cigarettes.*

We appreciate that cigarette-smoking has a very strong hold on a large section of the population and that no government can appear to be excessively authoritarian in its measures to eradicate it. None the less, international comparisons have shown that Britain is particularly weak in the policies it has pursued. For example, in 1976 Britain was seventeenth among twenty European countries in provision of non-smoking facilities and bans on smoking in public places (ASH, 1976; and see also House of Commons Expenditure Committee report, *Preventive Medicine*, 1977). We wish to stress the relevance of an anti-smoking campaign to any measures at district or national level to reduce inequalities in health.

4. Screening programmes

In this country, general screening programmes have usually been offered to, and accepted by, special high-income groups such as business executives, in whom compliance tends to be higher than average. The question naturally arises whether extension of such programmes to other groups would carry a high priority. On balance, the cost of population screening and the possible production of anxiety might well outweigh any likely benefits, even where there is a known higher incidence of disease in lower-income groups. A similar view on unselected screening is expressed by the Royal Commission on the National Health Service in para. 5.7 of their report.

Screening for particular disorders suffers from similar weaknesses. However there are exceptions. One is ante-natal screening, and we recommend that steps should be taken to educate women of child-bearing age in the importance of reporting suspected pregnancy at the earliest possible stage so that ante-natal care can be provided early in pregnancy. With early attendance at ante-natal clinics there are practicable programmes for screening for Down's syndrome and neural tube defects in the foetus.

The other exception is screening for hypertension in adults, which is both relatively simple and also becoming a more common practice.

In the light of the present state of knowledge we recommend that ante-natal screening for Down's syndrome and for neural tube defects (especially in high-risk areas) on the one hand, and in relation to adult disease for serious hypertension on the other, should be made generally available.

Before leaving this topic we should make it clear that this action programme is not complete and there is plenty of scope for local and voluntary initiatives. In particular we hope that Community Health Councils might be invited to monitor developments in their areas. What is most important is that standards of health, and knowledge about health, should be raised through face-to-face contacts and local group practices, clinics, day centres and schools.

A programme for ten special areas

What might be called an 'area deprivation' strategy has not so far been formally adopted in health policies although it has been followed up in the policies of other central departments, the Department of Education, the Home Office and the Department of the Environment, in the last twelve years. The concepts of 'Educational Priority Area', 'Community Development Project', 'Housing Action Areas' and 'Inner Cities' have become well known and the idea of 'positive discrimination' has been pursued with enthusiasm though with some loss of clarity and coherence.

We are conscious of both the advantages and disadvantages of different forms of 'positive discrimination'. The term itself can be misleading. It implies or rather tends to be taken to mean that individuals, groups or populations are singled out for preferential or above-average treatment to redress their deprivation. In practice, close examination suggests that new programmes are attempting only to bring services in a small number of places closer to the national standard by exceptional, supplementary action. There have been difficulties in selecting areas of deprivation because of lack of certain kinds of information. And the programmes have rarely been related either to the possibility of putting experimental schemes subsequently into wider practice or integrating them fully into the administration of services in their areas. On the other hand, when money is tight there is some advantage from developing demonstration, experimental and compensatory projects.

The argument is three-fold: (i) *for purposes of demonstration.* When resources are scarce the beneficial effects of adopting additional measures generally can be demonstrated for a few places; (ii) *for purposes of experiment.* When there are doubts about the best methods of developing certain features of services – for example early ante-natal attendance or collaboration in assessment and visiting of disabled or elderly people by the statutory and voluntary services – alternatives need to be tried and evaluated; (iii) *for purposes of developing reasoned priorities.* Comparatively little is known about the relationship between health service inputs and outputs and it is becoming more and more important to discover what additional developments, and rearrangements of service, are most economically related to high standards of health in a population and the reduction of inequalities in health.

We therefore recommend that the government should finance a special health and social development programme in a small number of selected areas, costing about £30 m. in 1981–2 (the figure given in Table 37). The following ten areas have the highest death rate, standardized for population and age/sex structure (see also Table 38, p. 141):

Salford
Tameside
Gateshead
Liverpool
South Tyneside
Tower Hamlets
Durham
Bolton
Wirral
North Tyneside

It should be pointed out that *within* these areas wide variations in mortality rates are to be found. In Gateshead, for example, the ratio of infant mortality in some wards to that in others in the mid-1970s was 3:1, but the wards with highest mortality were also wards with the smallest proportions of population in classes I and II.

We propose that in each of the ten areas experimental programmes within the three priority spheres should be introduced. We envisage that a proportion (say at least £2 m.) of the £30 m. should be reserved for evaluative research and statistical and information units, and that the remaining sum should be divided among the ten areas for development of the types of services listed below.

In order to gain a better sense of the problems to be found in these areas, two, Tower Hamlets and Gateshead, were visited by members of the Working Group. Gateshead is in fact already one of the three beneficiaries of the Comprehensive Community Programme. There is no doubt that the health and personal social services, and especially the community health services, in such areas of high mortality where there are also other indicators of severe health and social problems deserve additional government aid.

It is perfectly true of course that many innovations in service provision on a local basis, such as mobile clinics, are already being attempted in areas like the ten listed above. Many of these may indeed be proving successful in reaching those in particular need (the mobile clinic may well be an example), but these innovations are rarely (if ever) the subject of rigorous experimental assessment. It is this essential element of experimental assessment, the equivalent of the randomized clinical trial of clinical procedures, that we wish to stress, certainly in relation to child health, but also in relation to disabled people. Without this not only can change be on no more than an intuitive basis, but learning by one area from another is inhibited. Although the precise form of the proposals will need to take specific aspects of the local situation into account, and there is inevitably an element of overlap among our three spheres of activity, the following would appear to be among the candidates for action:

Making clinics more responsive to needs

i. Developing clinics in group practice and dispensing with hospital clinics dealing with large populations;

ii. Providing child play facilities;

iii. Combining child welfare and ante-natal clinics;

iv. Providing evening and weekend clinics;

v. Setting up counselling services for mothers, covering pregnancy, infant and child care and family health;

vi. Provision of detailed nutritional counselling to pregnant women by trained nutritionists;

vii. Additional or special clinics for (1) lone and/or young mothers (2) handicapped children.

viii. Experiments to enable mothers to keep in touch with each other independently of ante-natal and post-natal appointments by such developments as Young Family Centres and the provision of facilities to enable mothers and babies to meet together regularly.

Domiciliary services

i. More health visitors to (a) follow up all missed clinic appointments; (b) undergo special training in helping ethnic minorities; (c) provide better services at home for severely disabled people.

ii. Liaison between GPs and health visitors: GPs should notify health visitors of all pregnancies promptly, and all pregnant women should be visited. GPs can be encouraged either in existing partnerships or health centres, or, if single-handed, collaboratively, to set up special maternity and infant care groups (possibly, through notification of first births, for first-time mothers and, through child benefit registrations or schools, for mothers of four or more children).

iii. Active development of community nursing services so that nurses are trained to work in the community as well as hospital and prevent certain hospital admissions as well as provide services for disabled or chronically sick people when discharged;

iv. Planned joint services with: (a) social service departments; (b) voluntary bodies. Schemes should include attachment of social workers to primary care teams and use of voluntary visitors on a 'preventive' basis for the disabled.

v. Special counselling services (including services on income rights, heating and housing problems) for severely disabled (especially elderly and mentally handicapped) people and their relatives.

School health

i. Special programme of assessment of health of school children;

ii. Special health education programme in schools as an integral part of the curriculum.

Food

i. Special welfare food provision on greatly increased scale;

ii. Enhanced (free) school meals programme.

Smoking

Experimental anti-smoking programmes (educational and therapeutic).

Screening

Experimental services aimed specifically at older mothers and middle-aged people.

It should not be supposed that an additional area programme would simply add to existing resource allocation. It would contribute to a better balance between necessary and less necessary services and hence would contribute to the more economical satisfaction of the aims of the health and personal social services.

Conclusion and summary

We have identified three objectives for the administration of health and personal social services and recommend their adoption by the Secretary of State. They are:

i. To give children a better start in life.

ii. For disabled people, to reduce the risks of early death, to improve the quality of life whether in the community or in institutions, and as far as possible to reduce the need for the latter.

iii. To encourage good health among a larger proportion of the population by preventive and educational action.

We believe that if these three objectives are pursued vigorously inequalities in health can be reduced. To fulfil them we recommend a shift in the allocation of resources (Table 37). However, this in itself is not enough. It must be combined with an imaginative, and in part necessarily experimental, approach to the nature and delivery of care. District action programmes, by which we mean general programmes for the health and personal social services to be adopted nationwide and involving necessary modifications to the structure of care, should be developed in each area; and an additional experimental programme should be funded in ten areas of high mortality and adverse social conditions.

We have argued for changes in the planning of the development of health services and especially resource allocation. We believe that allocation of resources should be based on need. We recognize that there are difficulties in assessing need, but we agree that standardized mortality ratios (SMRs) are a useful basis for broad allocation at regional level. At district level, further indicators of health care and social needs are called for. These should be developed as a matter of urgency, and appropriately to reinforce, supplement or modify allocation according to SMRs.

Resources within the National Health Service and the personal social services should be shifted more sharply than so far accomplished towards community care, particularly towards ante-natal, post-natal and child health services, and home help and nursing services for disabled people. We see this as an important part of a strategy to break the links between social class or poverty and health.

In building up revenue targets it is not the current distribution of expenditure between services which should be used, but that which is aimed at in the planning of services. In particular, this process should reflect a higher share of resources for community care.

While we are aware of the problems of conceptualizing and measuring 'need', we consider there is no better alternative conceptual basis for developing a coherent rationale for the allocating of health care and resources, and recommend accordingly.

Our main recommendations for a district action programme can be listed under the three objectives set out above.

(A) *Health and welfare of mothers, pre-school and school children*

i. A non-means-tested scheme for free milk should now be introduced, beginning with couples with their first infant child and infant children in large families.

ii. Areas and districts should review the accessibility and facilities of all ante-natal and child health clinics in their areas and develop plans to increase utilization by mothers, particularly in the early months of pregnancy.

iii. Savings from the current decline in the school population should be used to finance new services for children under 5. A statutory obligation should be placed on local authorities to ensure adequate day care in their area for children under 5, and a minimum number of places (the number being raised after regular intervals) should be laid down centrally. Further steps should be taken to reorganize day nurseries and nursery schools so that both meet the needs of children for education *and* care.

iv. Every opportunity should be taken to link revitalized school health care with general practice, and intensify surveillance and follow-up both in areas of special need and for certain types of family.

Some necessary developments apply to other groups as well as children and mothers.

v. The professional associations as well as the Secretary of State and the health authorities should accept responsibility for making improvements in the quality and geographical coverage of general practice, especially in areas of high prevalence of ill-health and poor social conditions. Where the number or scope of work of general practitioners is inadequate in such areas we recommend health authorities to deploy or re-deploy an above-average number of community nurses, attached where possible to family practices. The distribution of general practitioners should be related not only to population but to medical need as indicated by SMRs, supplemented by other indicators, and the per capita basis of remuneration should be modified accordingly.

vi. An assessment which determines severity of disablement should be adopted as a guide to health service priorities, and this should be related to the limitation of activities rather than loss of faculty or type of handicap.

Although we attach priority to the implementation of this recommendation in the case of disabled children we believe that it must ultimately apply to all disabled people. We are aware that since 1977 most local councils have adopted classification of severity of disablement of people on their registers of the handicapped. We hope that this can be extended to people with all types of handicap and to patients in the health services.

(B) *The care of disabled people in their own homes*

i. A Working Group, to include representatives of voluntary organizations concerned with relevant client groups, should be set up to review: (a) whether sheltered housing should be a responsibility of social service or housing departments, and to make recommendations; and (b) the present functions and structure of hospital, residential and domiciliary care for the disabled elderly in relation to their needs, and to decide the best and most economical balance of future services.

ii. Joint funding should be developed and further funding of a more specific kind should be introduced, if necessary within the existing NHS budget, to encourage joint care programmes. A further sum should be reserved for payment to authorities putting forward joint programmes to give continuing care to disabled people – for example post-hospital follow-up schemes, pre-hospital support programmes for families, and support programmes for the severely incapacitated and terminally ill.

iii. Clear criteria for admission to, and continuing residence in, residential care should be agreed between the DHSS and the local authority associations, and steps taken to encourage rehabilitation and in particular to prevent homeless elderly people from being offered accommodation only in residential homes. Priority should be given to expansion of domiciliary care for those who are severely disabled in their own homes.

iv. The functions of home helps should be extended to permit a lot more work on behalf of disabled people; short courses of training, specialization of functions and the availability of mini-bus transport, especially to day centres, should be encouraged.

(C) *Prevention: the role of government*

i. An enlarged programme of *health education* should be sponsored by the government, and necessary arrangements made for optimal use of the mass media, especially television. Health education in schools should become the joint responsibility of LEAs and health authorities. However, we do not believe that an effective programme of preventive health can be a matter entirely for personal initiative and responsibilities. Commitment on the part of government is required, and has not so far been demonstrated, especially in so far as it involves (as it must) departments other than the DHSS. For example, there has been no major attempt at making more adequate provision for physical recreation in inner city area developments, as recommended by the Expenditure Committee in 1977. Additionally, the decline in recourse to vaccination and immunization (as in the case of polio) is worrying. Doctors and others in the NHS must be encouraged to convince members of the public of the importance of these preventive measures.

ii. *National health goals* should be established and stated by government after wide consultation and debate. Measures that might encourage the desirable changes in people's diet, exercise, and smoking and drinking behaviour should be agreed among relevant agencies.

Legislation, and fiscal and other financial measures, may be required and a wide range of social and economic policies involved. We see the time as now opportune for a major step forwards in the field of health and prevention.

iii. Stronger measures to *reduce cigarette smoking* must be adopted. Our recommendations here should be seen not only as a priority in themselves, but as illustrative of the determined action by government necessary in relation to all essential elements of a strategy for prevention. Measures should include those listed on pp. 154–5.

We have already recommended that steps be taken to increase utilization of ante-natal clinics, especially in the early months of pregnancy. Given early attendance there are practical programmes for screening for Down's syndrome and for neural tube defects in the foetus. In relation to adults screening for severe hypertension is practicable, and effective treatment is available.

iv. In the light of the present state of knowledge we recommend that ante-natal screening for neural tube defects (especially in high-risk areas) and Down's syndrome on the one hand, and in relation to adult disease for severe hypertension on the other, should be made generally available.

Additional funding for ten special areas

We recommend that the government should finance a special health and social development programme in a small number of selected areas, costing about £30m. in 1981–2. At least £2m. of this sum should be reserved for evaluation research and statistical and information units. The object would be both to provide special help to redress the undeniable disadvantages of people living in those areas, and also to permit special experiments to reduce ill-health and mortality, and provide better support for disabled people. Some possibilities have been illustrated particularly in connection with the development of more effective ante-natal services.

Chapter 9

The Wider Strategy

While the health care service can play a significant part in reducing inequalities in health, measures to reduce differences in material standards of living at work, in the home and in everyday social and community life are of even greater importance. We have in mind not simply a general reduction of inequalities in living standards, but a marked relative improvement in the living standards of the poorest people, together with measures to prevent new technologies, new working procedures, changes in styles of urban and rural living and the emergence of new social and political associations from undermining the existing living standards of some groups. Like the strategy we proposed for the health care system, the strategy to be adopted outside that system needs to be comprehensive and interlinked.

We therefore outline how a broad strategy might be made up and make certain specific proposals for inclusion in it. Specifically, we shall first indicate the general need for an anti-poverty strategy and then discuss and recommend selected measures, especially for families with children and disabled people.

A comprehensive anti-poverty strategy

Despite increases in GNP during the 1960s and 1970s successive governments have recognized the wide extent of poverty in the United Kingdom. In 1966 the report of a government survey of retirement pensioners estimated that up to 750,000 elderly people were living below national assistance standards – most of whom were eligible to draw national assistance and were not claiming it (Ministry of Pensions and National Insurance, 1966, p. 20). In 1967 a further report on a survey of families with children estimated that there were 160,000 families with half a million children who were living under the new supplementary benefit scale rates (Ministry of Social Security, 1967, p. iv). Further reports from the DHSS in the early 1970s tended to confirm the large numbers of people with incomes below the scale rates and yet who were in, or were dependants of people who were in, full-time employment.

(See for example, Howe, DHSS, 1971.) In Table 32 (p. 108) we showed, on the basis of DHSS estimates, that in 1977 over 14 million people (or 26.6 per cent of the population) had incomes of below or not more than 40 per cent above the supplementary benefit level (a cut-off chosen in recent government and independent studies). About a third were employed, or were dependants of people who were employed, and about two fifths were on retirement pensions. (Because of the under-representation of elderly, sick and disabled people, the use of a measure of 'normal' instead of 'current' income for people who have been sick or unemployed for less than three months, and the exclusion of those receiving supplementary benefit from the data, numbers with incomes below SB level are underestimated (Townsend, 1979, pp. 275–276 and 908–9).) At these levels of income there is evidence of multiple deprivation in diet, housing and environmental amenities, leisure activities and at work. Because of changes in earnings and numbers of dependants, the movement of people into and out of poverty is considerable, and while there is no hard evidence covering a long span of individual life it may be inferred, from survey or cross-sectional data, data about incomes currently and for the previous year, and New Earnings Survey data followed through for several years, that a very high proportion of manual workers experience poverty, or exceptionally low living standards, for a substantial part of the life-cycle.

There are differences of view about what in fact constitutes poverty. The main question is how far a definition acceptable to the government should depend on needs as assessed in contemporary society and how far on needs as measured by some historical bench-mark. Today's poor in Britain have more purchasing power than the poor of the depression years of the 1930s because of the growth of national prosperity. But they are living in a different kind of society, in which they have, and are held to have, different and often *additional* obligations as workers, parents, householders, friends and citizens. We therefore take the view that any historical standard of need becomes more and more unreal with the passage of time in a changing and especially growing economy even when it is repriced in accordance with rises in the cost of living. An effort has to be made every few years to redefine the standard itself in accordance with changing social conditions. As long ago as 1812 Adam Smith recognized the need for such redefinition, declaring that 'by necessities I understand, not only the commodities which are indispensably necessary for the support of life, but whatever the custom of the country renders it indecent for creditable people even of the lowest order to be without'. One of the last reports from the Supplementary Benefits Commission (*Annual Report for 1978*, 1979) expresses the point as follows: 'Poverty in urban industrial countries like Britain is a standard of living so low that it excludes and isolates people from the rest of the community. To keep out of poverty they must have an income which enables them to participate in the life of the community.'

We believe a comprehensive anti-poverty strategy must fall into two parts. The first is a fairer distribution of resources. Successive governments have supposed that they did not so much have to intervene in the initial production and determination of the structures of wealth and of gross incomes in the first place, as redistribute through taxation a slice of gross income to make up minimum subsistence incomes for the poor. But attempts to raise the relative living standards of the poor have been largely frustrated by growing opposition to progressive taxation as well as the diminution of its practical effects, and the steady growth relative to the employed population, of a dependent population. Different examples might be given of this growth. Between 1951 and 1976 the number of social security beneficiaries, excluding those receiving family allowances, grew from just over 7.5 million to 14.25 million, or by 88 per cent, while the total population increased from 51 million to 56 million, or by only 10 per cent. The government expects the number of social security beneficiaries to grow to over 15.5 million by 1982/3, even on an assumption of no growth in unemployment (*Social Trends*, 1979).

Governments have tried to meet this developing problem by lowering the tax threshold, so that people start paying tax on lower incomes, and shifting the balance from direct to indirect taxation. They have also tried to reduce the growing costs of categories already defined as dependent, as well as meeting the additional costs of new categories, by relying increasingly on the supplementary benefit and other means-tested schemes.

Even this solution, however, has now reached a dead end. In the 1980s either the living standards of the poor will not be maintained relative to the rest of the population as their numbers grow, or if living standards are maintained or efforts are made even to improve them, then radically new methods of financing them from the prosperous sections of the population will have to be devised.

We believe that a new approach to the fairer distribution of resources needs to be developed on the following basis. It starts with a recognition that the dispersion of resources *is* very unequal, and that the long-term objective of reducing by a moderate amount the proportionate share of, say, the top 30 per cent of income recipients would substantially augment the sum redistributed at present to the poor. If the share of disposable income of the top 30 per cent, as given in Report No. 5 (p. 75) of the Royal Commission on the Distribution of Income and Wealth, were only moderately reduced, the sum available for distribution in social security benefits, for example, could be doubled.

It follows that although it will be politically difficult, we shall need to develop greater restrictions on the amount of wealth which may be inherited and accumulated, together with more effective measures to inhibit the growth of top incomes and reduce present differentials in incomes. Quite how this might be done and how it might be democratically agreed and enforced is not something we can cope with here. But we believe it may be desirable to establish national minimum *and* maximum earnings (and family income) as indispensable elements of a nationally approved framework of incomes. Within statutory limits local and industrial or occupational wage-levels might be negotiated. Below we shall recommend certain measures to be included in such a strategy.

The second part of a comprehensive anti-poverty strategy is to encourage self-dependence and a high level of individual skill and autonomy as a basis for creating a more integrated society. We believe that this is possible only by raising the standards and broadening the content of education so that the need for advice or supervision from professionally trained personnel in medicine, nursing, law, housing, child care or administration is less marked and the capacity to undertake a range of skills is greater. This includes improving individual access to information about, and control over, what goes on in the immediate community as well as society generally, and conferring rights to employment and occupation and creating corresponding opportunities for such employment. There are of course possibilities of augmenting formal education and of introducing into the curriculum more studies of such subjects as health and nutrition, and (some believe) political education. Methods of enabling adults to have better access to knowledge, theoretical and practical, are equally important.

Most important, of course, is the right to fulfilling employment. Among a variety of possible measures there are two which deserve special mention. One is the energetic sponsorship of new industrial enterprise, based upon newly emerging technologies. In the face of a world recession in trade and severe foreign competition the nation cannot afford to be timid. The other measure is to expand employment within different branches of community service. Up to the present time the youth opportunities programme and similar schemes have done little more than provide some people who would otherwise count as unemployed with temporary, and ill-paid, employment. There are thousands of other men and women who have been unemployed for many months and whom it costs the state nearly as much to support as it would to employ in useful work.

Within this broad outline there are a number of specific measures which need to be picked out and given priority. In the rest of this chapter we shall develop certain priorities outside the health service which correspond with those picked out for the health care system.

A major concern must be families and children. Top priority must be given to measures which will enhance family living standards and reduce the high risk of children suffering those forms of deprivation and poverty which inhibit healthy development. In drawing this conclusion we are conscious in particular of two facts of the utmost importance:

i. There is evidence of substantial deprivation among young children (for example, Wilson and Herbert, 1978; Bone, 1977) and, after people of advanced age, they run the highest risk of all age groups of being in poverty (Townsend, 1979, p. 285);

ii. Those in middle and late middle life (mostly couples without dependants) have a standard of living, measured in relation to supplementary benefit scale rates, far higher than that of families in which there are young children (Townsend, 1979, Figure 7.1, p. 288). This difference between the young and the middle-aged appears to have grown more marked in recent years, partly because the rearing of children has been completed after the first twenty or twenty-five years of adult life by more married couples in each succeeding cohort, but partly because more married women have re-entered employment, non-manual occupations with strongly defined incremental pay scales have grown disproportionately, and more of the middle-aged have had access to cheap housing, through the completion of mortgage repayments or a relative fall in the real value of repayments, because of inflation. The implication for policy is therefore both that a need exists to direct more resources towards children and that checks might be placed on the tendencies for people in middle life without dependants to attract an undue share of additional national resources, so that adequate measures for young children might with less difficulty be financed. A complex programme covering financial well-being, education, nutrition and housing must be developed. In this chapter we have selected some principal measures to give effect to such a programme.

A policy for families and children

It is our view that *the abolition of child poverty should be adopted as a national goal for the 1980s*. We recognize that this requires a redistribution of financial resources far beyond anything achieved by past programmes, and is likely to be very costly. We recognize also that with the growth in national income it will become easier to find the resources for such an anti-poverty strategy.

The recommendations which we make below are presented as a modest *first step* which might now be taken towards such an objective.

1. Child benefit

The history of child benefit has proceeded through two stages and is now entering a third. The first was the campaign to establish family allowances, culminating in the Family Allowances Act 1945. History demonstrates the different motives of the participants in the campaign.

Family allowances were supported in the early days as a means of reducing inequalities between rich and poor, and between men and women. To socialists and feminists these were worthy ends in themselves but were not regarded as legitimate ends for government social policy until the Second World War. Broader support from Liberals and Conservatives was forthcoming only when family allowances became linked with other problems: a declining birth rate, poverty and malnutrition among children, the maintenance of work incentives and the need to curb inflation. These problems were established concerns of government and thus, by association, the legitimacy of family allowances was enhanced. (Land, 1975, p. 227)

The government agreed to pay 25p (less than the 40p recommended by Beveridge) per week for every dependent child excluding the first.

The second was the re-kindling, in the mid 1960s, of a campaign to extend family allowances to the first child in the family and simultaneously increase the real value of all family allowances, partly in exchange for the phasing-out of child tax allowances. This stage culminated not so much in the Child Benefit Act of 1975 as the completion of its phasing-in during the two years from April 1977 up to the budget of 1979.

Yet throughout this entire period government support for family allowances was never more than luke-warm. (For the recent history see *The Great Child Benefit Robbery*, 1977; Land, 1978; Field, 1978.) Between 1946 and 1978 pensions and other major social security benefits were increased on seventeen occasions: family allowances were increased only six times. This poor record must have some bearing on the relatively large numbers of wage-earning families found in national surveys and by statistical comparison with other countries to be living in poverty or on its margins, and on such indicators as the failure of infant mortality rates to decline as rapidly as those in some other countries.

Over the last half-decade the position has not substantially altered. Improvements introduced in the last years of the 1970s have done little more than restore the levels of the late 1960s, and inflation continues to eat into these 'improved' rates.

The importance of a properly endowed child benefit programme to the future health of the children of this country cannot be exaggerated. In its report for 1973 the Supplementary Benefits Commission stated: 'The adequacy of family benefits in general, and the new child benefits in particular, seems to us to be the most urgent concern of the whole field of social security' (Cmnd 6615, p. 17). This was reiterated in the next report, and in its response to the review which preceded the reorganization in 1979–80 of supplementary benefits, the Commission went on to affirm: 'Further improvements in child benefit and help for the unemployed – particularly in the form of better opportunities for work – are the most urgent of our proposals' (*Response of the SBC*, 1979, p. 40). From our different remit we endorse those priorities. *We recommend as an immediate goal the raising of the level of child benefit to 5.5 per cent of average gross male industrial earnings – in November 1979 equivalent to the rate for a dependent child of a sick or unemployed person (£5.70 including child benefit).* [The latter sum would have to be increased to about £7.00 by April 1981 to keep pace with earnings.] In the longer term, we recommend that larger child benefits be paid for older children, perhaps with age bands corresponding to those used by the SBC. Also in the longer term we should like to see age-related child benefit rates index-linked to average gross male industrial earnings, or, because an increasing number of women are entering employment and because in many cases both husband and wife have earnings, to some other perhaps more appropriate standard (such as average net disposable personal income). Otherwise it will be difficult to maintain the 'tax equity' as well as the 'need-serving' functions of child benefit. One-parent families present special problems, and in our view their financial needs too would be better met through an increase in child benefit.

2. Infant care allowance

A re-grouping of resources on behalf of young mothers with infants is required. In principle, needs at child-birth are met through the maternity benefit and maternity grant. But the grant has not been maintained during inflation and would need to be raised to *about £100* from the present £25.00, which has not been changed since 1969, to restore its value to that equivalent to the payment when first introduced. We recommend that *the grant should be increased to £100 to acknowledge the high cost to parents of child-birth.*

The special responsibilities of caring for young children, other than through the married man's tax allowance, are, however, not yet recognized in Britain. Some countries – Hungary is one example – have introduced infant care allowances in addition to child benefit. The case for the introduction of a home responsibility payment has been made in Britain:

The benefit would be paid to all families in which there were children or other dependants needing home care, except those where the social insurance benefit included a dependant's allowance for the wife. In the case of children such a benefit could presumably be paid simply by paying an addition to the child benefit payable for the eldest dependent child in the family, and it might be better presented in this way. The payment for the care of adult dependants would then be a separate benefit, a development of the present invalid care allowance. (Meade Report, p. 287. See also pp. 498–9)

The Child Poverty Action Group has proposed a more differentiated scheme, whereby women with children under 5 would receive twice as much as those with dependent children of school age (Select Committee on Tax Credit, Vol. II, pp. 325–30). The allowance could be phased in, beginning with all births after a particular date. *We recommend the introduction of an infant care allowance of approximately the same level as of child benefit, to be paid to mothers of children under 5 years of age, to be phased in over a period of five years.* As suggested later (p. 182), the cost might be met not so much from new resources as by restricting the scope of the married man's tax allowance to wives with dependants.

Beyond these initial elements of an anti-poverty strategy, a number of other steps need to be taken.

3. Pre-school education and day care

In Chapter 8 we recommended that local authorities should be under a statutory obligation to ensure an adequate provision of day care facilities (taking this term to include not only places in day nurseries but also in nursery classes, and with trained and registered childminders). To emphasize the importance we attach to this recommendation as well as its central place in any policy devoted to meeting the developmental needs of the under-5s, we further elaborate on it at this point.

It is well known that the desire for day provision on the part of parents of under-5s greatly exceeds what is currently available. A survey in 1977 found that 'provision was wanted for twice as many children as were receiving it, so that whilst 32 per cent of children were using facilities, they were desired for 64 per cent (Bone, 1977). The survey also found that this unmet need was class related (see Table 40) and that cost was a significant factor in inhibiting usage of such facilities by the children of working-class parents.

The same survey also looked at the demand for facilities judged on the basis of the number of 'disadvantaged' children who might benefit from them. The need criteria used, which more or less correspond to those leading to priority admission to day nursery, were as follows:

Need Group A

Child had only one parent

or

Child had two parents but father's income was less than 150 per cent of long-term SB level

or

Child's household accommodation was two or more bedrooms less than standard

or

Child's household accommodation was inadequate in four ways

or

Child was definitely handicapped (definite diagnosis)

Need Group B

Child already allocated to need group A

or

Child's mother was worried he might be handicapped (no definite diagnosis)

or

Child was 3 or 4 years old and soiled himself more than twice a week

or

Child's mother classified as 'depressed' or 'anxious'

or

Child had behaviour difficulties (on standard scaling)

On this basis, 15 per cent of all pre-school children fell into need group A and 36 per cent into need group B (which includes A). In fact only 28

Table 40: *Desire for day provisions for under-5s by occupational class**

	Occupational class				
	I	*II*	*IIINM and IVNM*	*IIIM*	*IVM and V*
Day provisions used	40	40	32	29	24
Not used but desired	22	26	36	33	39
Day provisions not desired	37	33	31	36	33
Total percentage†	100	100	100	100	100

*This survey used a different social class breakdown including a 'semi-skilled non-manual' (IVNM) category.

† Includes a few instances of 'not known'.

Source: Bone, 1977, Table 3.2.

per cent of all children in need group A were making use of any facilities for day provision and 30 per cent in need group B. All these figures are, perhaps, rather crude and we were unable to make a more detailed calculation of the need for day provision, but clearly the unmet need is substantial. What has to be remembered is that although the poorest children experience multiple forms of deprivation a very large proportion of children can be said to experience one or more forms of it. It is difficult to distinguish between deprived and non-deprived children and there are degrees of gradation, but by any calculation the unmet need is very substantial indeed. On the most conservative of estimates, the difference between the 36 per cent of children whose health and cognitive and psychological development (or financial circumstances, with the risks that might ultimately be entailed) make their need for day care overwhelming, and the 27 per cent of all under-5s who currently receive some provision (9 per cent of some $3\frac{1}{2}$ million under-5s in England and Wales), amounts to a minimum need of some 300,000 places. (This of course is based on the impossible assumption that all current places are taken up by children in need.) If the criterion of parental *desire* for some day provision were to be adopted, then the number of places available would have to be doubled, according to Bone's survey. This implies the creation of some 900,000 extra places in England and Wales.

The health and developmental needs of children, especially children rendered at risk by their environments, lead us to emphasize the importance of day facilities for under-5s catering for *both* these needs, and provided on an adequate scale. The precise pattern of such provision will necessarily vary with local conditions. It is clear that all available resources in the community must be used to their utmost: childminders, voluntary organizations and parents. More efficient use of existing facilities, such as nursery schools and classes, is also required. We are eager to see local authorities sponsoring collaborative arrangements between parents and others in the local community to complement the extended statutory services for the under-5s. This represents the principle of prevention at the local level. To reiterate the recommendation we have already made in Chapter 8: *We recommend that a statutory obligation should be placed on local authorities to ensure adequate day care in their area for children under 5, and that a minimum number of places (the number being raised after regular intervals) should be laid down centrally.*

Before leaving this topic it should also be made clear that different forms of provision – day care, nursery classes, playgroups, childminders etc. – cater for different needs. Local authority day nursery places are largely restricted to children regarded by social workers as 'at risk', or living in poor housing, or where a single parent is anxious to go to work. Staffed by nursery nurses they are less specifically concerned with the child's cognitive development than are nursery schools or classes. Our own view of the close relationship between health, social well-being and cognitive development in children leads us to argue for much greater integration between these forms of provision. This is of course widely acknowledged (as in the joint DES/DHSS circular *Co-ordination of Provision for the Under-Fives* of January 1978). So too is the need for more flexible provision of nursery education which caters better for the needs of working mothers (CPRS, 1978). It must be borne in mind that not only is the proportion of under-5s with mothers in paid employment rising (25 per cent in 1976) but that empty school places (due to the decline in the population of school age) represent an inefficient use of resources.

4. Nutrition: School milk and meals

In Chapter 6 we drew attention to the importance of the nutrition of children for their development. The DHSS booklet *Eating for Health* stated:

> If all were to enjoy the best possible diet, the variation in average height and weight of different socio-economic groups in the United Kingdom would probably be less marked. The attained height of adults depends to some extent on nutrition during growth as children and in particular during the most rapid period of growth as babies. Any persistent restriction of diet in a young child may impair growth to such an extent that the affected child never reaches its full hereditary endowment of height. (DHSS, 1978, pp. 12–13)

This booklet goes on to point out the remarkable gains, notably in perinatal mortality, which followed wartime food rationing, despite the overall shortages of food, and the introduction of such welfare foods as cod-liver oil and welfare orange juice: 'The unequal distribution of food, which had restricted the diet of families with low incomes, was made equitable by this system which included food subsidies on and control of the price of meat, bread, sugar, milk, potatoes, butter, margarine, cheese' (p. 16). The wartime scarcities which led to these policies fortunately no longer exist. It nevertheless remains important to *ensure* that all children are adequately nourished, if all are to achieve their potential for healthy growth.

In 1967 the Committee on Medical Aspects of Food Policy commissioned a nutritional survey of pre-school children, which was carried out in 1967–8 and eventually published in 1975. The acknowledged under-representation of large families, poor families and immigrant families in this survey must to some degree reduce the confidence which can be placed in the assessment of the adequacy of nutrition among these 'at risk' groups. The study nevertheless showed a clear decline in vitamin intake (A, C, D) with rising family size, and declining occupational class and income. Protein consumption rose with income though there was no trend with family size or occupational class. Calcium intake showed no trend. Total energy consumption actually rose with increasing family size, declining social class and falling income (except among the poorest families) – but some of this trend was certainly due to extra consumption of 'added sugar' – sweets, biscuits, soft drinks etc. – in poorer, larger working-class families (DHSS, *Reports on Health and Social Subjects*, No. 10, 1975).

Although the report concluded that there is 'no evidence that our pre-school children were underfed', it was hard to reconcile this with some of the statistics revealing under-nutrition and deprivation among some poor minorities. The proportions of children found to have intakes below 80 per cent of the recommended levels of specific nutrients varied from 20 to 30 per cent in some cases of energy, total protein and iron and around half were below that level for vitamin C (p. 27). The survey also showed the importance of milk in the diet of children. Although this was age-related, even at the age of $3\frac{1}{2}$ to $4\frac{1}{2}$ milk continued to provide, on average, 16 per cent of total energy intake, 26 per cent total protein and 62 per cent calcium and 42 per cent riboflavin.

A study of a sample of about 1,000 children resident in Kent aged 8–11 and 13–15, carried out between September 1968 and March 1970, throws some light on the nutritional status of older children. The sample was weighted to include larger numbers of children from occupational classes IV and V, large families, and families lacking fathers, and included a dietary assessment over a one-week period. Important conclusions were that: there was no clinical evidence of nutritional deficiency, and significant differences in average daily nutrient intake were not associated with class, number of siblings, or whether or not the mother worked. However, the *quality* of the child's diet (expressed in nutrients per 1,000 kcals) was class-related, falling with declining occupational class (Cook *et al.*, 1973). The study also showed that differences in nutrient intake and quality of diet were not explained by income differences when other class-related factors were held constant (Jacoby *et al.*, 1975).

Few today would therefore dissent from the view that given the importance of adequate nutrition for a child's development, and in the absence of a comprehensive food policy, attention quite properly focuses on school milk and meals. Between 1946 and 1968, one third of a pint of milk was available free every school day to all school children. From 1968 it ceased to be provided to secondary school pupils. In 1971 it was stopped for all children after the end of the school year of their seventh birthday, except where the school doctor recommended otherwise. Late in 1978 local authorities were once more permitted, though not obliged, to provide milk for 7–11-year-olds. In 1971, when the reduced availability of school milk was accompanied also by an increase in the price of school meals, the Committee on Medical Aspects of Food Policy (COMA) was asked to monitor the effects of these changes. Its Sub-Committee on Nutritional Surveillance issued an interim report in 1973 in which it indicated the dimensions on which effects would be monitored: height, obesity and dental caries were central.

So far as provision of milk to primary school children aged 7+ is concerned, the evidence, though not clear-cut, does not indicate a significant effect on growth. The earlier study of Kent children to which we referred above, conducted in 1968–70, found that, among 8–11-year-olds, those who regularly drank school milk had significantly higher intakes of energy, calcium and animal protein, but that this was not associated with height or other measures of nutritional status (Cook *et al.*, 1975a). The same research group, conducting a national surveillance study of a longitudinal kind under COMA auspices, found that between 1972 and 1973 the *growth* of 6–7-year-olds was not influenced by availability of school milk. The same held true of a special sample of children from occupational classes IV and V (formed by aggregation of successive age cohorts) (Cook *et al.*, in press). A study of 7–8-year-olds in South Wales, employing a sample deliberately weighted in favour of large families and occupational classes IV and V, also found that growth over twenty-one months was unaffected by provision of school milk (Baker *et al.*, 1978). Cook *et al.* summarize by stating 'the availability of school milk has no real effect on group well-being where drinking milk at home is almost universal'. It has however been suggested that linear growth may not be a wholly adequate measure of the benefits of milk consumption. Reed, for example, has referred to the need also to take account of bone status (Reed, 1978).

Moreover, current policy towards provision of school milk has to be judged, and developed, in the light of the continuing fall in household consumption of liquid milk revealed by the National Food Survey. In 1977 this average household consumption was 4.54 pints per person per week, compared with 4.71 pints in 1976 and 4.76 pints in 1975 (*National Food Survey*, 1977, p. 7). Moreover, the survey shows that in 1977 of 7–9-year-olds in lower-income families with three or more children, 12 per cent consumed less than 2 pints per week in the home, and over 25 per cent less than 3 pints.

It is clear that current policy must therefore be kept continuously under review, in the light of these trends, and also in the light of further research on growth and development.

The evidence in relation to provision of schools meals is more clear-cut. School meals are intended to provide about one third of the daily allowance of nutrients and energy for a child, and are recommended to contain, on average, 29g total protein, 880 kcals energy, and 32g fat. We have no evidence on the range in nutritional quality of the meals in practice provided. We have no doubt that this meal is the principal source of essential nutrients for many low-income children. Many may be offered a poor-quality evening meal, and many come to school without breakfast. (This sixteen hour 'fast' may well affect the child's powers of concentration, and hence his ability to profit from his schooling.) It should be regarded as a matter of importance – on education *and* health grounds – to ensure that all children receive a school meal or an adequate substitute at least during term time. To leave school children, especially young school children, to make their own free choices of what food is to be purchased would be wrong. Children will frequently prefer to consume foods high only in sugar and other sources of energy. As an inadequate substitute for a nutritious meal, this is likely to lead to increases in obesity and in dental caries.

Certainly, great importance has been attached to the nutritional variety and adequacy of school meals by a number of official committees. For example, the Working Party on the Nutritional Aspects of School Meals has commented: 'We do not think it is safe to assume that all children necessarily receive a satisfactory diet at home. We are especially concerned that all children should receive enough protein at school since any shortfall in the midday meal might easily not be made up in other meals or snacks and drinks consumed outside school' (DES, 1975, p. 8).

The survey of Kent children aged 8–11 and 13–15 offers some support to these views (Cook *et al.*, 1957b). Consumption of school meals (about 80 per cent overall) proved to be higher among children without fathers, with working mothers, etc. Distinguishing children who had all five, or no, school meals in the test week, the study found that younger children who had school meals had higher lunchtime intakes of nearly all nutrients (and more nutrients per 1,000 kcals) than those who did not. It also found that children from classes IV and V taking school meals obtained a very much higher proportion of their total weekday nutrient intake from their lunches than did children from the same classes who did not. The same was not consistently true of class I/II children.

Taking these findings together with known biases in the information, it is possible to conclude, with the authors, that

families without a father, those in lower social classes, and with large numbers of children relied to a greater extent than others on the intake of nutrients important for growth from school meals. This reliance may or may not depend on a conscious decision. The present study took place before recent large increases in the cost of protein-rich foods and such families may now rely even more on the food intake from school meals.

Yet the percentage of pupils receiving school meals (whether free or paid for) is falling: from 70 per cent in 1975 to 62 per cent in 1977. There are a number of explanations for this, partly cost, partly poor quality and partly administrative inertia.

At present local authorities administer a government scheme making school meals free for children of parents receiving supplementary benefit or parents whose income is below certain limits laid down in national regulations. In May 1978 about 15 per cent of school children were getting it. The limits are revised regularly, normally when supplementary benefit scales are increased. In recent years the Department of Education has estimated that about three quarters or four fifths of children eligible to receive school meals free are in fact receiving them. Others consider the right figure may be no higher than 60 per cent. Part of the problem arises in fluctuating incomes and frequent assessments or reassessments, but also in the fluctuation in standards of living brought about by changing household dependencies. Experimental campaigns by the government, especially in 1967 and 1968, have shown that take-up can be increased substantially through letters addressed directly to parents and through advertisements. But because of the numbers of children passing through the schools and fluctuations in family living standards, quite apart from the effect of inflation, higher take-up rates do not endure. Twice in 1977 and again in 1978 the Secretary of State for Education was asked to renew the approach adopted in 1967 and 1968 and issue a simple letter to all parents advising them about free school meals. Although an estimated half a million children were not obtaining free dinners although entitled to them, this invitation was not accepted. Whatever the exact short-fall, there is no doubt that it is substantial and there have been a large number of research studies demonstrating that means-tested exemption from charges for school meals is not a satisfactory way of helping poor families (Field, 1975; Field and Townsend, 1975; Townsend, 1979). A recent study has shown that there are even wide variations among areas with similar characteristics. 'This type of analysis can help to identify areas where there may be low take-up to inadequate efforts by local authorities and central Government' (Bradshaw and Weale, November 1978, p. 22).

In our view any reduction in the provision of school meals, or in eligibility for free meals, would mean putting further at risk the development of significant numbers of children. A study carried out by a team from St

Thomas's hospital showed that children receiving free school meals are significantly shorter than those who do not. Though the study was not designed to assess the value of school meals in terms of growth, the indicators are 'that free school meals are going to the right group of children and that withdrawal might well prejudice their future development' (Rona *et al.*, 1979).

Moreover from the perspective of this report it is clear to us that expansion in such provision, elimination of inequalities in provision, and elimination of the barrier to take-up which means-testing represents, are essential aspects of a policy designed to break the continuing association between social class and health in its broad sense. We are aware that much of what we have said about school meals is very different from current government policy and much orthodox opinion in the teaching profession. Nevertheless, in our view the evidence strongly supports a change of direction.

We believe that the number of schools with facilities for providing meals for all or most of their pupils can be increased, and that more consultation with parents about the organization and administration of meals would be an important element in raising quality. Children from families living in poverty sometimes attend schools lacking facilities for meals, and although others go home at mid-day for meals because their parents believe they can provide a more nutritious meal for them, there is no doubt that some would get meals at school if they were an automatic right.

At the same time the attitude of a school does seem to influence the consumption of school meals and the eating habits of children generally. It is therefore important that teachers should understand the importance of adequate nutrition for a child's physical development and concentration in school. Moreover meals are also a social occasion when some of the intentions of an education can be consolidated. School staff are apt to underestimate the value of social relationships that can be developed.

We accordingly recommend:

i. *That the provision of nutritionally adequate meals at all schools should be required of local authorities and that the service should be extended in areas where there is under-provision;*

ii. *That there should be regular consultations between local authority representatives, community dietitians, and parents and teachers from each school in turn, over the provision and quality of school meals;*

iii. *That meals be provided in schools without charge.*

5. Accidents to children

In Chapter 2 we drew attention to the fact that the steepest gradients in childhood mortality are found with accidents, a fact all the more disturbing now that accidents account for one third of deaths of children. Moreover there has been little improvement in this class differential over the period 1959–63 to 1970–72. It is remarkable, given these facts and given that there is a known course of action which could be put into effect rapidly without great cost to the public, that so little has been done.

Although accidents in the home are not the largest single group of accidents to children it is probably in the home that major progress could be made most quickly. Regulations could be introduced immediately to produce a safer home environment, and these could be applied stringently to public housing. Risks of falls from roofs and staircases can be reduced without great cost by safer design, and the positioning of windows could make a substantial difference. Much could also be done to reduce the dangers from household equipment, especially the dangers from fire and burning. There is still a great deal which can be done to reduce the risks of poisoning by the clearer packaging of dangerous substances. Although important work has been done by RoSPA and the Health Education Council in educating the public, it is likely that 'safety devices built in as a constant feature of the environment are more effective than attempts to alter people's behaviour'.

The problem, as elsewhere in preventive health, is that there is no focus for government action, and although the new voluntary Joint Committee on Accident Prevention may help, a clear initiative is needed from a powerful Minister if adequate co-operation is to be forthcoming from the Department of Environment, the Department of Trade and the local authorities.

Outside the home, traffic accidents are the single most serious factor. Despite the laudable attempts of town planners to separate traffic from pedestrian ways there are still over 700 children killed on the roads each year. Although it is important to give due recognition to the accident prevention campaign in schools and elsewhere, the only reliable long-term answer is to give children safe areas in which to play. Moreover, if there is a need to step up safety education it is the motorists, especially young drivers, who should be the target. Motorists need to be made more sensitive to the presence of children in the areas they drive through, and conscious of the way in which children behave on the roads.

Apart from the specific dangers of road traffic it is likely that the working-class child lives in a more dangerous physical environment than middle-class children. Derelict slum housing about to be cleared, deserted canals, mineshafts and factories, railway lines, rubbish tips; all these present potential dangers to the child in the urban-industrial area. Given the ingenuity and sense of adventure of children it is difficult to conceive of such areas ever being made danger-free, but more could be done by environmental health authorities to monitor the risks and keep the owners of such properties up to the required standards of safety protection.

When accidents happen there is no lack of concern for the child to see he gets the best treatment possible, but unfortunately public attitudes soon return to their normal complacency. If childhood accidents are to be reduced and the gradients between social classes minimized, the issues must be kept before the public gaze. The voluntary organizations both local and national have the important role here in stimulating the political will for action.

We recommend that the Health Education Council should be provided with sufficient funds to mount child accident prevention programmes in conjunction with the Royal Society for the Prevention of Accidents. These programmes should be particularly directed at local authority planners, engineers and architects.

6. Paying for the programme

The annual cost of our proposals might be roughly as follows:

1. increase in child benefit from £4 to £5.70 for each child	£970 m.
2. infant care allowance (on assumption that there are 600,000 births per annum)	£180 m. in first full year (rising to £870 m. after five years)
3. expansion of day provision	£150 m.
4. free school meals	£200 m.

We do not regard it as our function, nor are we technically equipped, to make specific recommendations as to how the costs of our proposals might best be met. We would suggest, however, that the additional tax allowance now made to married couples without dependants be considered as a source of savings to be set against the proposals we have made for increasing the well-being of families and children.

The wider community

1. A comprehensive disability allowance

Evidence suggests that disabled people are more likely than their able-bodied contemporaries to be living below or on the poverty line (Table 41). There are also indications that among disabled people income is inversely related to severity of disability (Townsend, 1979, Chapter 20; Harris *et al.*, Vol. III, 1972).

As a result of such findings, a strong case developed in the late 1960s and early 1970s for the introduction of a comprehensive allowance scheme for all disabled people. It was felt that equally disabled people were very unequally treated under different income security schemes. While there were fairly elaborate provisions for the war-disabled and those disabled in industry, those who were injured in home accidents, people who were congenitally handicapped, disabled housewives and disabled elderly people had little or no entitlement to additional income. But in 1974, while adopting different positive proposals for improvement of income benefit, both major political parties failed to commit themselves in principle to the phased introduction of a comprehensive scheme. Today major anomalies still exist and have been documented at length (Royal Commission on the Distribution of Income and Wealth, Report No. 6 (1978), Chapter 4, pp. 115–19, 152). The Snowdon Working Party stated (1976): 'The evidence clearly demonstrates the need for the fundamental methodical reforms advocated (by DIG and the Disability Alliance) to rectify the anomalous structure of disablement benefits whereby two people with equal handicaps and needs may end up with widely differing financial help to meet them' (p. 9).

After allowing for savings because of existing schemes, the introduction of a disablement allowance by stages has been costed at a little under £500 m. (Disability Alliance, 1978). Included in this estimate of costs are disabled elderly people. We believe that the establishment of such an allowance represents a major means of reducing inequalities of health and restoring equity between disabled and non-disabled people and we recommend accordingly that *a comprehensive disablement allowance for people of all ages should be introduced by stages at the earliest possible date*. There are of course other supporting measures, especially in improving the employment and wage rates of disabled people, which are important. We believe that the first step must be to establish equity for the most severely disabled people of all. At the present time there is a choice between introducing an allowance at a low rate, say £6, for all severely disabled children and adults in sup-

Table 41: *Numbers and percentage of total and disabled population living in poverty or on the margins of poverty (1977)*

Level of income	Total population		All ages (000s)	Disabled over pensionable age (000s)	Sick and disabled under pensionable age (000s)	Disabled of all ages (000s)
	Over pensionable age (000s)	Under pensionable age (000s)				
Below supplementary benefit level	760	1,270	2,020	250	70	320
Receiving supplementary benefit	2,000	2,160	4,160	790	240	1,030
At or up to 40 per cent above supplementary benefit level	3,010	4,830	7,840	860	400	1,260
More than 40 per cent above supplementary benefit level	2,750	35,960	38,720	690	1,380	2,070
Total	8,520	44,220	52,740	2,590	2,090	4,680
Below supplementary benefit level	8.9	2.9	3.8	9.7	3.3	6.8
Receiving supplementary benefit	23.5	4.9	7.9	30.5	11.5	22.0
At or up to 40 per cent above supplementary benefit level	35.3	10.9	14.9	33.2	19.1	26.9
More than 40 per cent above supplementary benefit level	32.3	81.3	73.4	26.6	66.0	44.2
Total	100	100	100	100	100	100

Note: The estimate of sick and disabled persons under pension age applies to those sick or disabled for three months or more and includes dependants in the income unit.

Source: DHSS (SR3), Analysis of FES 1977 for columns 1, 2, 3 and 5. The distribution of column 4 is based on evidence about those of pensionable age 'appreciably or severely incapacitated' in Townsend, 1979, p. 712 (and survey printout).

plementation of other income benefits and developing a scheme parallel to the main features of the war pensions and industrial injuries disablement pension schemes (into which the mobility allowance might be merged), introducing first a 100 per cent rate of payment (equivalent to the rate of £38 per week payable from November 1979 under the war and industrial injury disablement pension schemes). Even if the aggregate national sum available under either option were the same we believe the latter would be the right option. The net cost of establishing an allowance for 100 per cent disablement (the first stage) for people of all ages and causes of disablement would be approximately £24 m. at November 1979. (At November 1978 the cost was estimated by the Disability Alliance at £20 m.)

2. Improving working conditions

In our studies of inequalities in health we have been struck by the ill-developed nature of conceptions of deprivation at work. Although the hazards of working in particular industries have been carefully documented in the past, and detailed studies made of hours of work and conditions in which strikes and other conflicts between management and labour have occurred, generalizations of working conditions or work situations across industries have not been pursued very far. The point can be made by analogy. Generalization about diets, clothing, leisure-time pursuits, housing conditions and even environmental conditions are readily made, and standards of overcrowding, facilities and amenities are defined nationally for housing and are commonly understood and discussed. As a consequence, discussion about remedial measures is based upon statistics about the members who live in overcrowded or slum housing and lack particular amenities. Such standards do not exist for the world of work. There are no measures of the number in employment who have bad or deprived conditions of work, the industries or areas in which they are to be found and the degree to which they also experience bad housing conditions and low incomes.

So far as health is concerned the emphasis has been on safety and specific identifiable risks of accident or of contamination by toxic substances. For example, the Robens Committee, set up by the government in 1972 to look at health and safety at work, did not attempt to collect evidence about safety and health in relation to general working conditions. Neither did it attempt to pursue the interrelationship between fatal accidents, deaths and injuries arising from prescribed industrial diseases and occupational mortality and morbidity, for each of which independent sets of statistics exist. The importance of reports on occupational mortality to a better understanding of the work situation as well as to the circumstances outside work remains to be plumbed.

In Table 42 the wide differences between some occupations are illustrated. The marked gradient from sedentary non-manual to heavy unskilled manual work, which with some exceptions the table shows, is accompanied by wide variations between the mortality rates for specific occupations within each occupational class.

Table 42: *Mortality by occupation unit: men aged 15–64 (selected examples)*

Occupations units	Direct age-standardized death rate (per 100,000)	SMR
Relatively low death rate		
University teachers	287	49
Physiotherapists	297	55
Paper products' makers	302	50
Managers in building and contracting	319	54
Local authority senior officers	342	57
Company secretaries and registrars	362	60
Ministers of the Crown, MPs, senior government officials	371	61
Office managers	377	64
Primary and secondary school teachers	396	66
Sales managers	421	70
Architects, town planners	443	74
Civil service executive officers	467	78
Postmen	484	81
Medical practitioners	494	81
Relatively high death rate		
Coalminers (underground)	822	141
Leather products' makers	895	147
Shoemakers and shoe repairers	898	156
Machine-tool operators	934	156
Watch repairers	946	154
Coalminers (above ground)	972	160
Steel erectors, riggers	992	164
Fishermen	1028	171
Deck, engineering officers and pilots, ship	1040	175
Labourers and unskilled workers, all industries	1247	201
Policemen	1270	109
Deck and engine-room ratings	1385	233
Bricklayers' labourers	1644	274

Specific and well-known work hazards, characteristic of many manual occupations and differing from one to another, are one factor. But in the light of the analysis of this report, we consider that in addition to these hazards, and associated risks of accidents and of certain occupational injuries and diseases, a wider variety of job characteristics may be implicated. These would include security and material rewards of employment, patterns of work (such as shift-work), conditions of work and welfare and other amenities. However, the *extent* to which work conditions, interpreted in this broad fashion, are responsible for differences in rates of occupational mortality remains uncertain and requires further research (although the work of Fox and Adelstein, 1978, suggests that other and more general elements of the 'class' factor may also be important).

Nevertheless, reduction in inequalities between occupations in their work conditions may be of importance in reducing inequalities in health. *We recommend that representatives of the DHSS, the Department of Employment, the Health and Safety Commission, together with representatives of the trade unions and CBI, should draw up minimally acceptable and desirable standards of work; security; conditions and amenities; pay; and welfare or fringe benefits.*

A national study found that in 1968, 20 per cent of the employed population, representing over 4½ million people, had poor conditions of work (Townsend, 1979, p. 453) and a list of individual examples from a random sample called attention 'both to the diverse hazards and frequent poor conditions of manual work'. They also suggested uncertainty or ignorance on the part of many about the hazards involved with dust, noise and chemicals. Doctors, for whatever motives, as well as employers, may withhold information, and the importance of the role of union safety representatives (the legal right to which workers have enjoyed since October 1978) is clear. There is still a tendency to accept poor working conditions as an inevitable accompaniment of particular jobs, and attention needs to be devoted to the question of enlightened standards which *can* be introduced, as in public housing and town planning. Among the matters which we hope will attract more attention are facilities for meals, warmth and shelter from bad weather, a dry and secure place for outer clothes and other belongings, access to a telephone, availability of first aid and first aid equipment, 'unsocial' hours, warmth, humidity, light, noise, availability of machinery to avoid or reduce the physical stress of the work, washing and toilet facilities, and facilities for changing clothes. In many of these instances regulations under current legislation are non-existent, or partial, or complex and confused (TUC, 1978).

What we are calling for is more preventive work by government departments, employers and unions and would hope to see a shift of emphasis in the work and functions (as defined by legislation) of the Health and Safety Commission and Executive, and the Employment Medical Advisory Service. It is fair to say that although there are provisions for both bodies to follow positive policies they are at present restricting their activities to specific hazards and general questions of safety. The need for legislation defining acceptable working conditions and basic employer welfare benefits is urgent.

3. Housing

Housing conditions are associated with health status in a variety of ways. Inadequate heating (or a form of heating which is too expensive for a resident) can give rise to hypothermia in old people (Wicks, 1978). Over-crowding can produce respiratory and other diseases (some of the studies are reviewed by Benjamin, 1965, who, however, pointed out that class explained more of the inter-area variance than housing). It can also produce adverse psychological responses and may give rise to mental illness.

High-rise living is known to have deleterious consequences for children. In some areas (such as Tower Hamlets) TB is common among the homeless vagrants and represents a real problem for the health authorities.

It is families with children, and especially large poor families with many children, who are most likely to be living in overcrowded conditions. Over-crowding adds to the health risk under which working-class children labour, and the extent to which such children, and especially those born into larger families, are being brought up in overcrowded conditions is unacceptable. Bone's survey of pre-school children found that 10 per cent of them inhabited dwellings inadequate on at least one of four criteria: overcrowding; no separate unshared bathroom; shared WC; no sole use of permanent fixed water supply (Bone, 1977, p. 26). But this percentage was highly class-related: 3 per cent in class 1 increasing to 29 per cent in classes IVM and V. For some of these children there is a risk of ill-health throughout life, because chronic respiratory disorder (for example) in childhood is an all too effective predictor of adult suffering. Such considerations tend not to weigh as heavily with housing departments as they should.

We showed in Chapter 2 (on the basis of the new OPCS longitudinal study) that there is an association between tenure and SMR, independent of the occupational class of the household head. Of course, this does not demonstrate that being a tenant *causes* ill-health. But we wish to stress that the rights and privileges which are so unequally associated with housing tenures *are* associated with health both in the negative sense of freedom from ascertainable clinical disease and in the positive sense of welfare. Fear of eviction is the sort of situation which has been related to clinical depression in women (Brown and Harris, 1978). Security in housing does have health benefits and should be equally available for all. Accessible play areas for young children are vital and owner-occupation often meets this need, by virtue of garden space available. Gardening is one of the most popular outdoor leisure pursuits for people in Britain who have access to a garden, and we have already indicated the health benefits attaching to active outdoor recreation. We believe that there must be a much greater extension of the rights and privileges associated with owner-occupation to the tenants both of local authorities and private landlords. Health considerations are certainly among the factors which justify such extension.

In order to allow good housing policy to play its part in promoting health we consider the *most essential step is to co-ordinate policies in the council and owner-occupied sectors*. The changing pattern of housing tenure has been leading to problems of access to housing for the poor and mobile, which have gradually become more acute in recent years. Only in part has that been due to the decline of the privately tenanted sector. In part it has been due to rigidities in the management of council housing, together with a very uneven flow of new housing. There needs to be a more vigorous programme of rehabilitating rented housing which is obsolescent. This includes many thousands of council housing units. Comparisons need to be made between the tenures so that priorities in improvement policies and the allocation of resources, but also new standards of space, amenities and access to play areas, including gardens, can be determined. *We therefore recommend a substantial increase in local authority improvement spending under the 1974 Housing Act.*

But broad equity between the sectors must be achieved in other ways as well. The previous administration tended over-optimistically to reiterate the view that there was no longer any overall shortage of housing, while allowing local authorities to refuse housing to such groups as homeless single and childless couples. Secondly, the rights and opportunities of tenants need to be reviewed in the light of conditions enjoyed by owner-occupiers. The previous administration experimented with a 'Tenants Charter', but in some respects this was half-hearted, and among the most important measures to be introduced are freedom of movement, freedom to carry out minor improvements and repairs (and benefit from them in the terms under which the tenancy may be passed on subsequently), greater freedom in the rules of residence and more effective representation in the management of housing estates.

A number of housing charities believe that local authorities have been interpreting their obligations under the 1977 Housing Act rather too loosely. Some councils are exploiting the loop-hole of 'intentional' homelessness while others have taken advantage of the fact that the Act does not impose any standard for homeless accommodation. Moreover the Act allows local authorities to refuse accommodation to single homeless and childless couples.

We believe the legislation on homelessness deserves strengthening along the lines recommended by the housing charities. With the dwindling of the private rented sector, local authorities must provide rented accommodation for a wider range of households, including the single and childless, who are unable to enter owner-occupation. *We recommend, therefore, that local councils should increasingly be encouraged to widen their responsibilities to provide for all types of housing need which arise in their localities.*

We also believe that the sale of council houses badly needs to be placed in the changing context of the relationship between the different housing sectors. If, in the long run, a better balance could be struck in the conditions enjoyed in the two sectors, objections in principle to interchange of stock could be minimized. But indiscriminate sales may worsen housing opportunities for families needing to rent; they may reduce the quality and attractiveness of the council housing stock; and, by introducing a new basis to the relationships in many estates, they may affect the cohesion of existing communities.

Finally, a further aspect of the relationship of housing to health concerns the housing of the disabled. If the institutionalization of disabled people is to be avoided, as we have recommended, there must be sufficient provision of sheltered and adapted housing. This implies a much better working relationship than is frequently the case today between social service and health authorities and housing departments, so that necessary adaptations to dwellings can be obtained easily. We have elsewhere recommended that serious consideration should be given to the possibility that social service departments assume responsibility for the management of sheltered housing. A second aspect of such collaboration concerns policy over the re-housing of disabled people, which seems generally to be inadequate. The Working Party on Housing of the Central Council for the Disabled wrote in its (1976) report, of local authority policy:

... unless the disabled person *also* happens to be living in overcrowded accommodation with few amenities, his position on the waiting list is likely to be low indeed, even if he has the maximum medical points possible ... But the housing difficulties that are peculiarly associated with disability ... require a separate type of solution ... the priority given to disabled people should not be decided at an individual level – as tends to happen at present – but should be decided within an overall strategy of priorities within the housing policies of the authority as a whole.

... [T]he existing system means that a disabled person may not be rehoused until the situation has reached a desperate pitch. By that time the move may really be too late: his physical condition may have deteriorated too rapidly – possibly aggravated by his inadequate housing – so that he is not in a position to settle into a new environment ... Where a disabled child is concerned, to move the family to suitable housing when the child is grown and the situation has reached breaking point may work against the educational development of the child and his ability to learn to cope independently ... (Working Party on Housing of the Central Council for the Disabled, *Towards a Housing Policy for Disabled People*, 1976, pp. 58–60)

We therefore recommend that special funding on the lines of joint funding for health and local authorities should be developed by the government to encourage better planning and management of housing, including adaptations and provisions of necessary facilities and services for disabled people of all ages by social service and housing departments. This recommendation is on the same lines as that made by the Snowdon Working Party, which argued that one immediate priority was 'to develop a real choice of life-style for the severely disabled through joint planning and financing by the Department of Environment and the Department of Health and Social Security'. We also endorse that Working Party's plea for the 'urgent establishment of schemes for non-institutional accommodation for severely disabled people living in every area of the country' (Report of the Snowdon Working Party, 1976, p. 32).

Towards a co-ordinated government policy

We believe that an improvement in the nation's health should be a priority for government. The evidence of various indicators of mortality shows that in this respect Britain's record in recent years has not compared well with other countries. We should like to see drastic reduction in rates not only of perinatal and infant death, but of the extent of chronic and acute sickness and of physical and mental handicap, much of which develops in the period around birth, as well as promotion of health in its positive sense of 'well-being' and functional capacities.

The costs of sickness – the direct costs of the National Health Service, of supporting care, and of sickness benefits, as well as the indirect costs of sickness for productivity – though not easily calculated *in toto*, are very great. Acute care provided in hospitals demands an increasing share of national resources. The financial costs of bouts of ill-health, chronic sickness and handicap to individuals and families – especially poor families – are frequently immense. These private costs are not fully captured in financial terms. The alarming prevalence of depressive illness, especially among working-class women, cannot be without profound effect on family life and child-rearing, irrespective of the misery the women themselves suffer.

It is also our view that the attempt to reduce, and ultimately eliminate, the social inequalities in health which we have documented offers the greatest opportunity for achieving this overall improvement. It is surely no accident that, as we showed in Chapter 5, those countries such as Sweden and Norway which have particularly low mortality rates also seem to have greatly reduced inequalities in health. This argument is quite separate from the argument – to which we also attach great weight – that simple justice demands that this attempt be made.

Part of what is required involves attention to those regions and small areas, for example in the inner cities, where concentrations of sickness are high and levels of service provision low. Another part involves attention to improvements that can be made and new measures that can be introduced for families in all areas of the country. A third part involves attention to the vicious cycle by which, through a variety of mechanisms, poor families are locked into material, educational, environmental and social disadvantage for a lifetime and even sometimes for generations, with all that this implies for their health.

Our analysis has shown that inequalities in health have complex, multi-causal explanations. They seem to be rooted in the general nature and conditions of activity, both in work and outside work, and in the styles and standards of living of different occupational classes. Some factors have a clear causal association with ill-health: inadequate access to and use of (particularly preventive) health services; the hazards attaching to certain occupations; overcrowded and damp housing, and smoking. But there remains much that is probably not explicable in any direct fashion and meanwhile must be attributed to the pervasive effects of the class structure.

It follows, and our recommendations reflect this fact, that a reduction in health inequalities depends upon contributions from within many policy areas. Our recommendations have involved reference to community and preventive health services, to the personal social services, to health education in a very broad sense including the promotion of physical recreation, to social security measures, to uptake of school meals, to improvement in working conditions, to housing and to measures directed specifically at minority groups and notably in inner city areas. Clearly such a range of services and policies involves many departments of central government: DHSS, DOE, DES, DE (and the Health and Safety Executive), MAFF, the Department of Transport and the Home Office, as well as the Welsh

Office and the Scottish and Northern Ireland Offices. Our objectives will be achieved *only* if each department makes its appropriate contribution and this in turn, we believe, requires a better degree of co-ordination than presently exists. The fact is of course that housing, leisure, education and other relevant policies have important objectives traditionally associated with them: there is always the danger that this potential contribution to the reduction of health inequalities will receive little attention in departmental decision-making.

Machinery of government

For this reason, *we propose recourse to Cabinet Office machinery*, in order to ensure that this does not happen. A broadly based programme of work needs to be explicitly adopted, and seen to be adopted. Our analysis is very much within the spirit of the Joint Approach to Social Policy (JASP), and we envisage that a Ministerial and, secondly, an Officials Committee, corresponding to those established under JASP, would provide appropriate fora: we would certainly wish the Central Policy Review Staff to be involved. It would then be for these committees regularly to consider developments and to propose developments in relevant policies from the perspective of health inequalities. Major initiatory responsibility would be vested in the Department of Health and Social Security, and we envisage the two committees being chaired respectively by a Minister and by a senior DHSS official having major responsibilities for health and prevention. They should have before them relevant statistical material, provided by government statisticians, and relating to changes in uptake and provision of services, changes in relevant distributional aspects, and evaluation of policies. New methods of transmitting the information reviewed would have to be adopted, not least because it would need to reach a wider, public audience.

There would have to be local counterparts of national co-ordinating machinery, and a joint approach to health policies would be necessary at local level to a greater extent than at present. This might take a number of forms – inter-departmental action, for example, to reduce environmental pollution and squalor and redistribute skilled manpower to communities where the risk to health was high, acceleration of joint funding schemes, and the establishment of joint committees for planning and for the monitoring and supervision of hazards to health.

The need for a joint framework for social policies has been increasingly acknowledged in recent years. Of course, a co-ordinated approach could achieve a variety of objectives. One would be simply to warn central departments earlier than at present of forthcoming plans of individual departments.

Another would be to work out more smoothly than at present the over-lapping functions of two or more departments (a good example is nursery education and day nurseries – in the interests of child health). But others would include large-scale reallocation of priorities, for example a decision to reduce the rate of expansion in expenditure of one major social service, such as education, and greatly increase the rate of expansion of another, such as health. For this, however, support independent of central administration may be required, as we argue below. We appreciate that there are a wide range of possibilities, and that a joint approach could mean a great deal or very little. But considering that the government accepted, in the early 1960s, the need for plans for hospitals and for community care and that since then there have been a stream of plans of wider and lesser scope, developments in the actual co-ordination of social policies, as distinct from the reorganiza-tion of individual services, has been slow. (The progress since the JASP initiative has been traced by Plowden, 1977.) No doubt this is attributable to the precedence currently given not only by the government but by other bodies to economic over social objectives in policy, to a failure to appreciate the interrelatedness of policies, but above all to the stultifying effects of public expenditure control which has dominated all attempts of planning during the mid- and late-1970s. In the last fifteen years social planning has been, for the central government, predominantly one of control of public expenditure (Diamond, 1975; Glennerster, 1976; Heclo and Wildavsky, 1976). It would be wrong to suppose that this form of control could be changed overnight, because it has penetrated administrative practice at every level, or that there will not be financial and institutional constraints on more imaginative social planning. But the formulation of new social objectives by the government can only be sustained if certain changes are also made in the mechanisms of planning and administration.

A Health Development Council

Finally, and distinct from this machinery, although with the same objective in mind, we *propose the establishment of a Health Development Council*. This would be an independent body, with a small staff of seconded civil servants. Strictly its functions would be advisory, but the Council would, we recommend, play a key role in social planning. It would be invited to consider and spell out longer-term strategies to reduce inequalities of health and improve general family living standards, evaluate progress in relation to this aim, with particular reference to the roles of particular government and local authority departments and services, marshal a range of outside expertise, consult the public at every stage and play a major part in explaining the need for certain developments. Opportunities should be afforded to it of commenting on, and contributing to, plans, including expenditure programmes, which are to be published by the government on matters relevant to its concerns.

Although we are aware of the arguments against proliferation of such standing advisory bodies, we make this proposal for three particular reasons. First, the existence of the Council would provide some guarantee that, when initial enthusiasm had abated, the attempt at inter-departmental co-ordination through a Cabinet sub-committee did not 'run out of steam', as some would say happened with the original JASP initiative. Second, by virtue of its public existence such a body could serve both to keep the issue of health inequalities in the public eye, and enlist widespread support. This is essential, and the development of comparable machinery at the local level (perhaps based on existing Health and Local Authority Joint Consultative Committees) could be invaluable. Third, the Council would be in a position to assist Ministers in formulating longer-term strategies.

Conclusion and summary

In discussing actions outside the health care system which need to be taken to diminish inequalities of health we have been necessarily selective in this chapter. We have attempted to pay heed to those factors which are correlated with the *degree* of inequalities. Secondly, we have tried to confine ourselves to matters which are immediately practicable, in political, economic and administrative terms, which will none the less, properly maintained, exert a long-term structural effect. And thirdly, we have continued to feel it right to give priority to young children and mothers, disabled people and measures concerned with prevention. Above all we consider that the *abolition of child poverty should be adopted as a national goal for the 1980s.* We recognize that this requires a redistribution of financial resources far beyond anything achieved by past programmes and is likely to be very costly. Our recommendations here are presented as a modest first step which might be taken towards this objective.

i. As an immediate goal the level of child benefit should be increased to 5½ per cent of average gross male industrial earnings, or £5.70 at November 1979 prices.

ii. Larger child benefits should be progressively introduced for older children, after further examination of the needs of children and consideration of the practice in some other countries.

iii. The maternity grant should be increased to £100.

iv. We recommend the introduction of an infant care allowance over a five-year period, beginning with all babies born in the year following a date to be chosen by the government.

Beyond these initial elements of an anti-poverty strategy, a number of other steps need to be taken.

v. Provision of meals at school should be regarded as a right. Representatives of local authorities and community dietitians should be invited to meet representatives of parents and teachers of particular schools at regular intervals during the year to seek agreement to the provision and quality of meals. Meals in schools should be provided without charge.

vi. The Health Education Council should be provided with sufficient funds to mount child accident-prevention programmes in conjunction with the Royal Society for the Prevention of Accidents. These programmes should be particularly directed at local authority planners, engineers and architects.

vii. A comprehensive disablement allowance for people of all ages should be introduced by stages at the earliest possible date, beginning with people with 100 per cent disablement.

viii. Representatives of the DHSS and DE, HSE, together with representatives of the trade unions and CBI, should draw up minimally acceptable and desirable conditions of work.

ix. Government departments, employers and unions should devote more attention to preventive health through work organization, conditions and amenities, and in other ways. There should be a similar shift of emphasis in the work and functions of the Health and Safety Commission and Executive, and the Employment Medical Advisory Service.

x. Local authority spending on housing improvements under the 1974 Housing Act should be substantially increased.

xi. Local authorities should increasingly be encouraged to widen their responsibilities to provide for all types of housing need which arise in their localities.

xii. Policies directed towards the public and private housing sectors need to be better co-ordinated.

xiii. Special funding, on the lines of joint funding, for health and local authorities should be developed by the government to encourage better planning and management of housing, including adaptations and provision of necessary facilities and services for disabled people of all ages by social service and housing departments.

Our recommendations reflect the fact that the reduction in health inequalities depends upon contributions from within many policy areas, and necessarily involving a number of government departments. Our objectives will be achieved *only* if each department makes its appropriate contribution. This in turn requires a greater degree of co-ordination than exists at present.

xiv. Greater co-ordination between government departments in the administration of health-related policies is required, by establishing interdepartmental machinery in the Cabinet Office under a Cabinet subcommittee along the lines of that established under the Joint Approach to Social Policy (JASP), with the Central Policy Review staff also involved. Local counterparts of national co-ordinating bodies also need to be established.

xv. A Health Development Council should be established with an independent membership to play a key advisory and planning role in relation to a collaborative national policy to reduce inequalities in health.

Summary and Recommendations

1. Most recent data show marked differences in mortality rates between the occupational classes, for both sexes and at all ages. At birth and in the first month of life, twice as many babies of 'unskilled manual' parents (class V) die as do babies of professional class parents (class I) and in the next eleven months nearly three times as many boys and more than three times as many girls. In later childhood the ratio of deaths in class V to deaths in class I falls to 1.5–2.0, but increases again in early adult life, before falling again in middle and old age. A class gradient can be observed for most causes of death, being particularly steep in the case of diseases of the respiratory system. Available data on chronic sickness tend to parallel those on mortality. Thus self-reported rates of long-standing illness (as defined in the General Household Survey) are twice as high among unskilled manual males and $2\frac{1}{2}$ times as high among their wives as among the professional classes. In the case of acute sickness (short-term ill-health, also as defined in the General Household Survey) the gradients are less clear.

2. The lack of improvement, and in some respects deterioration, of the health experience of the unskilled and semi-skilled manual classes (class V and IV), relative to class I, throughout the 1960s and early 1970s is striking. Despite the decline in the rate of infant mortality (death within the first year of life) in each class, the difference in rate between the lowest classes (IV and V combined) and the highest (I and II combined) actually increased between 1959–63 and 1970–72.

3. Inequalities exist also in the utilization of health services, particularly and most worryingly of the preventive services. Here, severe under-utilization by the working classes is a complex result of under-provision in working-class areas and of costs (financial and psychological) of attendance which are not, in this case, outweighed by disruption of normal activities by sickness. In the case of GP, and hospital inpatient and out-patient attendance, the situation is less clear. Moreover it becomes more difficult to interpret such data as exist, notably because of the (as yet unresolved) problem of relating utilization to need. Broadly speaking, the evidence suggests that working-class people make more use of GP services for themselves (though not for their children) than do middle-class people, but that they may receive less good care. Moreover, it is possible that this extra usage does not fully reflect the true differences in need for care, as shown by mortality and morbidity figures Similar increases in the use of hospital services, both in-patient and out-patient, with declining occupational class are found, though data are scanty, and possible explanations complex.

4. Comparison of the British experience with that of other industrial countries, on the basis of overall mortality rates, shows that British perinatal and infant mortality

rates have been distinctly higher and are still somewhat higher than those of the four Nordic countries and of the Netherlands, and comparable with those of the Federal Republic of Germany. Adult mortality patterns, especially for men in the younger age groups, compare reasonably with other Western industrialized countries: the comparison for women is less satisfactory. The rate of improvement in perinatal mortality experienced by Britain over the period since 1960 has been comparable to that of most other countries. In the case of infant mortality (which is generally held to reflect social conditions more than does perinatal mortality) all comparable countries – especially France – have shown a greater improvement than has Britain. France, like Britain and most other countries considered (though apparently not Sweden), shows significant class and regional inequalities in health experience. It is noteworthy that through the 1960s the ratio of the post-neonatal death rate (between four weeks and one year) in the least favoured social group to that in the most favoured fell substantially in France. Also important probably has been a major French effort to improve both attendance rates for ante-natal care and the quality of such care. Very high rates of early attendance are also characteristic of the Nordic countries; so too are high rates of attendance at child welfare clinics, combined with extensive 'outreach' capacity. In Finland, for example, whenever an appointment at a health centre is missed, a health visitor makes a domiciliary call. We regard it as significant also that in Finland health authorities report not on the volume of services provided, but on the proportion of all pregnant women and of all children of appropriate ages who register with Health Centres.

5. We do not believe there to be any single and *simple explanation* of the complex data we have assembled. While there are a number of quite distinct theoretical approaches to explanation we wish to stress the importance of differences in material conditions of life. *In our view much of the evidence on social inequalities in health can be adequately understood in terms of specific features of the socio-economic environment:* features (such as work accidents, overcrowding, cigarette-smoking) which are strongly class-related in Britain and also have clear causal significance. Other aspects of the evidence indicate the importance of the health services and particularly preventive services. Ante-natal care is probably important in preventing perinatal death, and the international evidence suggests that much can be done to improve ante-natal care and its uptake. But beyond this there is undoubtedly much which cannot be understood in terms of the impact of so specific factors, but only in terms of the more diffuse consequences of the class structure: poverty, working conditions, and deprivation in its various forms. It is this acknowledgement of the *multicausal* nature of health inequalities, within which inequalities in the material conditions of living loom large, which informs and structures our policy recommendations. These draw also upon another aspect of our interpretation of the evidence. We have concluded that early childhood is the period of life at which intervention could most hopefully weaken the continuing association between health and class. There is, for example, abundant evidence that inadequately treated bouts of childhood illness 'cast long shadows forward', as the Court Committee put it.

6. We have been able to draw upon national statistics relating to health and mortality of exceptional quality and scope, as well as upon a broad range of research studies. We have, however, been conscious of certain inadequacies in the statistics and of major lacunae in the research. For example it is extremely difficult to examine health experience and health service utilization, in relation to income and wealth.

7. Moreover, we consider that the *form* of administrative statistics may both reflect and determine (as the Finnish example quoted above suggests) the way in which the adequacy and the performance of a service is understood: hence it acquires considerable importance. We also consider systematic knowledge of the use made of the various health services by different social groups to be inadequate: though this is less the case in Scotland than in England and Wales. While conscious of the difficulties in collecting and reporting of occupational characteristics within the context of administrative returns, we feel that further thought must be given to how such difficulties might be overcome. We argue that the monitoring of *ill-health* (itself so imperfect) should evolve into a system also of monitoring *health* in relation to social and environmental conditions. One area in which progress could be made is in relation to the development of children, and we propose certain modifications to community health statistics.

(1) *We recommend that school health statistics should routinely provide, in relation to occupational class, the results of tests of hearing, vision, and measures of height and weight. As a first step we recommend that local health authorities, in consultation with educational authorities, select a representative sample of schools in which assessments on a routine basis be initiated.* (Chapter 7, p. 127)

8. *Accidents* are not only responsible for fully one-third of child deaths, but show (with respiratory disease) the steepest of class gradients.

9. We should like to see progress towards routine collection and reporting of accidents to children indicating the circumstances, the age and the occupational class of the parents. In relation to traffic accidents there should be better liaison between the NHS and the police, both centrally and locally.

(2) *We therefore recommend that representatives of appropriate government departments (Health and Social Security, Education and Science, Home Office, Environment, Trade, Transport), as well as of the NHS and of the police, should consider how progress might rapidly be made in improving the information on accidents to children.* (Chapter 7, p. 128)

10. The Child Accident Prevention Committee, if suitably constituted and supported, might provide a suitable forum for such discussions, to be followed by appropriate action by government departments. Further,

(3) *We recommend that the Health Education Council should be provided with sufficient funds to mount child accident prevention programmes in conjunction with the Royal Society for the Prevention of Accidents. These programmes should be*

particularly directed at local authority planners, engineers and architects. (Chapter 9, p. 182)

11. While drawing attention to the importance of the National Food Survey as the major source of information on the food purchase (and hence diet) of the population, we are conscious of the scope for its improvement.

(4) *We recommend that consideration be given to the development of the National Food Survey into a more effective instrument of nutritional surveillance in relation to health, through which various 'at risk' groups could also be identified and studied.* (Chapter 7, p. 128)

12. We have already referred to the difficulties in examining health experience in relation to income and wealth. In principle this can be done through the General Household Survey in which the measure of income now (since 1979) corresponds to the more satisfactory measure employed in the Family Expenditure Survey. However,

(5) *We recommend that in the General Household Survey steps should be taken (not necessarily in every year) to develop a more comprehensive measure of income, or command over resources, through either (a) a means of modifying such a measure with estimates of total wealth or at least some of the more prevalent forms of wealth, such as housing and savings, or (b) the integration of income and wealth, employing a method of, for example, annuitization.* (Chapter 1, p. 41)

13. Beyond this, we feel that a comprehensive research strategy is needed. This is best regarded as implying the need for careful studies of a wide range of variables implicated in ill-health, in their *interaction over time*, and *conducted in a small number of places*. Such variables will necessarily include social conditions (and the interactions of a variety of social policies) as well as individual and behavioural factors. Any major advance in our understanding of the nature of health inequalities, and of the reason for their perpetuation, will require complex research of a multi-disciplinary kind.

(6) *The importance of the problem of social inequalities in health, and their causes, as an area for further research needs to be emphasized. We recommend that it be adopted as a research priority by the DHSS and that steps be taken to enlist the expertise of the Medical Research Council (MRC), as well as the Social Science Research Council (SSRC), in the initiation of a programme of research. Such research represents a particularly appropriate area for departmental commissioning of research from the MRC.* (Chapter 7, p. 129)

14. We turn now to our recommendations for policy, which we have divided into those relating to the health and personal social services, and those relating to a range of other social policies. Three objectives underpin our recommendations, and we recommend their adoption by the Secretary of State:

– To give children a better start in life.

– To encourage good health among a larger proportion of the population by preventive and educational action.

– For disabled people, to reduce the risks of early death, to improve the quality of life whether in the community or in institutions, and as far as possible to reduce the need for the latter.

Thirty years of the Welfare State and of the National Health Service have achieved little in reducing social inequalities in health. But we believe that if these three objectives are pursued vigorously inequalities in health can now be reduced.

15. We believe that *allocation of resources* should be based on need. We recognize that there are difficulties in assessing need, but we agree that standardized mortality ratios (SMRs) are a useful basis for broad allocation at regional level. At district level, further indicators of health care and social needs are called for. These should be developed as a matter of urgency, and used appropriately to reinforce, supplement or modify allocation according to SMRs. *However, a shift of resources is not enough: it must be combined with an imaginative (and in part necessarily experimental) approach to health care and its delivery.*

   (7) *Resources within the National Health Service and the personal social services should be shifted more sharply than so far accomplished towards community care, particularly towards ante-natal, post-natal and child health services, and home-help and nursing services for disabled people. We see this as an important part of a strategy to break the links between social class or poverty and health.* (Chapter 8, p. 136)

   (8) *The professional associations as well as the Secretary of State and the health authorities should accept responsibility for making improvements in the quality and geographical coverage of general practice, especially in areas of high prevalence of ill-health and poor social conditions. Where the number or scope of work of general practitioners is inadequate in such areas we recommend health authorities to deploy or redeploy an above-average number of community nurses attached where possible to family practice. The distribution of general practitioners should be related not only to population but to medical need, as indicated by SMRs, supplemented by other indicators, and the per capita basis of remuneration should be modified accordingly.* (Chapter 8, p. 145)

16. Moreover, we consider that greater integration between the planning process (and the establishment of priorities) and resources allocation is needed. In particular the establishment of revenue targets should be based not upon the current distribution of expenditure between services, but that distribution which it is sought to bring about through planning guidelines: including a greater share for community health.

   (9) *We recommend that the resources to be allocated should be based upon the future planned share for different services, including a higher share for community health.* (Chapter 8, p. 142)

17. Our further health service-related recommendations, designed to implement the objectives set out above, fall into two groups.

18. We first outline the elements of what we have called a District Action Programme. By this we mean a general programme for the health and personal social services to be adopted nationwide, and involving necessary modifications to the structure of care.

19. Second, we recommend an experimental programme, involving provision of certain services on an experimental basis in ten areas of particularly high mortality and adverse social conditions, and for which special funds are sought.

District action programme

Health and Welfare of mothers and pre-school and school children

(10) *A non-means-tested scheme for free milk should now be introduced beginning with couples with their first infant child and infant children in large families.* (Chapter 8, p. 134)

(11) *Areas and districts should review the accessibility and facilities of all ante-natal and child-health clinics in their areas and take steps to increase utilization by mothers, particularly in the early months of pregnancy.* (Chapter 8, p. 143)

(12) *Savings from the current decline in the school population should be used to finance new services for children under 5. A statutory obligation should be placed on local authorities to ensure adequate day care in their area for children under 5, and that a minimum number of places (the number being raised after regular intervals) should be laid down centrally. Further steps should be taken to reorganize day nurseries and nursery schools so that both meet the needs of children for education and care.* (Chapter 8, p. 146 and Chapter 9, p. 174)

(13) *Every opportunity should be taken to link revitalized school health care with general practice, and intensify surveillance and follow-up both in areas of special need and for certain types of family.* (Chapter 8, p. 147)

20. Some necessary developments apply to other groups as well as children and mothers.

(14) *An assessment which determines severity of disablement should be adopted as a guide to health and personal social service priorities of the individual, and this should be related to the limitation of activities rather than loss of faculty or type of handicap.* (Chapter 8, p. 147)

21. Though we attach priority to the implementation of this recommendation in the care of disabled children, we believe that it must ultimately apply to all disabled people. We recognize that such assessments are now an acknowledged part of 'good practice' in providing for the disabled – we are anxious that they should become standard practice.

The care of elderly and disabled people in their own homes

22. The meaning of community care should be clarified and much greater emphasis given to tendencies favoured (but insufficiently specified) in recent government planning documents. (See Recommendation 7.)

(15) *A Working Group should be set up to consider:*

i. *the present functions and structure of hospital, residential and domiciliary care for the disabled elderly in relation to their needs, in order to determine the best and most economical balance of future services;* (Chapter 8, p. 151) and

ii. *whether sheltered housing should be a responsibility of social service or of housing departments, and to make recommendations.* (Chapter 8, p. 149)

(16) *Joint funding should be developed and further funding of a more specific kind should be introduced, if necessary within the existing NHS budget to encourage joint care programmes. A further sum should be reserved for payment to authorities putting forward joint programmes to give continuing care to disabled people – for example, post-hospital follow-up schemes, pre-hospital support programmes for families, and support programmes for the severely incapacitated and terminally ill.* (Chapter 8, p. 152)

(17) *Criteria for admission to, and for continuing residence in, residential care should be agreed between the DHSS and the local authority associations, and steps taken to encourage rehabilitation, and in particular to prevent homeless elderly people from being offered accommodation only in residential homes. Priority should be given to expansion of domiciliary care for those who are severely disabled in their own homes.* (Chapter 8, p. 149)

(18) *The functions of home helps should be extended to permit a lot more work on behalf of disabled people; short courses of training, specialization of functions and the availability of mini-bus transport, especially to day centres, should be encouraged.* (Chapter 8, p. 152)

Prevention: the role of government

23. Effective prevention requires not only individual initiative but a real commitment by the DHSS and other government departments. Our analysis has shown the many ways in which people's behaviour is constrained by structural and environmental factors over which they have no control. Physical recreation, for example, is hardly possible in inner city areas unless steps are taken to ensure that facilities are provided. Similarly, government initiatives are required in relation to diet and to the consumption of alcohol. Legislation and fiscal and other financial measures may be required and a wide range of social and economic policies involved. We see the time as now opportune for a major step forwards in the field of health and prevention.

(19) *National health goals should be established and stated by government after wide consultation and debate. Measures that might encourage the desirable changes in people's diet, exercise and smoking and drinking behaviour should be agreed among relevant agencies.* (Chapter 8, p. 154)

(20) *An enlarged programme of health education should be sponsored by the government, and necessary arrangements made for optimal use of the mass media, especially television. Health education in schools should become the joint responsibility of LEAs and health authorities.* (Chapter 8, p. 153)

24. The following recommendation should be seen not only as a priority in itself but as illustrative of the determined action by government necessary in relation to many elements of a strategy for prevention:

(21) *Stronger measures should be adopted to reduce cigarette-smoking. These would include:*

a. *Legislation should be rapidly implemented to phase out all advertising and sales promotion of tobacco products (except at place of purchase);*

b. *Sponsorship of sporting and artistic activities by tobacco companies should be banned over a period of a few years, and meanwhile there should be stricter control of advertisement through sponsorship;*

c. *Regular annual increases in duty on cigarettes in line with rises in income should be imposed, to ensure lower consumption;*

d. *Tobacco companies should be required, in consultation with trades unions, to submit plans for the diversification of their products over a period of ten years with a view to the eventual phasing out of sales of harmful tobacco products at home and abroad;*

e. *The provision of non-smoking areas in public places should steadily be extended;*

f. *A counselling service should be made available in all health districts, and experiment encouraged in methods to help people reduce cigarette-smoking;*

g. *A stronger well-presented health warning should appear on all cigarette packets and such advertisements as remain, together with information on the harmful constituents of cigarettes.* (Chapter 8, p. 154)

We have already recommended that steps be taken to increase utilization of antenatal clinics, particularly in the early months of pregnancy (Recommendation 11). Given early attendance there are practical programmes for screening for Down's Syndrome and for neural tube defects in the foetus. In relation to adult disease, screening for severe hypertension is practicable, and effective treatment is available.

(22) *In the light of the present stage of knowledge we recommend that screening for neural tube defects (especially in high risk areas) and Down's Syndrome on the one hand, and for severe hypertension in adults on the other, should be made generally available.* (Chapter 8, p. 156)

Additional funding for ten special areas

(23) *We recommend that the government should finance a special health and social development programme in a small number of selected areas, costing about £30 m. in 1981–2.* (Chapter 8, p. 157)

25. At least £2 m. of this sum should be reserved for evaluation research and statistical and information units. The object would be both to provide special help to redress the undeniable disadvantages of people living in those areas but also to permit special experiments to reduce ill-health and mortality, and provide better support for disabled people. Some elements of such a programme are illustrated, particularly in connection with the development of more effective ante-natal services. (Chapter 8, pp. 157–9)

Measures to be taken outside the health services

26. In discussing actions outside the Health Care system which need to be taken to diminish inequalities of health we have been necessarily selective. We have attempted to pay heed to those factors which are correlated with the *degree* of inequalities. Secondly, we have tried to confine ourselves to matters which are practicable now, in political, economic and administrative terms, and which will none the less, properly maintained, exert a long-term structural effect. Third, we have continued to feel it right to give priority to young children and mothers, disabled people, and measures concerned with prevention.

27. Above all, we consider that the *abolition of child-poverty* should be adopted as a national goal for the 1980s. We recognize that this requires a redistribution of financial resources far beyond anything achieved by past programmes, and is likely to be very costly. Recommendations 24–27 are presented as a modest first step which might be taken towards this objective.

(24) *As an immediate goal the level of child benefit should be increased to 5½ per cent of average gross male industrial earnings, or £5.70 at November 1979 prices.* (Chapter 9, p. 171)

(25) *Larger child benefits should be progressively introduced for older children, after further examination of the needs of children and consideration of the practice in some other countries.* (Chapter 9, pp. 170–71)

(26) *The maternity grant should be increased to £100.* (Chapter 9, p. 171)

(27) *An infant care allowance should be introduced over a five-year period, beginning with all babies born in the year following a date to be chosen by the government.* (Chapter 9, p. 172)

28. Beyond these initial elements of an anti-poverty strategy, a number of other steps need to be taken. These include steps to reduce accidents to children, to which we have referred above (Recommendation 3). Further.

(28) *Provision of meals at school should be regarded as a right. Representatives of local authorities and community dietitians should be invited to meet representatives of parents and teachers of particular schools at regular intervals during the year to seek agreement to the provision and quality of meals. Meals in schools should be provided without charge.* (Chapter 9, p. 180)

(29) *A comprehensive disablement allowance for people of all ages should be introduced by stages at the earliest possible date, beginning with people with 100 per cent disablement.* (Chapter 9, p. 183)

(30) *Representatives of the DHSS and DE, HSE, together with representatives of trade unions and CBI, should draw up minimally acceptable and desirable conditions of work.* (Chapter 9, p. 187)

(31) *Government departments, employers and unions should devote more attention to preventive health through work organization, conditions and amenities, and in other ways. There should be a similar shift of emphasis in the work and function of the Health and Safety Commission and Executive, and the Employment Medical Advisory Service.* (Chapter 9, pp. 187–8)

(32) *Local authority spending on housing improvements under the 1974 Housing Act should be substantially increased.* (Chapter 9, p. 189)

(33) *Local authorities should increasingly be encouraged to widen their responsibilities to provide for all types of housing need which arise in their localities.* (Chapter 9, p. 190)

(34) *Policies directed towards the public and private housing sectors need to be better co-ordinated.* (Chapter 9, p. 189)

(35) *Special funding, on the lines of joint funding, for health and local authorities should be developed by the government to encourage better planning and management of housing, including adaptations and provision of necessary facilities and services for disabled people of all ages by social services and housing departments.* (Chapter 9, p. 191)

29. Our recommendations reflect the fact that reduction in health inequalities depends upon contributions from within many policy areas, and necessarily involves a number of government departments. Our objectives will be achieved *only* if each department makes its appropriate contribution. This in turn requires a greater degree of co-ordination than exists at present.

(36) *Greater co-ordination between government departments in the administration of health-related policies is required, by establishing inter-departmental machinery in the Cabinet Office under a Cabinet sub-committee along the lines of that established under the Joint Approach to Social Policy (JASP), with the Central Policy Review Staff also involved. Local counterparts of national co-ordinating bodies also need to be established.* (Chapter 9, p. 193)

(37) *A Health Development Council should be established with an independent membership to play a key advisory and planning role in relation to a collaborative national policy to reduce inequalities in health.* (Chapter 9, p. 194)

30. Within such co-ordinating machinery major initiatory responsibility will be vested in the Department of Health and Social Security, and we recommend that the Cabinet Committees we have proposed be chaired by a Minister, and by a senior DHSS official respectively, having major responsibility for health and prevention. Similarly it will be an important obligation upon the DHSS to ensure the effective operation of the Health Development Council.

Appendix of Tables

Table 1. *Percentage of economically active men in different occupational classes 1931, 1951, 1961, 1966, 1971 (England and Wales)*

Occupational class (Registrar General)	1931*		1951*		1961†	1966‡	1971
I	1.8	(2.2)	2.7	(3.2)	4.0	4.5	5.0
II	12.0	(12.8)	12.8	(14.3)	14.9	15.7	18.2
III	47.8	(48.9)	51.5	(53.4)	51.6	50.6	50.5
IV	25.5	(18.2)	23.3	(16.2)	20.5	20.6	18.0
V	12.9	(17.8)	9.7	(12.9)	8.9	8.8	8.4
Total	100.0	(100.0)	100.0	(100.0)	100.0	100.0	100.0
Number (thousands)	13,247		14,064		14,649	15,686	15,668

* Percentages have been weighted to allow for changes in classification between the 1931 and 1961 censuses: *The General Report, 1951* and *The General Report, 1961* allow the percentage change for each class between censuses to be calculated and the figures to be adjusted accordingly to bring both the 1931 and 1951 figures into line with the 1960 classification. Figures in brackets are based on the classification at that time. The estimates for 1931 and 1951 are necessarily crude – the latter partly for the reasons carefully listed in *The General Report 1961*, p. 193.

† Substantial numbers who were unclassified in 1961 (518,000) have been excluded. (Only 84,034 unclassified in 1971 have been excluded.)

‡ Percentages given are for economically active and retired males. Substantial numbers who were unclassified in 1966 have been excluded.

Sources: Census 1951, *General Report*, Table 66, p. 147; Census 1961, *General Report*, Table 55, p. 193; Census 1966, *Economic Activity Tables Part III*, Table 30, p. 416; Census 1971, *Economic Activity Tables Part IV*, Table 29, p. 96 (10 per cent sample).

Table 2. *Percentage of men aged 25 and over in five occupational classes in 1951, 1961 and 1971 (England and Wales), according to 1960 (and 1970) classification of occupations*

Age	Year	Professional I	Intermediate II	Skilled III	Partly skilled IV	Unskilled V
	1951	2.1	7 9	54.5	26.8	8.6
25–34	1961	5.3	12.9	55.9	18.4	7.5
	1971	7.5	18.1	53.2	15.2	6.1
	1951	2.1	12.6	49.0	26.7	9.8
35–44	1961	4.3	16.6	53.4	18.8	6.9
	1971	6.2	20.7	50.5	16.1	6.6
	1951	1.9	13.1	43.5	28.5	12.9
45–54	1961	3.3	18.8	48.5	21.1	8.2
	1971	4.8	21.3	48.8	17.9	7.3
	1951	1.8	14.0	39.9	29.5	14.7
55–9	1961	2.9	17.8	45.0	23.5	10.8
	1971	4.0	20.5	46.3	20.2	9.1
	1951	1.7	13.6	38.3	30.0	16.3
60–64	1961	2.6	17.5	42.7	24.5	12.7
	1971	3.7	18.7	45.3	21.4	10.9
	1951	1.9	13.3	42.6	29.1	15.0
65–9	1961	2.7	17.9	41.8	24.5	13.1
	1971	3.4	17.2	43.2	22.5	13 7
	1951	1.9	14.7	46.1	25.4	11.8
70+	1961	3.2	19.2	41.7	24.0	11.9
	1971	3.3	19.4	44.0	21.6	11.8
	1951	1.9	11.9	47.1	27.5	11.5
Total	1961	3.9	16.8	49.3	21.0	9.0
	1971	5.2	19.7	48.8	18.1	8.3

Note: An attempt has been made in this table to allow for changes of classification brought about after the introduction of the 1960 Classification of Occupations (there were only a few further changes in the 1970 classification and the figures from the 1961 and 1971 Censuses did not need to be adjusted before being compared). However, for 1951 we have changed the figures for each age-group by the proportion suggested for all age-groups in an exercise reported in *The General Report*, General Register Office, Census 1961, Great Britain, HMSO, 1968, p. 193. The 1961 data were re-classified for a sample using the 1951 classification and compared with the 1961 data classified according to the 1960 Classification of Occupations. We have worked back to the 1951 data for social classes and changed the figures for each class by the proportion suggested by the results of the exercise carried out by the GRO. The 1951 figures given above must be treated as approximate only. But they are more nearly comparable with the 1961 and 1971 Census results than the figures published in the 1951 Census reports.

The table gives estimates by age as well as class of the distribution in 1951, 1961 and 1971. For men aged 25 and over the percentage in class V declined from 11 to 8 and in class IV from 27 to 18 in the twenty years 1951 to 1971 (most of the corresponding increase taking place in class II, but also class I). However, the rate of change slowed down in 1961–71 and it can be seen that between a fifth and a quarter of those in the youngest age-groups continued to be found in classes IV and V. Overall, substantially more than a quarter of economically active men remained in class IV and V in 1971.

Sources: General Register Office, Census 1951, England and Wales, Occupation Tables, HMSO, 1956; General Register Office, Census 1961, England and Wales, Occupation Tables, HMSO, 1966, Table 20; Office of Population Censuses and Surveys, Census 1971, Great Britain, *Economic Activity Tables, Part IV*, HMSO, 1975, Table 29.

Table 3. *Two versions of trends in the distribution of wealth (Britain)*

Year	Inland Revenue data series B*				Atkinson and Harrison (assumption B3)†			
	Top 1%	Top 5%	Top 10%	Top 20%	Top 1%	Top 5%	Top 10%	Top 20%
1960	38.2	64.3	76.7	89.8	34.4	60.0	72.1	83.6
1964	34.4	59.3	73.5	88.4	34.7	59.2	72.0	85.2
1966	31.8	56.7	71.8	87.8	31.0	56.1	69.9	84.2
1968	32.7	59.0	73.8	89.4	33.6	58.6	72.0	85.4
1970	29.0	56.3	70.1	89.0	30.1	54.3	69.4	84.9
1972	29.9	56.3	71.9	89.2	32.0	57.2	71.7	85.3

* Assuming that persons not covered by the Inland Revenue estimates have no wealth.
† Assuming that the value of certain property not accounted for by estate data but estimated by means of the balance-sheet method is distributed between the population included in the estate data and the population excluded. This is their 'central estimate'.

Sources: Royal Commission on the Distribution of Income and Wealth, *Report No. 5 Third Report on the Standing Reference*, Cmnd 6999, HMSO, 1977, p. 76; A. B. Atkinson and A. J. Harrison, *Distribution of Personal Wealth in Britain*, Cambridge University Press, 1978, p. 159.

Table 4. *Distribution of personal income – study of the incidence of taxes and benefits (1961 to 1975, UK). Percentage shares of final income received by given quantile groups, and supplementary statistics (1961 to 1975). Income unit: households.*

Quantile group	Final income			
	1961	1965	1971	1975
Top 10 per cent	23.7	23.3	23.7	22.4
11–20 per cent	15.1	15.2	15.6	15.4
21–30 per cent	12.8	12.8	12.8	13.0
31–40 per cent	11.1	11.1	11.0	11.2
41–50 per cent	9.8	9.8	9.6	9.7
51–60 per cent	8.6	8.5	8.3	8.4
61–70 per cent	7.2	7.1	6.9	7.0
71–80 per cent	5.8	5.7	5.4	5.7
81–90 per cent	4.3	4.3	4.1	4.3
91–100 per cent	1.7	2.3	2.5	2.9
Difference as a percentage of the median between highest and lowest deciles	149	149	158	149
Upper and lower quartiles	75	77	83	81
Median £ pw	15	18	26	52
GINI coefficient %	32.9	32.2	33.0	31.1

Note: While this table shows no pronounced trend in the distribution of final income, it is also true that fringe benefits (employer welfare and public sector subsidies) have grown in importance, and probably this has been to the relative advantage of higher income groups. (See for example Royal Commission on Distribution of Income and Wealth Report, No. 13, Chapter 4 and Appendix H, 1975.)

Source: Royal Commission on the Distribution of Income and Wealth.

Table 5. *Recent trends in death rates by occupational class men aged 15–64 (England and Wales)*

Occupational class	Age-standardized death rate per 100,000 living at ages 15–64		
	1951	*1961*	*1971*
I	103	82	79
II	108	87	83
III	116	106	103
IV	119	108	113
V	137	134	123

Note: Adjustments have been made by the OPCS to improve comparability between censuses.

Source: OPCS, *Occupational Mortality, Decennial Supplement, 1970–72, England and Wales*, HMSO, 1978, p. 174 (supplemented by the OPCS).

The Health Divide

Preface

Reproduced below is the original preface to *The Health Divide*, which stirred strong reaction – favourable and otherwise.

This final report from the Health Education Council before its demise on 31 March 1987 is, in my opinion, an essential element in the public debate which must occur on health inequalities in the United Kingdom.

Such inequity is inexcusable in a democratic society which prides itself on being humane. To eliminate or even reduce it substantially would be a major contribution to the health of the people of this country.

DR DAVID A. PLAYER
Director General
Health Education Council, 1982–7

Foreword to the 1992 Edition

It is now exactly ten years since Penguin first published the Black Report and four years since it was joined by the publication of the first edition of *The Health Divide*. The interest in the subject has not abated over the years.

So much has happened in the intervening period that yet again I find myself collecting together the latest information from diverse sources and trying to put it into some sort of coherent order. I have been particularly struck by four trends during the course of this review.

Firstly, the dramatic changes that have taken place in the last four years in central and eastern Europe cannot be ignored. The statistics on health were routinely collected but in some countries they were kept secret, so it comes as a particular shock to be faced with newly released evidence of inequalities in health on such a large scale. The figures give a stark illustration of the effect of economic crisis and widespread pollution on the health of whole populations and reveal a growing health divide *between* countries in Europe. For the first time, we are also presented with evidence of the large inequalities in health and health care *within* these central and eastern European countries. If anyone needed convincing of the influence of socio-economic factors on health, they need look no further.

Secondly, more countries are reporting to the World Health Organization that a widening of inequalities in health has occurred within their own countries during the 1980s, and countries with excellent health profiles, such as Sweden and the Netherlands, are among them. This awareness of a growing problem has shifted the issue of inequalities in health further up the political agenda in some countries and has led to renewed calls for action.

Thirdly, here in Britain the contradictory nature of some of the policy developments is striking. On the one hand, there have been moves to give public health and prevention greater emphasis, with commitment to this goal secured right through from national to local level. Yet at the same time other policies have been introduced which appear to have been devised with no consideration of the impact they will have on public health in general, and on the health of the most disadvantaged groups in society in particular. Consequently the situation for many has worsened over the decade. Perhaps if we had more 'equity impact assessments' *before* policies were introduced, we would avoid some of the worst pitfalls.

Fourthly, and ironically, these negative trends offer a ray of hope for the future, because at last there are indications that inequalities are beginning to be taken seriously. There has been a subtle but profound change in official attitudes over the past two years. Not only is there official recognition that inequalities in health actually exist, but there are also signs that more policy-makers are asking what can be done about them. That is the major challenge for the 1990s.

July 1992   Margaret Whitehead

Chapter 1

Setting the Scene

The first edition of *The Health Divide* came to be written because of the pressing need for an update on inequalities in health as the number of studies on the subject mounted at a quite extraordinary rate. Now, in 1992, there are literally hundreds of new studies published since 1988 in Britain alone and a growing number from abroad, especially Europe. This chapter explains the purpose behind this report. It describes some of the terms and measures used and outlines the main questions the body of the report sets out to answer.

The purpose of the report

In 1980 the research Working Group chaired by Sir Douglas Black produced an authoritative report documenting inequalities in health in Britain since the war. As soon as it was published it stimulated a widespread response from the research community both here and abroad and since then much more evidence has accumulated on several different fronts. By the end of 1985 it was obvious that the non-specialist would find it difficult to keep abreast of all the developments. Additionally, there was a growing desire to know what the picture on inequalities in health looked like in the 1980s, as the Black Report, because of the time-lag in analysing official statistics, drew much of its data from the early 1970s.

For these reasons the Health Education Council in early 1986 commissioned an update of the evidence. The original aims of *The Health Divide* were to draw together and summarize the wide-ranging new evidence and to describe what had happened and could happen, in policy development. It was felt that the report needed to be sufficiently detailed and fully referenced to be useful both as an insight into the literature for those wishing to study the subject further, and a resource for those working in diverse fields who wanted more of an overview of the subject. The story of its development and reception is, of course, told in the introduction to this volume. Four years later, it is now time for a further update as the evidence unfolds and policies move on.

Equity and health

Before going any further it is necessary to be clear about the meaning of some of the terms and about precisely what is being measured. It is widely accepted that there are natural differences in health in the population – human beings vary in health as they do in every other aspect of life. What is being addressed in this report is the extent of unfair or unacceptable inequalities: what some would call 'inequities'. Deciding what is fair and just comes down to a subjective judgement in the end, but the working definition outlined in a recent World Health Organization discussion paper has met with widespread support:

In health terms, 'ideally everyone should have a fair *opportunity* to attain their full health potential and, more pragmatically, none should be disadvantaged from achieving this potential if it can be avoided' (Whitehead, 1990).

In health care, the principle of equity 'leads to equal access to available care for equal need, equal utilization for equal need and equal quality of care for all.'

One of the major issues is whether we have anything approaching equity in health in the UK. Are there groups in the population who are disadvantaged to such an extent that it affects their opportunity to achieve good health? For instance, does a person's financial resources, social position, ethnic origin or gender affect their chances of good health? Are certain areas of the country or certain neighbourhoods unduly disadvantaged in health terms? Are the unemployed disadvantaged compared with those in work? Does the health care system treat some people more favourably than others? Are the resources available to the NHS fairly distributed around the country? These are the sorts of issues that arise when trying to answer the question of whether equity in health has been achieved. There are two quite different orientations in the studies in this field: those concerned with inequalities in health and those concerned with deprivation and health. Those dealing with *inequality* consider the gradient in health over the whole population through the various grades from top to bottom of the social scale. Those focusing on *deprivation* single out the most disadvantaged subgroup whose welfare falls below the average or below a reasonable minimum standard of the society in which they live. Both types of study are included here in an attempt to give a broad overview, though it should be borne in mind that each may have quite different policy implications. Policies related to deprivation may be targeted exclusively to the worst-off. Policies to reduce inequalities may be wide-ranging and encompass changes at all levels of society.

Measuring health

Work on clarifying the meaning of health and health promotion has moved forward since 1980. The World Health Organization in particular has been active in helping to define these terms for practical policy-making purposes. A consensus is emerging from WHO discussions in which *health* is conceived as 'the extent to which an individual or group is able, on the one hand, to realize aspirations and satisfy needs and on the other hand, to change or cope with the environment. Health is therefore seen as a resource for everyday life, not the objective of living: it is a positive concept emphasizing social and personal resources as well as physical capacities' (WHO, 1984).

Expressed in this form, health is a complex rather than a simple concept, with several dimensions to it which may not all be capable of measurement. Two reviews have given clear accounts of the measurement of the various aspects which go to make up the concept of health (Macintyre, 1986a; Blaxter, 1990).

Traditionally, the negative end of the health spectrum concerned with death and disease has been most extensively investigated. The expected length of life is calculated from death rates and the relative chances of death at a stated age are expressed as a ratio – the Standardized Mortality Ratio (SMR), used extensively in the chapters which follow. Short-term (acute) and long-term (chronic) disease rates are calculated from medical records or self-reports of complaints. It should be noted that statistics based on the use of health services or absence from work are not valid measures of the extent of disease in the population because they are influenced by different administrative arrangements and individual circumstances (Blaxter, 1987a).

However, the last ten years have seen a concerned effort to document other dimensions of health, including ones which consider the more positive end of the spectrum, incorporating various 'quality-of-life' measures. Whether people feel ill in themselves is considered an important dimension, affecting their quality of life and influencing subsequent behaviour. *Illness* is defined as the subjective experience of symptoms of ill-health, and has been measured in the Health and Life-style Survey, for example, by a symptom check-list to obtain an 'illness score' (Cox *et al.*, 1987). Paradoxically, people can be diseased without feeling ill and feel ill without having a medically recognizable disease. Studies using the Nottingham Health Profile have brought in the physical, social and emotional effects illness can have on an individual's everyday life (Hunt and McEwen, 1980). More use has also been made of measures like the General Health

Questionnaire to assess minor psychiatric illness in the community and a modified form of this score has been used to assess psycho-social well-being/malaise. Growth and development, especially in babies and children, has been measured by height, weight, percentage of babies of low birth-weight and so on.

There is a certain amount of scepticism from the medical profession about the validity of health measures based on a lay person's own reported experience. However, when checked against doctors' records or other clinical measurements, the self-reports are found to agree remarkably well. Studies using these additional measures are introduced wherever possible in the pages that follow and the techniques employed are described in greater detail in Chapter 8. These new measures are intended to supplement rather than replace traditional indicators.

Measuring social factors

In order to compare the health of people in different social circumstances in society, a variety of indicators has been employed in the studies quoted. The two most frequently used are based on the occupation of the head of the household. The first is the Registrar General's scale of five social or occupational classes, based on the skills and status of the job, ranging from professionals in class I to unskilled manual workers in class V (the full scale is outlined on p. 228). The second is the scale of socio-economic groups which brings together people with similar skills and life-styles. A condensed scale of six or seven catergories is normally used:

Socio-economic groups
1. Professional
2. Employers and managers
3. Intermediate/junior non-manual (sometimes split into two groups)
4. Skilled manual
5. Semi-skilled manual and personal service
6. Unskilled manual.

Both are taken as a rough guide to the way of life and living standards experienced by the separate groups and their families. They correlate fairly well with other components of social position, like education and income. Measures based on occupation have their limitations though, which are discussed in more detail in Chapters 3 and 8. Increasingly, information from this source is being supplemented by data from other measures. For example, three categories of housing tenure – local authority tenant, private tenant and owner-occupier – are being used as a guide to resources available to individuals. Car ownership is also used as an indirect indicator of poverty or affluence. Employment status has been used in several studies examining the difference between those who are employed, unemployed, retired, permanently sick, housewives, etc. It is also now much easier to use the census data to study basic amenities and housing conditions in quite small areas to assess the degree of material and social deprivation in an area. These have been used in the regional studies quoted in Chapter 2, and the details and merits of some of the major deprivation indicators are discussed in Chapter 8.

Limited data on ethnic origin are obtained from the country of birth as recorded on death certificates and from the mother's country of birth which appears on birth certificates. Surveys in which people are asked to define their own ethnic origin and colour are increasingly being used.

Summary

The purpose of this new edition of *The Health Divide* is to bring together and review the array of studies published between 1980 and 1992 on the issue of social inequalities in health in Great Britain, and to document promising initiatives which have been taken to tackle this pressing problem.

In line with the social and ecological concepts of health, evidence quoted looks not only at mortality but also at the growing body of evidence on other dimensions of health which can have a profound influence on the quality of life of individuals and groups. The existence of long-standing disease and the experience of illness, restrictions on day-to-day living and measures of psycho-social health are included, as are measures of growth and development and of health-related behaviour.

The Registrar General's occupational class scale is still the most frequently used indicator of social inequalities in this report. But research on social inequalities has been greatly extended over the last few years into areas concerned with unemployment, income, housing, and material and social deprivation in small areas. There is also more discussion about gender and ethnic inequalities. For ease of reference *The Health Divide* follows a very similar format to that of the Black Report, with an updated chapter on each of the topics covered by Black for Chapters 2 to 6. The remaining chapters are concerned with policy issues. Chapter 7 outlines the growing consensus on the direction in which policy should be developing. Chapter 8 looks at information needs and research developments. In

Chapter 9, the contribution of the caring services is discussed, and in the final chapter strategy on a broad front beyond the health care sector is examined.

Chapter 2

Health Inequalities Today

Does everyone in Britain have the same opportunity to attain the highest level of health? Are some unduly disadvantaged? This chapter makes a start at answering these questions by looking first of all at the present pattern of health across groups in the population with differing social circumstances. It considers for instance the latest evidence on how health varies with occupational class, employment status, household characteristics, gender and ethnic origin and asks if certain areas of the country or neighbourhoods are disadvantaged in health terms. Evidence on trends and possible causes of inequalities in health will help complete the picture in later chapters.

Occupational class and mortality

Much of the evidence on social differences in health in Britain is measured in terms of social or occupational class. Occupation is recorded in the census, on birth and death certificates and on some, but not all, health records. From that information the Registrar General classifies people into the five social classes listed below. Men and single women are classified by their own occupation, children by the occupation of the head of the household, and married women by their husband's occupation, though their own occupation is available for analysis now and is used in some studies.

It is important to realize that although this classification is based on occupation it is not just a measure of working conditions. The intention is to group together people with broadly similar living standards and way of life indicated by their occupation. When the scale was first devised it was intended to reflect both the wealth or poverty and the culture associated with each class. Although it is obviously not a very precise measure it is still, even today, useful as a general guide to social position (see p. 351 for its limitations and alternatives).

The five classes consist of the following:

I. Professional (for example lawyer, doctor, accountant)

II. Intermediate (for example teacher, nurse, manager)

IIIN. Skilled non-manual (for example typist, shop assistant)

IIIM. Skilled manual (for example miner, bus driver, cook)

IV. Partly skilled manual (for example farm worker, bus conductor)

V. Unskilled manual (for example cleaner, labourer).

Using this scale, clear evidence emerges of occupational class differences in mortality in the 1980s and early 1990s. This applies at every stage of life from birth, through to adulthood and well into old age. From Fig. 1, for instance, it can be seen that in 1990 rates of stillbirth and death in the first year of life increased progressively from occupational class I to V. Thus babies whose fathers had unskilled jobs ran approximately twice the risk of death under one year than babies whose fathers worked in the professions. These figures are based on legitimate births only, as equivalent figures for all births are not available every year. However, a special analysis combining the 1987 and 1988 figures showed that the differential in death rates between social classes was even greater when births outside marriage (jointly registered) were included. This arises because babies born outside marriage who are jointly registered by both parents have death rates on average 40 per cent higher than those of babies of the same social class but with married parents. The addition of births outside marriage (jointly registered) to those born inside has little effect on the within-marriage mortality rates for social classes I, II and IIIN as births inside marriage still form more than 85 per cent of all births in these classes. However, jointly registered births outside marriage form 25 per cent of births to social classes IIIM and IV, and 40 per cent of births to class V. Therefore mortality rates are increased by the addition of the births outside marriage. As a result, the differential between the bottom and top of the scale is increased by combining births inside and outside marriage (OPCS, 1991a).

The evidence on children and adults in Fig. I is taken from the Registrar General's latest Decennial Supplement covering the years 1979–83 (OPCS, 1986b and 1988). Figures for the years around the 1991 census will be available in the mid 1990s. Death rates are expressed as Standardized Mortality Ratios (SMRs) to show the relative chances of death at a given age. The average for the population as a whole is 100, so SMRs below 100 indicate lower than average chances of death and SMRs above 100 indicate higher than average. The distinct gradient in mortality in children and adults can be seen to increase in a stepwise fashion from class I to class V, so that, for example, unskilled workers run at least twice the risk of death as professionals, and so do their children. In terms of expectation of life, this means that, for example, a man aged 20 in social classes I or II can expect to live over five years longer than a counterpart in classes IV or V (Haberman and Bloomfield, 1988). Furthermore, if all infants and children up to age 15 enjoyed the same survival chances as the children from classes I and II, then over 3,000 deaths a year might be prevented (Whitehead, 1988a). In addition, bringing all adults aged 16–64 up to the mortality experience of class I would mean 39,000 fewer deaths per year (Scott-Samuel and Blackburn, 1988).

Note that the Decennial Supplement records a very high SMR for class V. For technical reasons related to the reclassification of occupations by the Registrar General in 1980, it is thought that class V figures may be artificially raised and data from the OPCS Longitudinal Study may provide more reliable figures for this class. The OPCS Longitudinal Study selected a 1 per cent sample of the population of England and Wales from the 1971 census and has continued to follow vital events in the sample and the associated families by use of flagged birth, death and cancer registrations. The study looked at mortality by occupational class in broad age-groups, and Fig. 2 shows that from this second, independent study a clear social gradient in adult mortality is again evident, with a twofold difference between the top and bottom of the social class scale for people of working age. Even at ages after retirement there are clear mortality gradients for men which are almost as steep as those found in the latter stages of working life. Thus even in old age, men from occupational class V had more than 50 per cent higher death rates than those in occupational class I (Fox *et al.*, 1986).

When the causes of death are investigated it becomes apparent that the social gradient in death is not limited to one or two specific causes but applies to a wide range of conditions. In order to make use of the mass of information in the latest Decennial Supplement and overcome the technical difficulties, it is necessary to group all the manual classes together and compare them with all the non-manual classes. Alternatively, data on classes I and II can be combined and then compared with data on combined classes IV and V, to compare the health of the richest and poorest classes. Several analyses of this nature are now available. For example, Marmot and McDowall (1986) carried out a careful study of some of the major causes of death for men and married women in the two distinct categories: manual and non-manual. Table 1 shows the results of this study and reveals that, for all the causes analysed, non-manual workers in 1979–83 had a lower risk of death than manual workers. This

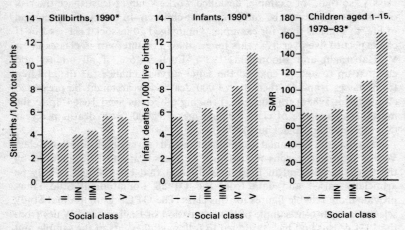

*England and Wales

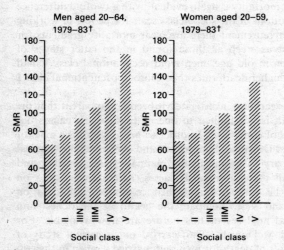

†Great Britain

Figure 1. *Occupational class and mortality in infants, children and adults.* (*Source: OPCS, 1986b, 1988, and 1992.*)

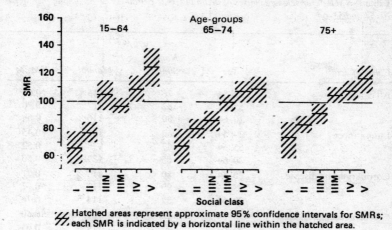

Figure 2. *Mortality of men by social class and broad age-groups, 1976–81.* (*Source: Fox* et al., *1986, OPCS Longitudinal Study. Crown Copyright.*)

was particularly striking in the younger age range, and married women showed a similar pattern.

Another study of the 1979–83 data compared the two highest and the two lowest occupational classes. In 65 of the 78 disease categories for men, SMRs for classes IV and V were higher than for either class I or II. Only one cause, malignant melanoma, showed the reverse trend. This is a form of skin cancer associated with over-exposure to the sun. For women, 62 of the 82 categories of disease showed higher SMRs for classes IV and V and only 4 showed the reverse – cancer of the breast and the brain, malignant melanoma and chronic lymphoid leukaemia. The remainder showed no consistent pattern (Townsend *et al.*, 1988).

This work illustrates that most of the major and minor killer diseases now affect the poorest occupational classes more than the rich. This applies equally well to coronary heart disease, stroke and peptic ulcer, which are still sometimes misleadingly referred to as 'diseases of affluence' or 'executive diseases' when in fact they are more common in the manual classes. It is thought that the confusion has arisen partly because of misdiagnosis in the past and partly because these diseases are more common in developed or affluent societies than in developing ones. The fact that they

Table 1: *SMRs* for selected causes of death in Great Britain 1979–83 among men aged 20–54 and 55–64*

Cause of death	Age	1979/83 Non-manual	Manual	NM/M
All causes	20–54	76	115	0.66
	55–64	82	117	0.70
	20–64	80	116	0.69
Lung cancer	20–54	60	133	0.45
	55–64	67	128	0.52
	20–64	65	129	0.50
Coronary heart disease	20–54	80	113	0.71
	55–64	90	117	0.77
	20–64	87	114	0.76
Cerebro-vascular disease	20–54	73	121	0.60
	55–64	77	119	0.65
	20–64	76	120	0.63

* For each cause, and within each age-group, the SMR for all men in 1979/83 is 100.

Source: Marmot and McDowall (1986).

predominantly affect the poor in affluent societies has been overlooked. Clearly in this country nowadays 'diseases of affluence' have all but disappeared and what is left is a general health disadvantage of the poor.

Evidence from a second major longitudinal study has become available since the publication of the Black Report and sheds light on another important point: whether the national data under-estimate or over-estimate the social class gradient. The Whitehall study of civil servants examined over 17,000 office-based civil servants in London from 1967 to 1969 and followed the health of men in different grades of the service for more than a decade. The study found that the lower the grade, the higher the mortality for every cause of death except genito-urinary disease. There was a greater than threefold difference between the highest and the lowest grade: a much steeper gradient than the occupational class gradient found in the national data (Rose and Marmot, 1981; Marmot *et al.*, 1984b).

Other studies of single occupations have also found steeper gradients. For example, a study of mortality from coronary heart disease in different ranks in the British Army in 1973–7 found increasing mortality with decreasing rank, with a sixfold difference between the highest and lowest rank (Lynch and Oelman, 1981).

The social class gradient is also more pronounced when 'years of potential life lost' is used as a measure of mortality instead of SMR. This takes into account the fact that deaths in younger people will lead to a greater loss of years of life than deaths in people nearer or after retirement. This measure of mortality shows a threefold difference between social class I and V men of working age compared with a 2.5-fold difference using SMR. For women, the measure shows a 2.2-fold difference between top and bottom of the scale, compared with a 1.9-fold difference in SMR (Blane *et al.*, 1990). This contrast arises partly because accidents and violence often occur relatively early in life, so claiming more years of life, and death by this cause is more prevalent in lower social classes. The authors note that in terms of loss of potential life, accidents and violence are as important as heart disease and cancers in the 15–64 age-group, and this emphasizes the need for public health policy and the development of accident services to take this more fully into consideration (Blane *et al.*, 1990).

It seems that the national gradients may underestimate the real differences between social groups, because each class is made up of occupations with a range of mortality rates. Studies on single occupations are more homogeneous and can reveal a sharper distinction between top and bottom groups.

Occupational class and health

However, death rates measure only one dimension of health. Fortunately in recent years much more information has emerged about other dimensions, like the experience of illness, restrictions on everyday activity, and the levels of fitness and well-being in different groups. When these are investigated it appears that not only do lower occupational classes have higher death rates, but they also experience more sickness and ill-health throughout their lives. Indeed Blaxter (1989) argues that morbidity or general health status are more important indicators of inequality now that people are living longer and degenerative disease is becoming more prominent. One of the main sources of information on morbidity is the annual General Household Survey in which people are asked about both chronic and acute sickness. For such purposes six or sometimes seven socio-economic groups are used, which correspond fairly well to the Registrar General's scale (see p. 224). Rates of sickness by socio-economic group have shown the same pattern each year throughout the 1980s, revealing great inequalities between the groups (OPCS, 1991b). The gradient is steepest for limiting long-standing illness, where the rates in the unskilled manual group are more than double those of the professional group for both men and women. It is not quite as steep, but still marked, for long-standing illness without limitation; while for acute sickness the differential is only evident at ages over 45. When days of restricted activity are counted, however, the gradient reappears.

In the 1988 and 1989 General Household Survey, additional information was collected on the nature of the reported illness. Data for the two years were combined to calculate Standardized Long-standing Illness ratios (SLI ratios), to remove the effect of different age structures in different social groups (the equivalent of SMRs for mortality). This showed that the three most common causes of long-standing illness were conditions of the respiratory, musculoskeletal and circulatory systems. As Fig. 3 shows, there is a clear gradient in all three, with higher rates in lower socio-economic groups (OPCS, 1991b).

Another important study, the Health and Life-style Survey of 1986 investigated several dimensions of health and well-being and came to similar conclusions. The study is unusual in using physiological measurements, such as blood pressure and lung function, in addition to in-depth interview techniques, and in measuring income, education and housing as well as social class. A remarkably regular and in some cases steep social class gradient was found with a variety of measures of morbidity and fitness. For example, with self-perceived health the percentage of men believing their own health was only fair or poor increased from 12 per cent of class I to 36 per cent of class V. Analyses by income and education yielded similar results. Likewise when the experience of illness was assessed using a list of twenty-four common symptoms, the gradient appeared for a wide range of conditions from persistent cough and back trouble in men to headaches, palpitations, deafness and anxiety in women. When the prevalence of self-reported disease was assessed, lower social classes had higher rates of many common diseases like bronchitis, arthritis/rheumatism and varicose veins. With psychosocial health (ability to sleep well, to concentrate, etc.), high rates of 'malaise' were declared by lower social classes, with the steepest gradients found in middle age in women and older ages in men. Physiological measures of fitness, like weight, blood pressure and lung function, showed the same trend. The author of the study concluded that there was strong evidence of a high degree of inequality in health at the present time, not just in a particularly disadvantaged subgroup but throughout the social scale (Blaxter, 1987b; Cox *et al.*, 1987). This study was repeated in 1991 and when analysed should provide further valuable information.

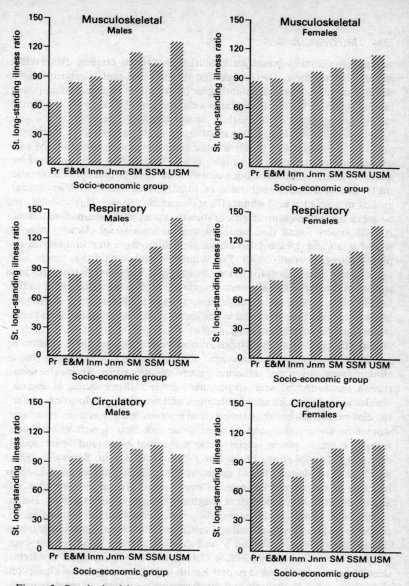

Figure 3. *Standardized long-standing illness ratios for men and women in different socio-economic groups, Great Britain, 1988–9.* (*Source: OPCS, 1991b.*)

Numerous studies based on clinical observations confirm the overall picture. For example, OPCS data for 1990 showed that low birth-weight was still much more common in babies born into lower occupational class families (OPCS, 1992). (Low birth-weight is considered to be the single most powerful predictor of death in the first month of life.)

In contrast, in the 1980 national survey of heights and weights, childhood and adult obesity was a problem more common in men in class IIIM and women in classes IV and V (Knight, 1984). This finding was supported by a cohort study of children born in 1946. By 1982 (when the sample was thirty-six years old) higher rates of obesity were found in lower social groups in both men and women (Braddon *et al.*, 1986). Height, which can be taken as an indicator of general health, varies with occupational class. A 1985 survey found that men and women from social classes I plus II were 1.8 cm and 2.8 cm taller respectively than those in social classes IV plus V (Gregory *et al.*, 1990). The Whitehall study found that height was significantly related to grade in the Civil Service. For example, the administrators in the highest grade were on average 4.7 cm taller than men in the lowest grade. In the same study, men in lower grades in the Civil Service had higher blood pressure and lower levels of glucose tolerance than those in the top grades (Marmot *et al.*, 1984b).

The Whitehall II study, carried out between 1985 and 1988, selected a cohort of British civil servants aged 35–55, both men and women, for a clinical examination and self-administered questionnaire. An inverse association was found between employment grade and prevalence of angina, electrocardiogram evidence of ischaemia, and symptoms of chronic bronchitis. Self-perceived health status and symptoms were worse in men and women in lower-status jobs, as were some risk factors such as smoking, lack of exercise, poorer social circumstances at work and fewer social supports (Marmot *et al.*, 1991). The Welsh Heart Health Survey of 1985, which also employed clinical measurements, found that manual groups had two or three times the rates of non-manual groups for symptoms of angina, breathlessness, persistent cough and phlegm (Nutbeam *et al.*, 1987).

The adult dental health survey of 1988 found that the proportion of people from class I with no natural teeth was much lower than in the other classes, though classes IV and V had shown a marked improvement over the previous twenty years (OPCS, 1991c). The OPCS survey of children's dental health in 1983 found poorer health in lower occupational classes on several counts. For example, among 5-year-olds on average twice as many teeth were actively decayed among those from the manual classes compared with those from the non-manual classes. They also had more teeth missing as a result of decay (Todd and Dodd, 1985).

During the 1980s a number of surveys used the Nottingham Health Profile to study differences in self-perceived health and its impact on daily lives. The nature of ill-health is considered under six main headings: lack of energy, pain, sleep disturbance, physical immobility, emotional distress and social isolation. The profile was used in a survey in 1981 that found clear differences in perceived health problems between occupational classes, but only in the 20–44 age-group: the lower the occupational class the greater the amount and severity of perceived distress. For example, men from classes IV and V had scores twice as high as men in classes I and II in the sections measuring lack of energy and emotional distress, over three times as high in the section measuring sleep disturbances, and over four times as high concerning feelings of social isolation. For women the findings were similar, though less marked. After the age of 45 the differences were smaller (Hunt *et al.*, 1985). More recently the profile was used to collect data on a sample of local residents in three London boroughs, dividing the sample into manual and non-manual classes. The manual groups registered higher rates of tiredness, sleep problems, pain and emotional distress, in line with the findings above (Bucquet and Curtis, 1986). In a pilot study of several different measures of health, it was found that manual groups not only had higher rates of chronic disease and disability than non-manual groups, but also were more likely to register a lack of psychological well-being and to have poorer fitness scores (Blaxter, 1985).

The age factor

It is important to appreciate the variation in the pattern of inequalities in different age-groups and stages of the life-cycle.

For mortality the picture is clear-cut. The social class gradient; with increasing mortality with decreasing social class, has already been detailed on pp. 288–9 for babies and for children in each age-group from 1–15 (OPCS, 1988). Swedish data on children and young adults show similar patterns (Vågerö and Östberg, 1989). Distinct gradients in mortality have also been noted in adolescence from 16–20, in men and women of working age, and lately for both sexes beyond retirement ages, detailed on p. 229. It is clear that mortality gradients are evident from birth to old age.

However, for morbidity and other dimensions of health the picture is slightly more variable and there is a debate about the existence of social class gradients for certain health measures in adolescence. This debate is reviewed by West (1988) and Macintyre and West (1991), who argue that there is a lack of a gradient in adolescence, and by Blane *et al.* (1993) and Davey Smith *et al.* (1992), who argue for the existence of a gradient at all ages.

To support the first argument, evidence from the General Household Survey shows that for both males and females the gradient in prevalence of long-standing illness by socio-economic group was evident for each age-group, apart from children, and was most pronounced for those aged 45 and over (OPCS, 1990b). The Twenty–07 study in the west of Scotland failed to find evidence of an occupational class gradient for self-reported chronic illness for males or females at age 15. Weak gradients were observed for self-assessed health, accidents and lung function in males but not in females. Systolic blood pressure showed an opposite class pattern for each sex – lower in manual class males but higher in manual class females. Height was the only measure to display a consistent gradient for both sexes and for several different measures of social position (Macintyre and West, 1991).

The argument against this view is that most of the measures of health used, such as self-reported chronic sickness and self-assessed health, may not be appropriate for young, generally healthy populations, and for the more suitable measures, like accidents, there is evidence of under-reporting by lower social class families (Blane *et al.*, 1993). The same problem of under-reporting does not arise when accidents result in death, and mortality rates for accidents then show a sharp gradient in adolescence. Some conditions and disabilities, based on clinical measures, rather than self-assessed health, also show social class differences in children and these health problems will also carry through into early adulthood, for example cerebral palsy, hearing and visual impairment, dental decay and lead poisoning (Davey Smith *et al.*, 1992).

In later life, a striking phenomenon is evident – health deteriorates more rapidly in those who are socially disadvantaged (Blaxter, 1989). In the Health and Life-style Survey, for example, social class differences in morbidity did exist at the start of adult life, but they were small and not always regular for the different dimensions of health. By the middle years, however, differences for all the dimensions of health measured were wide and regular, and for the over-60s and over-70s there was the largest differential in psychosocial health. For fitness and disease symptoms the gap got smaller in old age (Blaxter, 1990). A study in Newcastle of people who died prematurely in different neighbourhoods showed that men and women in poorer areas were likely to have been chronically sick or disabled for longer before death and have suffered a greater number of distinct health problems than their counterparts in more affluent localities (Phillimore, 1989).

This deterioration in health has led researchers to calculate how many years free of disability different groups in the population could expect to live. A review of the evidence in Europe, Canada and the United States concluded that wealthier people not only live longer but they also spend a significantly smaller proportion of their life disabled. For example, data from Canada showed that the wealthiest fifth of the population could expect to live over six years longer than men in the poorest fifth of the population. They could also expect to be free from disability for fourteen years longer than men in the poorest fifth of the population. The gap between the wealthiest and poorest women was 2.8 years of life expectancy and 7.6 years of life free of disability (Robine and Ritchie, 1991).

Looking at survival rates from cancer and coronary heart disease in men and women in the OPCS Longitudinal Study, it was found that lower occupational class people with cancer had poorer survival prospects, confirming earlier studies (Leon and Wilkinson, 1989).

To sum up, the studies quoted above show that the risk of death for lower occupational classes in the 1980s was much higher than that of the highest occupational classes at every stage of life. Thus stillbirths, deaths in babies and children, deaths in adults of working age and deaths in old age show this gradient from lower mortality in the richer classes to higher mortality in the poorer classes. The evidence presented also shows that it is not just one or two specific causes of death which are to blame for the higher mortality, but that the full range of diseases, with very few exceptions, are affecting the poorer classes more than the rich. Only a wide-ranging general explanation could account for such a phenomenon. In addition, examples are given from the growing body of evidence showing that lower occupational classes experience much more illness and a poorer quality of self-perceived health during their lives, though in adolescence the pattern is under debate. The evidence has been extended into other dimensions of health concerned with the experience of illness, fitness and well-being, and into older age-groups, and still wide differences are found. People from higher social classes not only live longer but experience a smaller proportion of their lives sick or disabled.

Household classifications and health

Conclusions about the extent of inequalities in health are not based solely on occupational class studies. The Black Report has been criticized for relying too heavily on mortality data, on a limited age range of the population (mainly men below retirement age), and of concentrating on one measure of social position, namely occupational class (Illsley, 1986;

Strong, 1990). The preceding pages have already shown that the analysis has been extended since then into older age-groups and various dimensions of health in addition to mortality. This and the next sections show that evidence is now accumulating on alternative social classifications and on the health of women in different circumstances.

Measures based on household characteristics, such as housing tenure or access to a car, are increasingly being used to investigate the association between health and social position. Used singly or in combination with one or more other factors, they help to give a more complete picture. They are used as indirect indicators of wealth and command over resources.

Three tenure groups are identified from the census, depending on whether the house is owner-occupied, privately rented or local authority rented, and this reveals persistent differences in mortality and morbidity. For example, higher stillbirth and infant mortality rates have been found in babies born to private tenants compared with owner-occupiers (Macfarlane and Mugford, 1984). The National Child Development Study found marked and consistent differences between those in owner-occupied and local authority accommodation at ages 7 and 23 for five different health measures (height, 'malaise', self-reported health, hospital admissions and psychiatric morbidity), with the owner-occupiers having better health (Fogelman *et al.,* 1987).

In adults, the OPCS Longitudinal Study found that owner-occupiers had lower mortality than private tenants who in turn had lower mortality than local authority tenants (Fox and Goldblatt, 1982). This study is valuable in being able to look at mortality in relation to a range of socioeconomic indicators. Table 2 shows mortality of men and women in the ten years from 1971 to 1981 by their housing tenure, education and access to cars. The same pattern is seen in both men and women, with lower than average mortality in the most favoured groups like the owner-occupiers, degree-holders and car-owners, rising to above-average mortality in the least-favoured groups such as the local authority tenants, those with no qualifications and no access to cars (Goldblatt, 1990b).

Using social class alone under-estimates the number of men at the extremes of the mortality spectrum. For example, Table 3 shows mortality of men aged 15–64 by social class and by a combination of household-based and occupation-based factors. The percentage of expected deaths covered by each category is also shown.

It shows that the SMR ranges from 67 to 125 from social classes I to V, but only covers 5 per cent and 7 per cent of expected deaths respectively. Combining classifications identifies an advantaged group of men with SMR of 67 and a disadvantaged group with SMR of 123, but these cover

Table 2: *Mortality of men and women in 1971–81 by housing tenure, education and access to cars (England and Wales)*

Socio-economic indicator	Standardized Mortality Ratios	
	Men (aged 15–64 at death)	Women (aged 15–59 at death)
Housing tenure:[1]		
Owner-occupied	84	83
Privately rented	109	106
Local authority	115	117
Education:[2]		
Degree	59	66
Non-degree higher qualification	80	78
A levels only	91	80
None or not stated	103	102
Access to cars:[1]		
One or more cars	85	83
No access to a car	121	135

1. Aged 15 years and over in 1971. 2. Aged 18–70 years in 1971.

Source: Goldblatt (1990b).

17 per cent and 21 per cent of expected deaths respectively (Goldblatt, 1990a). This particular comparison is of considerable importance because it overcomes one criticism of using occupational class alone: that it only relates to very small groups at the extremes of the spectrum (Illsley, 1986; Stern, 1983). Goldblatt's evidence relates to substantial segments of the population and produces a differential of similar magnitude to that obtained with occupation-based classifications.

Further evidence from the Longitudinal Study on cancer survival during 1971–83 showed that council tenants had poorer survival than owner-occupiers for the combined group of all cancers, and for 11 out of 13 cancers examined in men and 12 out of 15 in women. The differences were found irrespective of age, cause of death or prognosis of cancer. Analysis of the length of follow-up indicated that council tenants were more likely to present for treatment at a later stage than owner-occupiers. This delay in seeking treatment was judged to be one of the main contributing causes of the survival differences (Kogevinas *et al.*, 1991).

In the Whitehall study of male civil servants, larger differentials in

Table 3: *Mortality of men aged 15–64 by alternative social classifications. Longitudinal Study 1976–81*

Social classification Social class	SMR	Percentage of expected deaths
I	67	5
II	77	20
III (NM)	105	10
II(M)	96	37
IV	109	17
V	125	7
Other	189	4
Men in social class I and II with car access and owner-occupied housing	67	17
Men in social classes I–V without access to a car and living in rented accommodation	123	21

Source: Adapted from Goldblatt (1990a).

mortality were observed when employment grade was combined with details of car ownership than when employment grade alone was used. For example, a greater than fourfold difference in mortality was observed between the lowest grade without access to a car and the administrators with a car. When employment grade was used alone, there was a threefold difference between the two grades (Davey Smith *et al.*, 1990a).

Differences in morbidity in different tenure groups were observed in the Health and Life-style Survey. Overall, owner-occupiers were in better health than council tenants, whether they were in non-manual or manual social classes. These differences were greater for women than for men, particularly between non-manual women in owner-occupied housing and the much poorer health of non-manual women in rented accommodation. For men, there was better health among manual workers in owner-occupied housing than among non-manual workers in rented housing (Blaxter, 1990).

Women's health and social circumstances

In the past few years, the once-neglected area of inequalities in women's health has been given more attention and good reviews are available (Roberts, 1990; Moser *et al.*, 1990b; Arber, 1991).

Life-expectancy estimates show that in 1991 new-born girls could expect to live nearly six years longer than new-born boys, to 78.8 years and 73.2 years respectively, an improvement of over two years since 1981 (Central Statistical Office, 1992). In addition there are higher levels of male deaths in every age-group from birth right through to adulthood, when the adult ratio of male to female deaths is approximately 2:1 (Hart, 1991). Furthermore, the causes of death vary between men and women for different age-groups. One striking difference in young people is in accidental deaths. Approximately 40 per cent of deaths in boys aged 1–14 are due to accidents and violence compared with about 25 per cent of deaths in girls. By middle age, circulatory disease had assumed prominence for men while cancer claimed a high proportion of lives in women.

In general the pattern of differences in morbidity is reversed. Overall, women consistently record higher levels of chronic and acute sickness.

The picture is not quite as simple, though, when other factors like age, type of illness, social class and employment status are considered separately or in combination. Then certain groups of women can be seen to have less illness than their male counterparts, and among women themselves the rates of illness differ greatly with their differing social circumstances, as is the case for men.

When different ages are considered, for example, boys and young men are found to have higher rates of serious illness than girls. The National Survey of Health and Development found that serious illness in 21–25-year-olds was significantly more common in young men (15.8 per cent) than in young women (11.8 per cent) and the relationship held within each social class (Wadsworth, 1986). In 1988–9 a higher proportion of women (38 per cent) than men (36 per cent) reported having a long-standing illness. However, there was little difference between men and women in the age-groups 16 to 74. The noticeable difference emerged in the over-75s, when 70 per cent of women and 61 per cent of men had long-standing illness (OPCS, 1991b).

Psychological well-being also showed different patterns with age in men and women. In a pilot study men showed a steady decline in well-being with age, though for women well-being was lower in young women under 30 and older women over 70, but was much improved in the years between 50 and 59 (Blaxter, 1985).

When social class, family circumstances and employment status are brought into the equation the picture becomes even more complex. In this context current work in the Longitudinal Study is focusing on inequalities in women's health to see if some combination of social indicators would provide a better measure of the social circumstances of women than occupational class alone (which for married women is based on the husband's occupation). For instance, mortality differentials have been examined using a woman's occupation and that of her husband (if married), as well as housing tenure and household access to a car. Three separate groups of women were considered: single with an occupational class, married with an occupational class, and housewives (Moser *et al.*, 1988). Distinct groups with more than twofold differences in mortality could be differentiated by these methods. For example, among single women those with non-manual jobs and a car had SMR of 69, those with manual jobs and no car had SMR of 178. Among married housewives, those living in owner-occupied housing, with a car and a husband with a non-manual occupation, had SMR of 65; those in rented housing, with no car and a husband with a manual occupation, had SMR of 161. Among married women with an occupation the differentials were not quite as marked, but still evident. Those with non-manual jobs with non-manual husbands who were owner-occupiers and car-owners had SMR of 70, while those who had manual jobs and manual husbands in rented housing with no car had SMR of 113. This approach has also shown that there are advantaged and disadvantaged groups of women with widely differing mortality rates even at ages 75 and over in a way that occupational class alone could not do (Goldblatt, 1990b).

Further work on the Longitudinal Study has investigated how much the life-cycle stage affects these socio-economic differentials in mortality (Moser *et al.*, 1990a and b). To do this, the analysis concentrated on three groups of married women: those with no children; those with dependent children (aged 0–16); and those with grown-up children (aged 17 and over). Added to the equation was their own and their husband's social class, and whether they were housewives, or in full-time or part-time employment. Table 4 shows mortality experience between the ages of 15 and 59 for these three different stages of the life-cycle, coupled with social class and employment factors.

Table 4 illustrates several points:

1. Socio-economic differentials in mortality in women persisted at each life-cycle stage, irrespective of whether women were classified by their own or their husband's social class.

2. Looking at women in employment, generally women in non-manual jobs had lower mortality than those in manual jobs. Among those in non-manual jobs, part-timers had lower mortality than full-timers. In contrast, there was no consistent difference between the mortality of women in

Table 4: *Mortality in 1976–81 of married women by life-cycle stage, economic activity, social class, and hours worked in 1971*

A. *Mortality (SMRs) of married women with no children*

| | In paid employment | | | | Housewives |
| | Non-manual (own social class) | | Manual (own social class) | | |
	Full-time	Part-time	Full-time	Part-time	
Husband's social class, non-manual	85	59	82	—	85
Husband's social class, manual	94	103	116	112	144
Total (*All = 101*)	89	78	110	90	119

92

B. *Mortality (SMRs) of married women with at least one dependent child*

| | In paid employment | | | | Housewives |
| | Non-manual (own social class) | | Manual (own social class) | | |
	Full-time	Part-time	Full-time	Part-time	
Husband's social class, non-manual	104	49	76	103	65
Husband's social class, manual	117	85	91	93	107
Total (*All = 89*)	110	64	89	95	90

88

C. *Mortality (SMRs) of married women with youngest child aged 17 +*

| | In paid employment | | | | Housewives |
| | Non-manual (own social class) | | Manual (own social class) | | |
	Full-time	Part-time	Full-time	Part-time	
Husband's social class, non-manual	71	66	32	88	81
Husband's social class, manual	79	51	108	99	136
Total (*All = 94*)	75	59	96	97	113

82

Source: Adapted from Moser *et al.* (1990a and 1990b).

manual jobs working full-time or part-time. In general, women in part-time non-manual jobs had the lowest mortality in each life-cycle stage.

3. Looking at women not in employment, high mortality was confined to those who did not have dependent children. Women with dependent children had mortality levels comparable to those in employment (SMR approximately 90). Large differences in mortality by husband's social class were apparent for housewives irrespective of life-cycle stage, with death rates over one and a half times as high in women married to manual workers as those married to men in non-manual occupations (Moser *et al.*, 1990a and 1990b). Differences by husband's social class were not as great for employed women.

This picture of greater class differences for housewives than for women in employment can also be seen when illness, rather than mortality, is studied (Arber, 1987). An analysis combining data from the 1985 and 1986 General Household Surveys found that for chronic sickness, housing tenure also showed inequalities in health of a similar magnitude for both women and men. Combining various factors concerned with employment status, family roles and household charateristics showed that occupational class and paid employment were strongly associated with chronic sickness for women and men. Family roles were also important for women. For example, women without children and previously married women had particularly poor health status, especially those not in paid employment and living in local authority housing (Arber, 1991).

How should these findings on paid employment and women's health be interpreted, particularly the favourable position of non-manual women who work part-time? Two alternative explanations have been put forward. One possibility is that part-time work may be directly beneficial to health for some women, for example by allowing them to increase their income, have a fulfilling job while still having some time for domestic responsibilities. Full-time work, on the other hand, may be detrimental to health because of the added stress of trying to fit in the multiple roles of housewife, mother and employee, except for those women in more fortunate circumstances who can pay for help with some of their responsibilities (Arber *et al.*, 1985).

An alternative explanation is that part-time non-manual work is an indirect marker for social advantage for women, just as car- and house-ownership can be considered as indirect indicators of affluence and command over resources. The argument in this case would suggest that the choice of non-manual part-time work is more readily available to women in more favourable social circumstances, who have better health because of these circumstances rather than because of some attribute of the part-time job as such. These two explanations are being investigated by the use of the OPCS Longitudinal Study (Moser *et al.*, 1990b).

The interaction of social support, socio-economic position and mental as well as physical health is also of importance to the study of women's health. One much-quoted study showed that working-class women living in urban areas run very high risks of depression, with a threefold difference between the rates for working-class and professional women (Brown and Harris, 1982). It has been suggested that one contributory factor in such findings may be the greater degree of social isolation and lack of supporting networks for women living in disadvantaged conditions. Certainly, there is growing evidence that social isolation and poor social support (in quality and quantity) are linked to poor mental and physical health, and that, conversely, a close or confiding relationship may be protective of health (Berkman and Syme, 1979; Berkman and Breslow, 1983; House *et al.*, 1988; Bowling *et al.*, 1991; Blaxter, 1990; Marmot *et al.*, 1991).

In summary, the familiar statement that men have higher mortality than women, but women suffer more illness is obviously an oversimplification and social circumstances of both men and women are important considerations. For women, alternative social classifications, using such factors as household characteristics, employment status and family roles, may yield much more useful information than classifications based on occupational class alone. These new techniques are beginning to reveal large inequalities in health between different groups of women in the population.

Regional and area-based differences

The Black Report commented on differences in mortality between the major regions of the UK, with mortality rates increasing from the South and South-East to the North and North-West of the country. These regional differences have persisted into the 1980s, as illustrated in Table 5.

Table 5 gives the age-standardized death rates for men and women of working age in various regions of Britain. The general North-West/South-East gradient is evident for men and married women, though it is not as distinct for single women. If anything, the relative position of the North may have worsened over recent decades and East Anglia continues to exhibit the lowest mortality. Likewise, analysis by cause of death shows the same broad pattern for most diseases with the notable exception of malignant melanoma, leukaemia, and cancers of the breast and prostate, which show higher mortality in the South and East (Britton, 1990).

Table 5: *Mortality of men and women in different regions of Britain (1979–80 plus 1982–3)*

| | *Direct age-standardized death rate per 1,000* | | |
| | Men (20–64) | Single women (20–59) | Married women (20–59) |
Region			
Central Clydeside	7.86	1.78	3.23
Strathclyde	7.14	1.66	3.06
North	6.43	1.56	2.50
North-West	6.37	1.69	2.52
Remainder of Scotland	6.13	1.47	2.58
Wales	5.86	1.43	2.34
Yorkshire & Humberside	5.83	1.48	2.32
West Midlands	5.72	1.54	2.26
East Midlands	5.28	1.40	2.14
South-East	4.88	1.29	1.97
South-West	4.82	1.32	1.93
East Anglia	4.37	1.14	1.79
Scotland	6.92	1.62	2.89
England & Wales	5.43	1.41	2.17
Britain	5.57	1.43	2.23

Source: Townsend *et al.* (1986b), derived from OPCS (1986b).

At a more local level of district, county and borough councils, the overall impact of the twenty most common causes of death was assessed by counting the number of times a locality featured with high mortality. The more frequently listed were clustered in inner-city areas including South Wales, Great Manchester, Merseyside, Tyneside, Teesside and Greater London – the only one in the South (Britton, 1990).

Variation in infant mortality in relation to birth-weight was analysed for 1983–5 (Botting and Macfarlane, 1990). The results showed a clear geographic gradient in neonatal mortality rates, with all the regional health authorities in the south of England and only Mersey in the north having rates below that for England and Wales as a whole. The rates for Yorkshire, West Midlands, Wales and Northern were considerably above the national level. For post-neonatal mortality, higher than average rates could still be seen in the mid 1980s for Yorkshire, North-Western, Wessex and South-East Thames, but there was no clear North/South divide.

At the more local level, health districts with exceptionally high infant mortality rates tended to have above average proportions of mothers born

Table 6: *SMRs for all causes, 1979–80, 1982–3, by region and occupational class* (*men aged 20–64 and women aged 20–59*)

	Men			Women		
Standard region/country	I & II	IV & V	IV & V as % of I & II	I & II	IV & V	IV & V as % of I & II
North	81	152	188	80	136	170
Wales	79	144	182	79	125	158
Scotland	87	157	180	91	141	155
North-West	83	146	176	86	135	157
Yorkshire & Humberside	79	134	170	78	120	154
West Midlands	75	127	169	77	113	147
South-East	67	112	167	71	100	141
East Midlands	74	122	165	73	110	151
South-West	69	108	156	70	96	137
East Anglia	65	93	143	69	81	117
Great Britain	74	129	174	76	116	153

Note: SMR for all men, and for all women, in Great Britain in 1979–80, 1982–3, is 100. Regions ranked by SMR for classes IV and V combined as a proportion of SMR for classes I and II combined. Women classified on own, or husband's occupation.

Source: Townsend (1988a), derived from OPCS (1986b).

in the New Commonwealth and Pakistan, and above average proportions of fathers in social classes IV and V.

The interaction between area of residence and occupational class is illustrated by Table 6 where distinct regional differences in the size of the health gap between the richest and the poorest occupational classes can be seen. As the table shows, it is in the North that the gap between the health of the rich and the poor is at its greatest – mortality in classes IV and V is 188 per cent of that for class I and II men, and for women the figure is 170 per cent (Townsend *et al.*, 1988).

Information on differences in death rates has now been supplemented by data on disease and fitness and these, on the whole, reinforce the familiar picture. For instance, the North and Midlands had higher rates of chronic disease than the South when the age composition of each region was taken into account, though Wales and Scotland did not have as high rates as expected. The North/South gradient showed up for most disease

Table 7: *Mortality in 1971–81 of males in selected clusters by housing tenure (1971)*

Cluster	Owner-occupied SMR	Privately rented SMR	Local authority SMR
	Housing tenure		
Residential retirement areas	83	97	104
New towns	78	78	112
Older industrial settlements with low stress	94	115	119
Inner areas with low-quality, older housing	112	137	134

Source: Fox *et al.* (1984), OPCS Longitudinal Study.

conditions, for example arthritis/rheumatism, bronchitis, stomach disease, depression and heart disease, though asthma rates showed the reverse trend. Indicators of fitness showed people in Wales and Scotland in a poorer state of health (Cox *et al.*, 1987).

Coupled with this, further insight into the pattern of regional differences has been gained by the series of small-area analyses which have flourished since 1980. Previous studies had examined differences at the level of large areas such as regions and counties. However, several authors have detailed the potential for studies based on smaller areas and a number of recent technical advances, explained in Chapter 8, have made such studies possible (Carstairs, 1981a). The OPCS Longitudinal Study has the advantage of being able to study the deaths of specific individuals, linking details of their area of residence and household characteristics to some of their medical records. For example, it has looked at the relationship between housing tenure and mortality in different types of local authority ward. Thirty-six distinct ward types have been identified in England and Wales, ranging from residential retirement areas to new towns and inner-city areas. In thirty-five of the thirty-six types of ward, owner-occupiers had lower SMRs than local authority tenants (Fox *et al.*, 1984). Table 7 gives the evidence on four different ward types illustrating the familiar tenure gradient. It also highlights another point: that in each tenure category there was quite a large variation in death rates in different areas. For example, owner-occupiers in residential retirement areas had much lower mortality ratios than owner-occupiers in inner-city areas.

Details of some of the major small-area studies are listed in Table 8. A number of general points can be made about the findings:

1. Large differences exist between communities within one administrative area. In Sheffield, for instance, there was a difference in men's life expectancy of over eight years between the most affluent and the most deprived wards (Thunhurst, 1985a). And as the Greater Glasgow Health Board reported in 1984: 'In several communities [in the GGHB area] death rates are as low as or even lower than in the healthiest countries in the world – whereas in many others death rates are among the highest anywhere.'

2. These large variations suggest that the concept of the North/South gradient in Britain is far too simplistic. In studies in the Northern Region and in Bristol, for instance, it was found that the healthiest areas in the Northern Region compared well with the healthiest areas in and around Bristol. Such evidence is masked when analysis is carried out at the County or Regional Health Authority level. This issue should be considered in the light of point 3 below.

3. Several of these studies have shown very clearly the association between poor health and various indicators of social and material deprivation. This may be the key to the North/South gradient. Although there are very affluent areas in Scotland and the North, there is also the greatest concentration of material deprivation. It is this factor which may determine the overall regional health profile.

4. Some studies have been able to examine in more detail which particular factors in a deprived area are linked to the poor health record. Occupational class, unemployment rate and housing tenure differences 'explained' some but not all of the observed differences in health. In the comparison of Scotland with England and Wales, material deprivation was much more common in Scotland and much of the excess mortality in Scotland and England and Wales was 'explained' by differences in deprivation factors (Carstairs and Morris, 1989).

In addition to the studies in Table 8, several areas have produced local 'Black Reports' in which health profiles for specific areas have been drawn up and in some reports strategies have been put forward for local action on inequalities in health. Areas for which reports have been produced include: Merseyside (Ashton, 1984); Coventry (Binysh *et al.*, 1985); Manchester (Manchester City Council, 1985); Grimsby (Cubbon, 1986); Glyndon, Greenwich (Betts, 1985); Moyard, Belfast (Ginnety *et al.*, 1985); Glasgow (Forwell, 1991; Greater Glasgow Health Board, 1984); and Stoke-on-Trent (Thunhurst and Postma, 1989).

Further small-area studies cover unemployment and hospital admissions in children (Stirland, 1985) and the mapping of childhood accidents in Haringey (Constantinides and Walker, 1985).

Table 8: *Deprivation and ill-health. Small-area analyses*

Study	Findings
Carstairs (1981b). 37 municipal wards in Glasgow, 23 in Edinburgh	Good evidence of greater mortality and morbidity in areas of greater deprivation (except for perinatal and infant deaths)
Carstairs and Morris (1989). All post-code sectors in Scotland and wards in England and Wales	Strong correlation between deprivation and mortality, particularly steep in young adults. Deprivation worse in Scotland
Thunhurst (1985a). 29 wards in Sheffield	Clear correlation between 'areas of poverty' and mortality for men and women. For men, life expectancy over eight years greater in most affluent wards compared with most deprived
Townsend *et al.* (1986a). 755 wards in London	Mortality rates in the most deprived wards nearly double that of the least deprived wards
Townsend *et al.* (1986b, 1988). 678 wards in Northern Region	Correspondence between ill-health and deprivation extremely close. The strongest association between health and deprivation variables was with lack of a car (proxy for low income)
Townsend (1988b). 210 wards in Greater Manchester	High correlation found between deprivation and poor health, and evidence in the 1980s of growing divide in living standards and quality of life
Fox *et al.* (1984). 36 geographic clusters of wards in England and Wales. Longitudinal study – individuals linked directly to data	Pattern of low mortality in high-status clusters and high mortality in low-status clusters

Employed or unemployed: the health difference

Another factor which has been used as a general indicator of poverty or social disadvantage is unemployment, and it has become of increasing concern with the recessions of the early 1980s and 1990s. Several reviews have been valuable in bringing together the evidence on particular aspects of the subject (Smith, 1987a; Platt, 1984; Macfarlane and Cole, 1985; Iversen, 1989; Starrin *et al.*, 1989; Bartley, 1990).

As in previous decades, the unemployed tend to have much poorer health than those in work, and areas of the country with high levels of unemployment have worse health records than areas with low levels of unemployment. For example, high death rates for unemployed men have been recorded in various British studies, including the British Regional Heart Study of 1978–80 (Cook *et al.*, 1982), and the OPCS Longitudinal Study which found particularly high levels of lung cancer, suicide, accidents and heart disease among the unemployed (Moser *et al.*, 1984 and 1990c; Fox and Shewry, 1988).

Many studies have confirmed this association between suicide (or attempted suicide) and unemployment. For instance, one study found that in each year since 1977 the unemployment rate in Great Britain had been positively and significantly correlated with the total suicide rate (Kreitman and Platt, 1984). A study in Edinburgh during 1968–82 found that the unemployed had a much greater risk of attempted suicide than employed men – of the order of 11:1 (Platt and Kreitman, 1984). The risk ratio increased sharply with the length of the spell of unemployment, as follows:

Duration of unemployment in 1982 (men)	*Ratio of risk of attempted suicide of unemployed to employed*
Less than 6 months	6 : 1
6–12 months	10 : 1
Over 12 months	19 : 1

Similarly, a study in Oxford in 1979–82 found that the attempted suicide rates for unemployed men were twelve to fifteen times higher than those for employed men, and again were particularly high for the long-term unemployed (Hawton and Rose, 1986). In a later study looking at both Edinburgh and Oxford in 1980–82, unemployed women had even higher rates of attempted suicide than unemployed men (Platt *et al.*, 1988). Studies of national economies and national health statistics have also shown consistent correlation between indicators of recession and mortality in several countries (Brenner, 1979, 1983).

The unemployed experience higher levels of illness, too. For example, age-standardized illness ratios have been calculated from the General Household Survey for 1985–6 to give an indication of the relative risk of limiting long-standing illness in different groups. Employed men were more than 20 per cent less likely to report limiting chronic illness than all men, while the unemployed were over 30 per cent more likely to report such illness. The retired and permanently sick had even higher ratios.

Unemployed women had chronic illness ratios 28 per cent above the average for all women, while the ratios for housewives were 10 per cent above average. When the data on employment status were combined with housing tenure, housewives and unemployed men and women living in council housing reported very poor health indeed (Arber, 1991).

Poorer health and development have also been found in the children of the unemployed. Using data from the 1981 census it was found that children living in deprived districts of Glasgow were nine times more likely to be admitted to hospital than children in non-deprived districts. Overcrowding and parental unemployment were the aspects of deprivation most strongly correlated with hospital admission rates (Maclure and Stewart, 1984). A study of births in the Greater Dublin area found a higher incidence of low birth-weight in babies with unemployed fathers than in those whose fathers were employed (Dowding, 1981). In addition, children with unemployed fathers, especially the long-term unemployed, tended to be shorter than those whose fathers were in work (Macfarlane and Cole, 1985).

In the face of such abundant evidence of inequality the problems of interpretation need to be borne in mind. Are people who are in poor health more likely to become unemployed, or does the experience of unemployment itself have an adverse effect on health? Is it unemployment or an associated factor which causes areas of high unemployment to have high mortality and morbidity rates? Is the poor health experienced by a nation in times of recession a result solely of unemployment or is it also the result of deteriorating safety standards and increased stress on those in work? Separating the effect of unemployment from these other factors has been difficult. Some recent studies, however, show promise in disentangling cause and effect.

For example, the British Regional Heart Study of 1978–80 investigated, in particular, cardiovascular disease in middle-aged men selected at random from general practices in twenty-four towns. The unemployed sample was subdivided into those who said they were unemployed because of ill-health (the 'ill unemployed'), and those who considered that their unemployment was not due to illness (the 'not-ill unemployed'). It found that the frequencies of bronchitis, obstructive lung disease and ischaemic heart disease were indeed higher in the 'ill unemployed' than in the employed group. The rates of ischaemic heart disease were also significantly higher in the 'not-ill unemployed' compared with the employed population. Although smoking and heavy drinking were more common among the unemployed, once adjustments to the data had been made to allow for social class and town of residence, only smoking was slightly higher among the unemployed. Overall the authors concluded that the ischaemic heart disease rate was significantly higher in the 'not-ill unemployed' than the employed, when standardized for age, social class, town of residence and cigarette-smoking. However, this evidence was subject to the limitations of cross-sectional research, and a longitudinal follow-up is under way (Cook *et al.*, 1982).

The OPCS Longitudinal Study has been following a sample of men who were 'seeking work' at the time of the 1971 census and their mortality was recorded over the next ten years. As mentioned previously, the study found that these men had high mortality rates (SMR of 136) compared with that of all men in the study (SMR of 100). Some of the excess was 'explained' by occupational class factors, as unemployment was concentrated heavily in classes IV and V; but when adjustments were made to control for occupational class, it still left a 21 per cent excess in mortality unexplained. Two factors argue against any suggestion that these men became unemployed simply because they were already unhealthy. Firstly, those labelled as 'seeking work' in 1971 would be selected for *good* health, since there were two 'sickness' categories in the census to describe those not working because of poorer health. Secondly, women whose husbands were 'seeking work' were found to have raised mortality rates too (SMRs of 120 when compared with 100 for all married women in private households), suggesting a real effect of unemployment on families (Moser *et al.*, 1984). Later evidence from the Longitudir.al Study, relating to men who were seeking work in 1981, shows a similar pattern. The high death rates of men seeking work in 1981 could not be explained by the state of their health or social class before unemployment. Taken together the results lend support to the argument that unemployment had a genuine effect on the mortality rates (Moser *et al.*, 1987). Further evidence from this source shows that ill-health, marriage breakdown, movement into local authority housing and downward occupational mobility *followed* unemployment in the 1970s (Fox and Shewry, 1988). In contrast, the DHSS cohort study of unemployed men could find no evidence of a deterioration in self-reported health with unemployment, using the simple question: 'Has your health got better, got worse, or stayed about the same since registration?' (Moylan *et al.*, 1984).

The evidence that unemployment causes a deterioration in mental health is extremely strong. Several studies of people moving in and out of work have shown a decline in mental health on becoming unemployed and an improvement following re-employment. For example, numerous studies of minor psychiatric illness using the General Health Questionnaire found significant improvements in mental health when the unemployed were in work again (Warr, 1985).

In a most significant study in 1982 the General Health Questionnaire was used to assess young people moving from employment to unemployment or vice versa. It was able to test the young people before they left school and at intervals afterwards. Psychiatric symptoms increased significantly in those who left school and became unemployed and decreased in those who found work. As there had been no significant difference in mental health between the two groups while they were still at school, this is the clearest evidence yet of unemployment being the *cause* of poorer health (Banks and Jackson, 1982). Studies which have adopted an in-depth case-study approach have been able to document the effect of unemployment on family life and have shown that wives and children of unemployed men can also suffer psychologically (Fagin and Little, 1984), and financially (Heady and Smyth, 1989).

In a study based on one general practice in England, researchers have been tracing the health of workers from a meat-product factory over the course of eight years. They found a significant increase in GP consultation rates and out-patient referrals when the workers were made redundant, while a control group in stable employment in neighbouring factories showed no such increase. Furthermore, the decline in health was evident two years prior to job loss, dating from the time when the threat of redundancy became apparent. The results suggested that the *threat* of redundancy may be a stress equal to the actual event (Beale and Nethercott, 1985, 1986a, 1986b).

To sum up, the unemployed population continues to have poorer health than those in work. Studies in Britain since 1980 have provided firm evidence that unemployment can cause a deterioration in mental health. The evidence that unemployment *causes* physical ill-health and suicide is less conclusive, though the OPCS Longitudinal Study provides evidence of excess mortality in the unemployed which cannot easily be explained away.

Health and ethnic origin

It is useful to define precisely what is meant by the terms in this section. Adopting Donovan's definition (1984),

'minority', 'ethnic', or 'ethnic minority' group is used to describe any group of people who share a cultural heritage, are not part of the majority, and may experience varying degrees of discrimination – the term 'black people' in general tends to refer to people of Asian or Afro-Caribbean descent who share the common experience of differentiation or racial discrimination in Britain because of the colour of their skin.

It is also important to point out that it can be misleading to lump all members of ethnic minorities into one disadvantaged category. There is great variation in health status among the ethnic minorities and it is more fruitful to examine in which areas specific disadvantages lie.

It is we believe mistaken to treat being black, or old and alone, or single parenthood as part of the definition of deprivation. Even if many among these minorities are deprived, some are not and the point is to find out how many *are* deprived rather than operate as if all were in that condition. It is the form their deprivation takes and not their status which has to be measured. (Townsend *et al.*, 1986b)

Unfortunately, studies in this area are hampered by the way in which health information on ethnic groups is collected. Researchers have to rely almost entirely on the country of birth recorded on documents such as birth and death certificates to infer ethnic origin. This means that, apart from infant mortality data, there is still very little information on the health of British-born children of ethnic minority groups. The Black Report made this point (p. 51) and it is still relevant today. However, a little more information has come to light since then.

There are a number of specific illnesses which are nowadays far more common in certain ethnic minorities than in the population as a whole – for example, rickets in children of Asian origin, sickle-cell anaemia in people of Afro-Caribbean descent, and tuberculosis in several immigrant groups. The evidence on these is reviewed by Donovan (1984), and a particular focus on health in childhood is given by the National Children's Bureau (1987). The wider evidence on health and health care for ethnic minorities is reviewed by McNaught (1985) and Grimsley and Bhat (1988).

In 1984 the first major Immigrant Mortality Study in England and Wales was published (Marmot *et al.*, 1984a). It focused on people born outside those two countries who were over twenty years of age. It therefore *excluded* British-born members of minority groups and *included* British subjects born abroad. The mortality rates for most immigrant groups were lower than that of their countries of birth, indicating that healthier than average individuals 'selected' themselves for immigration. The exception was for immigrants from Ireland whose mortality was higher than that in Ireland or in England and Wales. Table 9 summarizes the main findings. For many diseases the pattern of mortality varied considerably from that commonly found in the country as a whole. All immigrant groups had higher mortality than the average for England and Wales for tuberculosis and accidents, but lower than average for diseases like bronchitis. Immigrants from the Indian subcontinent also had low mortality from several

Table 9: *Summary of main findings of Immigrant Mortality Study* (*England and Wales, 1970–78*)

Mortality by cause	Comparison with death rates for England and Wales
Tuberculosis	*High* in immigrants from the Indian subcontinent, Ireland, the Caribbean, Africa and Scotland
Liver cancer	*High* in immigrants from the Indian subcontinent, the Caribbean and Africa
Cancer of stomach, large intestine, breast	*Low* mortality among Indians
Ischaemic heart disease	*High* mortality found in immigrants from the Indian subcontinent
Hypertension and stroke	*Strikingly high* mortality among immigrants from the Caribbean and Africa – four to six times higher for hypertension and twice as high for strokes as the level in England and Wales
Diabetes	*High* among immigrants born in the Caribbean and the Indian subcontinent
Obstructive lung disease (including chronic bronchitis)	*Low* in all immigrants in comparison with ratio for England and Wales
Maternal mortality	*High* in immigrants from Africa, the Caribbean, and to a lesser extent the Indian subcontinent
Violence and accidents	*High* in all immigrant groups

Source: Adapted from Marmot *et al.* (1984a).

cancers which are common in this country, but they had high mortality from liver cancer, ischaemic heart disease and diabetes. Those born in the African Commonwealth or the Caribbean had higher than average mortality from liver cancer, strokes, maternal conditions and (for the Caribbean only) diabetes.

In addition, a detailed analysis was carried out of deaths in England and Wales of people born in India, Pakistan or Bangladesh, for the years 1975–7 (Balarajan *et al.*, 1984). This confirmed the findings of the Immigrant Mortality Study described above and provided further insight into mortality differences. Observed mortality for these groups was higher than expected for infective and parasitic disease, diabetes, ischaemic heart disease, cerebrovascular disease and cirrhosis of the liver. Fewer than expected deaths were due to cancer (notably lung cancer) and chronic bronchitis. Comparing different groups from the subcontinent with each other, proportional mortality ratios for cancer were lower for Hindu groups than for Moslems, and lowest for Punjabis. The rate for ischaemic heart disease was highest in Moslems. Significantly more Punjabi men died from cerebrovascular disease and cirrhosis of the liver. Diabetes was commonest among Gujaratis.

A further study of ethnic differences using data from the Decennial Supplements of 1970–72 and 1979–83 found very similar patterns for ischaemic heart disease and cerebrovascular disease as the earlier Immigrant Mortality Study. In 1979–83, mortality from ischaemic heart disease was highest in men and women born in the Indian subcontinent, especially so for young Indian men. Other groups with raised mortality included Irish, Scottish and Polish-born immigrants. Those born in the Caribbean, the Old Commonwealth and USA had low death rates. Mortality declined between 1970–72 and 1979–83 by 5 per cent in men and 1 per cent in women for England and Wales as a whole. However, immigrant groups with raised mortality in the early 1970s showed little improvement over the decade, and mortality from ischaemic heart disease increased among Indians, by 6 per cent in men and 13 per cent in women. For cerebrovascular disease, mortality was highest in Caribbeans in 1979–83, followed by Africans, Indians and Irish, with low rates in West Europeans. Over the decade, mortality from stroke declined by 28 per cent overall with most ethnic groups showing a similar decline. Men from the Indian subcontinent, however, only showed a decline of 3 per cent (Balarajan, 1991).

Analysis of the 1978 and 1980 General Household Survey showed that smoking and drinking habits varied considerably by country of origin. Heavy drinking was significantly higher in Irish men, with the lowest levels in those born in the Indian subcontinent. Heavy smoking was significantly higher in both Irish and Scottish men, with the lowest levels again recorded in those born in the Indian subcontinent. Similar smoking patterns were found for women (Balarajan and Yuen, 1986).

Attention has been focused on the health of babies born to mothers coming from the New Commonwealth countries and Pakistan. Fig. 4 gives the OPCS statistics on outcome of pregnancy for 1990, showing stillbirth, perinatal, neonatal and post-neonatal mortality by country of birth of mother. Infant mortality rates are strikingly high for babies of mothers born in Pakistan and to a certain extent in babies of mothers from the Caribbean (OPCS, 1992). This illustrates a common pattern found in a major study in the mid 1980s (Britton, 1990). In this study, the differences in mortality were not the same for each period of infancy. The differences were generally larger in the perinatal period than in the post-neonatal period, and not always in a consistent direction. For example, although all immigrant groups showed excess mortality over the indigenous population around birth and in the first month of life, post-neonatal mortality was raised only for Caribbeans and Pakistanis. In the other immigrant groups, the rate was actually *lower* than the level for the UK group. The Caribbeans and Pakistanis were the only immigrant groups to show excess mortality throughout infancy (Britton, 1990).

A number of studies centred around maternity hospitals have tried to unravel the causes of these high rates. Terry *et al.* (1980) studied all births occurring in one hospital in Birmingham in 1979. Most mothers fell into the social class IV and V categories. A high proportion of the mothers of Indian origin would be classified in a low-risk group based on age and parity, but had the highest stillbirth and perinatal mortality rates. Congenital malformation rates were highest in the Pakistani and Bangladeshi groups. The study concluded that the difference in the perinatal mortality rate was apparently not related to maternal age, parity or social class. Lumb *et al.* (1981), studying babies born to mothers of Asian origin in Bradford over the five years from 1974 to 1978, found that the perinatal mortality rate was persistently higher than for babies of mothers born in the UK. Factors operating in favour of Asian-born women were fewer teenage pregnancies, lower rates of illegitimacy and fewer smokers. Increased risks for the Asian group included more women over thirty-five, lower social class, higher parity, shorter pregnancy intervals, previous perinatal deaths, shorter duration of antenatal care, anaemia and shorter gestation.

Gillies *et al.* (1984) followed up this study in Bradford in 1975–81, looking at all births and infant deaths occurring in one health district. They found large differences in mortality between babies of Asian-born mothers and those of mothers born in the UK, associated with congenital abnormality, largely independent of social class. Risk factors (which the authors suggest might explain the findings) included low maternal height, poor antenatal attendance, anaemia, high parity of Asian-born mothers, late childbearing, high number of low birth-weight babies and consanguinity (marriages between first cousins were apparently common in Pakistani marriages in Bradford in 1981).

Studies like these have raised questions about the causes of some of the high mortality rates observed. What, for instance, would explain the high

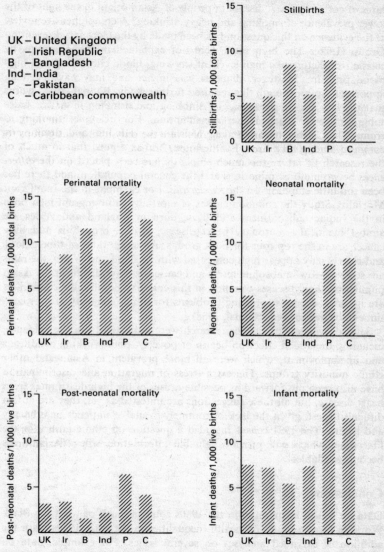

UK – United Kingdom
Ir – Irish Republic
B – Bangladesh
Ind – India
P – Pakistan
C – Caribbean commonwealth

Figure 4. *Outcome of pregnancy by mother's country of birth, England and Wales, 1990 (Source: OPCS, 1992.)*

rates of coronary heart disease in people of Asian origin in the light of the lower prevalence of smoking and heavy drinking? A comprehensive review of the evidence on this question has been made by the Coronary Prevention Group (1986). The high rates were not explained in Asian groups by classic risk factors like high levels of smoking, blood cholesterol and high blood pressure. However, diabetes was higher and may have been an important factor, though this required further study. Bhopal (1988) warns that the low overall prevalence of smoking and drinking in Asians hides subgroups with much higher consumption. For example, smoking is common in Asian men who are Muslims or Hindus, and drinking is common among Sikh men. Furthermore, he has argued that in much of the research literature too much emphasis has been placed on the *differences* between ethnic minorities and the general population, and there has been too little emphasis on the *similarities*. For example, in the Immigrant Mortality Study the common causes of mortality in immigrant men born in the Indian subcontinent and those born in England and Wales are almost identical – coronary heart disease, stroke, bronchitis and lung cancer are in the top four for both groups. Although rates of tuberculosis and rickets may appear high compared with England and Wales, the rates are still very low in absolute terms and cause far fewer deaths in the Asian population than diseases common in this country. Because the similarities are ignored, the most pressing problems for ethnic minority groups continue to be overlooked (Bhopal, 1988).

Several avenues for further research were indicated from the evidence, including the added effect on health of poverty, poor working conditions and unemployment, which were all more prevalent in Asian and other ethnic minority groups. The extra stress of migration and discrimination have also been put forward as possible causes of the high death rates from heart disease, but all these suggestions are untested as yet; they are in fact difficult to test, given the lack of routinely available statistics on ethnicity and health. The 1991 census included a question on ethnic group for the first time, which will provide valuable information when the analyses become available.

Conclusions

Data on health inequalities in the 1980s confirm much of what the Black Working Group found on health inequalities in the early 1970s, with the addition of extended analyses on several issues. For example, data on occupational class mortality have now been extended to ages over sixty-five, and still a substantial class gradient persists. The OPCS Longitudinal

Study has provided data free of numerator/denominator bias, and has confirmed a clear gradient under such conditions.

The experience of illness by occupational class has been extended into areas of self-perceived health and well-being. Lower occupational groups have been found to experience more illness which is both chronic and incapacitating. Although it is taken for granted that sickness will happen to almost everyone sooner or later, it seems that lower occupational groups experience it earlier and this must be seen as a major inequality in a welfare society.

Other indirect measures of affluence and poverty, such as household-based classifications and employment status, also highlight inequalities in health. Owner-occupiers continue to have lower rates of illness and death than private tenants, who in turn have lower rates than local authority housing tenants. It is well known, and confirmed in recent studies, that the unemployed have much poorer health than those with jobs. It is now also beyond question that unemployment *causes* a deterioration in mental health and there is increasing evidence that the same is true of physical health.

Women can expect to live longer than men and have lower mortality rates at every stage of life. However, women sometimes record higher levels of morbidity than men, depending on social and family circumstances. Research on inequalities in women's health is revealing fresh insights into the varied experience of women living in different conditions.

The overall North/South regional differences in health in Britain are still evident, but what is now becoming apparent is the great inequality in health which can exist between small areas in the same region. Areas suffering social and material deprivation have been found to have much poorer health profiles than neighbouring affluent areas. Furthermore, the gap between the health of the rich and the poor is greatest in the North.

Information on the health of ethnic minorities is mainly limited to studies of adult immigrants born outside England and Wales; there is hardly any information on the health of their descendants. A varied picture emerges. Mortality rates from lung cancer and chronic bronchitis, for example, are lower in most ethnic groups than in those born in the UK. On the other hand, deaths from coronary heart disease and accidents are disturbingly higher in many immigrant groups. There is strikingly high mortality from hypertension and strokes among people of Caribbean and African origin, and markedly higher mortality rates for babies of mothers born in Pakistan and, to a certain extent, for babies of mothers from the Caribbean. We need more information about the health of members of ethnic minority groups born in this country, but we already have sufficient to identify priorities for action.

Chapter 3

Recent Trends

There is no doubt that the health of the population as a whole has continued to improve over recent years, measured, for example, by life expectancy. In 1991 a new-born boy could expect to live to 73 years and a girl to nearly 79 – an improvement over the previous decade of over two years. Other measures of the population's health, like height and dental health, show steady improvements. As mortality rates from infectious diseases have continued to decline throughout the century, deaths in childhood have become less common, and a greater proportion of the population can now expect to live to middle and old age.

However, the news is not all good. Trends in the expectation of life without disability have not improved, despite improvements in life expectancy. This suggests that the added years of life are associated with disability and present a challenge to try to improve the quality of life of people in older age-groups. In addition, since the mid 1980s death rates among men and women aged 15–44 have stopped falling. An investigation of why this should have occurred found that some of the increase in deaths was due to the age structure of the population, with increasing numbers of 40–44-year-olds in the 15–44 age band. Allowing for this, the rates still remain level rather than declining, as increases in certain causes of death – AIDS/HIV, suicides and open verdicts in men – offset decreases in deaths from cancer and circulatory diseases. In women, deaths from cancer of the breast and cervix, digestive and nervous system diseases and open verdicts have increased and contributed to the overall trend in this age band (Dunnell, 1991).

Above all inequalities in health between different *social groups* within the population still exist on a substantial scale – as the evidence in Chapter 2 confirms. An important question now is whether these inequalities in health are increasing, decreasing or remaining the same. The Black Report, reviewing evidence from 1931 to 1971, concluded that the gap in health between different social groups had either stayed the same, or in some cases had widened. New evidence has been presented since then on trends over the past decade, and reassessments of the 1931–71 evidence have also been carried out; these will be discussed below, after an outline of some of the measurement problems.

Measurement problems

The seemingly simple task of following trends in health over time is fraught with difficulties, particularly in relation to occupational class comparisons. Some believe that the measurement problems related to occupational class are so serious that conclusions about trends cannot be made from such data (Illsley, 1986; Jones and Cameron, 1984). Others have reviewed the evidence and conclude that some analyses overcome these measurement problems (Wagstaff *et al.*, 1991; Davey Smith *et al.*, 1992; Wilkinson, 1986a and 1986b). From these reviews five main obstacles have been identified, which need to be borne in mind when assessing research on occupational class time trends:

1. *Numerator/denominator bias.* In the calculation of mortality rates the occupation of the deceased is taken from death certificates, while the total number of people in each class is calculated from occupations recorded in the ten-yearly national census. Misrecording of occupation in either source introduces bias into the calculation. OPCS points to a considerable increase in numerator/denominator bias in the latest Occupation Mortality Decennial Supplement based on the 1981 census. This census used the Registrar General's 1980 classification of occupations which changed the social class of some occupations. The recording of occupations on death certificates, however, is still much less precise and has not led to the same shift in occupations between classes. The social class mortality rates, in the form presented in the Decennial Supplement, may be misleading – especially for class V – unless analysed with care. Many believe that the data in the latest Decennial Supplement can be used by comparing manual with non-manual categories, or combining data on classes I and II and comparing it with data on classes IV and V combined. Another way to check results is to use the OPCS Longitudinal Study, which can link individuals with their mortality and socio-economic characteristics, and so does not have numerator/denominator bias.

2. *Reclassification.* Repeated reclassification of occupations at each census since 1931 has made it difficult to compare occupational classes over such a time-span, unless adjustments are made to allow for the reclassification. Acknowledging this, previous Registrars General have carried out bridging exercises to enable the old and new classifications to be compared and the effect of the changes to be gauged. Although this was not done for the

latest Decennial Supplement, the point can be checked by using the Longitudinal Study to identify individuals and code them by both 1971 and 1981 classifications to see if either affects the mortality gradients observed, (Goldblatt, 1989). Another way of overcoming this effect is to trace occupations which have stayed in the same class throughout the period under study.

3. *Changing size of classes.* The proportion of the population in each social class has changed over time. In particular, there is a smaller proportion of the population in class V and a larger proportion in classes I and II, because of an upward shift in occupations. It should be noted that class V is also being eroded by unemployment as well as by upward mobility into higher classes. Comparisons of class I with class V over thirty to fifty years are therefore not comparisons of similar-sized segments of the population. However, comparison of combined classes I and II with combined classes IV and V would compare large and roughly equal-sized slices of the population.

4. *Changing status.* Linked to the change in size of each class may be a change in the relative status of each class. For example, the status and lifestyle of the much smaller class I in 1921 or 1931 may have been very different from the status of the expanded class I in 1981, so again the studies may not be comparing like with like. At the other end of the spectrum, a shrinking class V may contain a very small section of the population, but they may have a very high risk of mortality. Again, one way to overcome this is to compare larger sections of the population by combining social classes or by using alternative social classifications to study equal and substantial sections of the population.

5. *Based on a small proportion of total deaths.* Some of the comparisons in the Black Report were based on the mortality of men aged 15–64. In 1921, deaths in this group accounted for 40 per cent of all male deaths, but by 1971 they only accounted for 31 per cent. Therefore only limited conclusions can be drawn from such data, though it is still true to say that they give a representation of premature adult male mortality. While it is true that conclusions are limited if based on deaths under the age of 65, these are a very important group, representing as they do premature or untimely deaths – and in some cases the most avoidable deaths. Many comparisons now include deaths in all working and unemployed men, their wives and babies, and have been supplemented by additional studies on women, the over-65s and on all social classes.

Recommendations have been made about which measures of inequality to use in future comparative studies (Wagstaff *et al.*, 1991).

Trends in infant and child health

Table 10 illustrates trends in deaths of babies in the first year of life, comparing combined classes I and II with combined classes IV and V. Since 1975 birth and infant death registrations have been linked, so there are no numerator/denominator problems with these figures. Over the fifteen years, although there was a general decline in death rates, the occupational class differences persisted for stillbirths and deaths in the first week of life (perinatal deaths). For example, the perinatal death rate of classes IV and V fluctuated at around 150 per cent of the rate for classes I and II during the whole period.

However, the picture for post-neonatal deaths (age one month to one year) is somewhat different. There was a clear narrowing of the mortality gap between classes I and II and IV and V in the early 1970s, though there has been little, if any, improvement since then. Trends in post-neonatal mortality since the Second World War have been traced. From 1949–50 to 1970–72 there was a rapid decline in death rates for classes I, II, III and IV, but as they reduced at the same pace the relative differential between these four classes remained the same. The decline in class V rates was much smaller, and therefore the differential between it and the other classes *widened* during that time. After 1970–72 there was another sharp overall decline in death rate but this time the greatest improvement was in class V, so the gap in mortality between the classes *narrowed* (Pharaoh and Morris, 1979).

From 1975 to 1988 post-neonatal death rates improved very little for non-manual classes, and from 1980 there was little improvement for manual classes either. The mortality gap thus remained fairly constant over the ten years, as illustrated in Fig. 5. Rates improved again for both classes in 1989 and 1990. The earlier improvement in class V rates has been attributed in part to the reduction in average family size, particularly in class V (Pharaoh and Morris, 1979; Macfarlane, 1986).

Regional differences in neonatal mortality are still evident (see p. 248). However, the regional differences in post-neonatal mortality of earlier decades, with higher rates in northern regions, disappeared by the mid 1970s, and noticeably higher rates remain in only four out of the fourteen regions: Yorkshire, North-Western, Wessex and South-East Thames (Botting and Macfarlane, 1990).

Trends in ethnic differences in infant mortality also showed some

Table 10: *Infant mortality by occupational class (1975–90)*

Deaths	1975	1977	1979	1981	1983	1985	1987	1989	1990
Perinatal deaths/1,000 total births									
Rate for classes I and II	15.0	12.6	11.4	9.3	8.1	7.6	7.0	6.6	6.2
Rate for classes IV and V	22.7	19.5	17.1	13.8	12.5	11.5	10.2	9.2	9.5
Rate for classes IV and V as % of rate for classes I and II	151	154	150	148	154	151	146	139	154
Post-neonatal deaths/1,000 live births									
Rate for classes I and II	3.1	2.9	2.9	2.8	2.8	2.7	2.7	2.1	2.0
Rate for classes IV and V	6.4	5.7	6.0	5.4	5.3	4.3	4.5	4.7	4.0
Rate for classes IV and V as % of rate for classes I and II	202	196	204	192	186	160	170	225	202

Source: Derived from OPCS data Series DH3, various years.

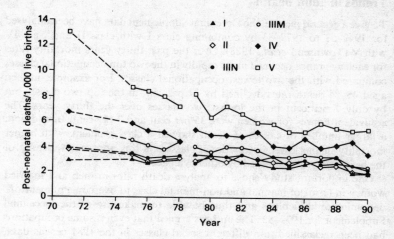

Figure 5. *Post-neonatal mortality by father's social class, England and Wales.* (*Source: OPCS Mortality Statistics, various years.*)

encouraging improvements between 1975 and 1985 (analysed by mother's country of birth). Infant mortality fell in all ethnic groups over the decade. By the mid 1980s the excess mortality for Indian, Bangladeshi and African infants seen during the 1970s had virtually disappeared. Infant mortality among West Indians and Pakistanis declined at almost the same rate as in the UK group; their excess over the UK group therefore remained virtually unchanged over the ten-year period. Trends in perinatal mortality show a significant narrowing of differentials. Although by the mid 1980s immigrant groups still showed excess mortality over the UK group, the excess was much smaller than in the 1970s. The Pakistani group was the only exception, showing the smallest improvement of all groups. In the post-neonatal period, what had been an excess mortality in the 1970s in Indian, Bangladeshi and African infants was transformed by the mid 1980s into a better rate than the UK group. Again, this improvement was not seen for Pakistani infants (Botting and Macfarlane, 1990).

For children aged 1–15, the 1959–63 social class gradient was largest for the 1–4-year-olds, and thereafter declined smoothly with age. In 1970–72 the gradient was largest for 5–9-year-olds, whereas by 1979–83 the 1–4-year-olds again had the largest gradient (OPCS, 1988).

Trends in adult health

To give a general picture, the Decennial Supplement data have been analysed for 1949–53 to 1979–83 by combining class I with class II and class IV with V (Townsend *et al.*, 1988). Over the past thirty years mortality rates for each age range declined more rapidly in the two top occupational classes compared with the two lowest occupational classes. For example, in men aged 45–54 death rates declined by 37 per cent in the top two classes but by only 7 per cent in the lowest two classes over the thirty years. The equivalent figures for women were 35 per cent and 7 per cent. In addition, a larger number of causes of death showed a class gradient, with higher mortality in the lower occupational classes. Is this apparent widening of the health gap substantiated by other evidence?

One important study chose to analyse death rates in men and married women in terms of manual and non-manual class to overcome numerator/denominator difficulties and thus be able to make use of the Decennial Supplement for 1979–83. The authors argued that even if some occupations had been reclassified into different social classes in the 1981 census data, there was no evidence that there would be any serious misclassification between these two very distinct groups. They also restricted their analysis to the recent past to avoid long-term complications (Marmot and McDowall, 1986).

The 1970–72 figures were standardized with the 1979–83 ratios to allow direct comparisons across time periods and classes. Fig. 6 summarizes the results and shows that all-cause mortality for 1979–83 fell in both groups in men and women, but because it had declined more rapidly in non-manual groups the social gap widened. When major causes of death were examined, the trends for cerebrovascular disease and lung cancer in men were similar to that for all-cause mortality. However, coronary heart disease (CHD) mortality in men in non-manual occupations fell by 15 per cent over the decade, whereas in manual occupations it increased by 1 per cent. For married women both lung cancer and CHD mortality increased in manual classes while decreasing in non-manual classes. The decline in CHD mortality was evident in non-manual men in every part of Great Britain, but only in Wales was there a noticeable decline in mortality for manual men.

The authors went on to consider what could account for this widening gap. Changes in disease classification over the ten years were examined and discounted, as was the changing size of the classes. Over the decade there was a 5 per cent decrease in manual classes and a 4 per cent increase in non-manual classes for men. They argued that a change of this order

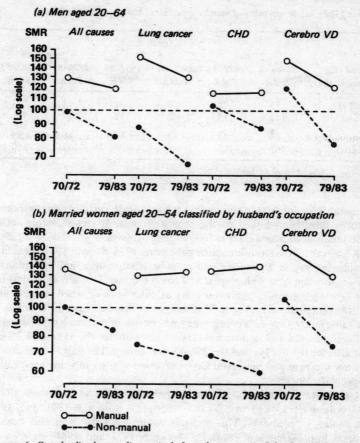

Figure 6. *Standardized mortality ratios* for select causes of death in Great Britain 1970–72 and 1979–83 for manual and non-manual groups. (Source: Marmot and McDowall, 1986. Copyright The Lancet).*

* For each cause the SMR in 1979–83 is 100 for each sex.

would not convert a 1 per cent rise in CHD mortality in manual men to a fall of 15 per cent to be in line with that of non-manual men. Their conclusion was that this reflected a genuine widening of the health gap, not influenced by statistical changes.

The OPCS Longitudinal Study is specifically designed to be free of

Table 11: *Trends in mortality of men by social class and age-group, 1976–83*

| Social class group in 1971 | Age at death | | | | | |
| | 25–64 | | 65–74 | | 75 and over | |
	1976–81 SMR	1981–83 SMR	1976–81 SMR	1981–83 SMR	1976–81 SMR	1981–83 SMR
I and II	75	78	79	81	82	81
IV and V	114	115	108	111	109	109
Non-manual	84	83	81	87	86	84
Manual	103	107	103	105	107	107

Source: Adapted from Goldblatt (1990a).

numerator/denominator bias as the sample's death certifications and other records have been linked to the census records. It can therefore retain individuals in the same class as follow-up progresses.

Results from the study comparing the years 1976–81 with 1981–3 confirm a widening gap in all-cause death rates between manual and non-manual classes for men of working ages, as Table 11 shows. It is less clear that the gap is widening for all-cause mortality at older ages, or when classes I and II are compared with IV and V. Changes in heart disease differentials in the same study showed a continuing and consistent widening of differences between manual and non-manual classes not only for the age range 25–64, but also for the 65–74s and the 75-and-over group. The gap in lung cancer did not increase and may even have narrowed slightly in some age-groups (Goldblatt, 1990a).

Using 'years of potential life lost' rather than SMR as a measure, Blane and colleagues looked at all-cause mortality from the 1971 and 1981 Decennial Supplements. This analysis confirmed that there had been a general improvement in mortality between 1971 and 1981 for men of working age, but for social class V men mortality expressed as 'years of potential life lost' had actually increased. When the three major causes of death were examined, years of potential life lost either remained stationary or increased for all three manual classes, not just class V. Any improvement was limited to social classes I, II and IIIN. In men aged 15–64, accidents and violence accounted for an increasing percentage of total years of potential life lost in *all* social classes between 1971 and 1981 (Blane *et al.*, 1990). A reworking of this analysis by plotting a concentration curve confirmed the increase in inequalities in potential life lost in the 1970s. (Wagstaff *et al.*, 1991).

So far the focus has been on trends in death rates, but illness rates also show some interesting changes. Trends in chronic illness recorded in the General Household Survey have been analysed for the years from 1972–1988 and are shown in Fig. 7 (OPCS, 1990b). These cover all ages from birth to old age. In contrast to the general fall in mortality, there is no sign of illness rates falling; rather they appear to be rising. From this analysis manual groups had higher rates of long-term illness than non-manual groups in every year, and the gap between the two groups widened over the sixteen-year period. The widening was apparent particularly between 1974 and 1984. From then until 1988 the differences did not increase further.

Another way of tackling the question is to look at trends in health measured by other socio-economic indicators which would not be subject to the same measurement problems. In the international study mentioned on p. 308 the level of education was used as an alternative measure of social position – ranging from groups with no qualifications to holders of degrees, aged eighteen and over. From this study, inequalities in mortality between different groups increased in England and Wales between the early 1970s and the 1980s because of an improvement in the higher education categories and little or no improvement in the lowest. This adds weight to the view that the widening health gap between top and bottom of the social scale is real and not dependent on the particular classification used (Valkonen, 1989).

So much for the trends over the last decade. The objections to comparisons over much longer time-spans are far more serious and need more sophisticated techniques to try to overcome them. Using widely differing statistical methods, some argue that inequalities in mortality have narrowed over the post-war period (Illsley and Le Grand, 1987; Le Grand and Rabin, 1986), while others argue that there has been a widening of differentials between social groups (Koskinen, 1985; Preston *et al.*, 1981; Pamuk, 1985). Even some statisticians get lost in the complexity of the exercise, but a current European Community project on equity in health care has brought some clarity to the issue. It has been reviewing the techniques used to assess how inequality can best be measured in studies on trends and cross-country differences (Wagstaff *et al.*, 1991). Table 12 summarizes the project's findings: the three minimum requirements of an inequality measure; the six measures in the literature to date; and an assessment of which measure is best suited to measuring health inequality. It can be seen that the range measure fails because it does not take account of the changes across all the social groups. The index of dissimilarity, the Gini coefficient and related measures fail because they do not actually

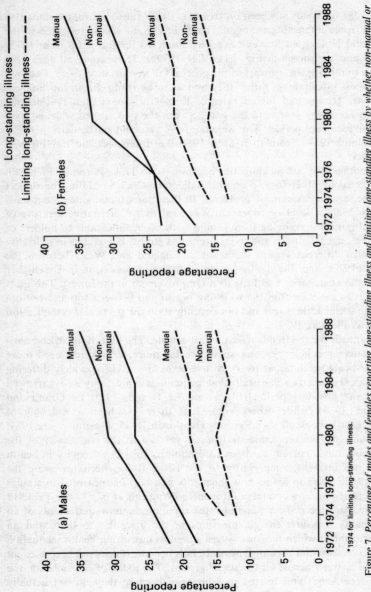

Figure 7. *Percentage of males and females reporting long-standing illness and limiting long-standing illness by whether non-manual or manual socio-economic group: Great Britain, 1972*, 1976, 1980, 1984 and 1988. (Source: OPCS, 1990b. Crown copyright.)*

*1974 for limiting long-standing illness.

measure socio-economic factors. Only the slope index of inequality (or its relative version) and the concentration index meet the three minimum requirements.

These conclusions call into question the studies which claim to have found a narrowing of inequalities since the war, as these used the Gini coefficient or related measures (Le Grand and Rabin, 1986; Illsley and Le Grand, 1987). Basically, these studies were not measuring the relevant parameters. It also calls into question some of the studies arguing for a widening of inequalities (Preston *et al.*, 1981; Koskinen, 1985), because of the unreliable techniques used. However, it provides strong support for the work of Pamuk (1985 and 1988). Pamuk used the slope index of inequality to look at social class inequality in mortality from 1921–72 in England and Wales. To overcome reclassification difficulties, 143 occupations were used, which could be traced consistently between 1921 and 1971. From this analysis the author concluded that class inequality in mortality among men declined in the 1920s but increased again during the 1950s and 1960s, so that by the early 1970s it was greater than it had been in the earlier part of the century. For married women there was a similar increase in inequality between 1949–53 and 1970–72. The class differentials in infant mortality declined dramatically in absolute terms, but still increased in relative terms, as did the adult trends (Pamuk, 1985 and 1988).

Therefore there is some support for a widening of social inequalities in health in this age-group over much of this century. The European Community project team pointed out that the data from some of the published studies can be reworked to include one of the more reliable measures – as they did for the study by Blane and colleagues quoted on p. 272. The team recommends that the relative index of inequality or the concentration index are easy to compute and should be reported in future alongside the results of comparative studies (Wagstaff *et al.*, 1991).

Have inequalities in health widened?

There are a number of fundamental problems in measuring health trends over time, but recent assessments indicate ways of overcoming them satisfactorily. The results of some studies give convincing evidence of a widening of health inequalities between social groups in post-war decades, especially in adults. In general, death rates in adults of working age have declined more rapidly in the higher than in the lower occupational classes, contributing to the widening gap. Indeed in some respects the health of the lower occupational classes has actually deteriorated against the background of a general improvement in the population as a whole. While death rates

Table 12: *Assessing measures of inequality in health*

Minimum requirements for a measure:

1. That it reflects the socio-economic dimension to inequalities in health.

2. That it reflects the experience of the entire population (rather than just the top and bottom of the scale).

3. That it is sensitive to changes in the distribution of the population across socio-economic groups.

The six measures from the literature:

- The range: fails requirements 2 and 3.
- Gini coefficient (and associated Lorenz curve): fails requirement 1.
- Pseudo-Gini coefficient (and associated pseudo-Lorenz curve): fails requirement 1.
- Index of dissimilarity: fails requirement 1.
- Slope index of inequality (and relative index of inequality): meets all requirements.
- Concentration index (and associated concentration curve): meets all requirements.

Source: Adapted from Wagstaff *et al.* (1991)

have been declining, rates of chronic illness seem to have been increasing, and the gap in the illness rates between manual and non-manual groups has been widening too, particularly in the over-65 age-group.

The exception to the widening trend was in relation to deaths in babies under one year. While there has been little change in the differential for deaths around birth and in the first month of life, great improvements have occurred in the post-neonatal period (age range from one month to one year). There was a dramatic decline in post-neonatal death rates during the 1970s in all classes, but especially for class V, and thus the gap in mortality narrowed considerably. Although there was very little further improvement at least until 1988 for manual or non-manual classes, the evidence does illustrate that the class differential is not inevitable and can be reduced. The regional differences in post-neonatal mortality, evident in earlier decades, had disappeared by the mid 1970s, though regional differences in neonatal mortality remain. Trends in ethnic difference in infant mortality also showed encouraging improvements between 1975 and 1985, though high rates in mothers born in Pakistan are still causing concern.

Chapter 4

Health Services: Fair and Equitable?

For many years, health services in this country have been based on the principle that health care should be available to all groups in the population according to their need, irrespective of their income or social position. One hundred per cent of the population has entitlement to the services of the National Health Service, which puts Britain in the top league in Europe and compares favourably with countries like the USA, where approximately 30 per cent of the population has inadequate or non-existent insurance cover for health care. However, entitlement in law does not always guarantee access to a service in practice and there has been concern that an 'inverse care law' might be operating. This was a phrase coined by Julian Tudor Hart in 1971 to describe the situation in which medical services were least available where they were most needed – an observation on the poorer provision of services in more deprived areas where mortality and morbidity were greatest (Hart, 1971).

This highlights a geographic access problem, but there may also be financial or cultural barriers preventing people from using services even if available. There may also be differences in the type or quality of care offered to different sections of the population, and all these aspects need to be brought into the equation when considering if health services are fair and equitable (Whitehead, 1990).

This chapter looks at the evidence on access, quality and uptake of services, before discussing attempts to allocate resources fairly at national and local level.

Access

Studies which have looked at availability of services in different geographical areas give a mixed picture of progress. For example, a study of the location and accessibility of GP surgeries in Aberdeen found that the location of the surgeries clearly favoured the longer-established middle-class districts of the city, and that the deprived areas were poorly served. When car ownership was considered as an additional factor, it was found that the high levels of car ownership in the owner-occupied outlying areas of the city extended accessibility to services quite markedly, while there continued to be very low levels of accessibility in the outlying local authority estates (Knox, 1979). Another study confirmed that transport difficulties to GP surgeries appeared to have a deterrent effect on the use of the service (Whitehouse, 1985).

In 1985 the availability of dental services in Newcastle upon Tyne was clearly greater in more affluent areas and poorer in officially designated 'priority areas' (Carmichael, 1985). In contrast, improvements were reported in the distribution of hospice care for terminally ill patients. A 1980 survey had shown considerable regional inequalities in provision, with the South-East generally much better off than the rest of the country. Since then the imbalance has been reduced by differential funding for hospices (Lunt, 1985).

An OPCS national survey in 1977 investigated access to primary health care in terms of ease of journey, use of appointment systems, doctors' approachability, ease of getting home-visits and so on. Most people found the services easily accessible. The proportion of people reporting difficulties was relatively small, between 5 per cent and 10 per cent of all informants, though the report did point out that this would represent over two million people nationally. As expected, those in rural areas were more likely to experience difficulties than urban dwellers, but age, sex and social class proved to be more important factors. Problems were most common among the elderly, especially manual-group women. People in social classes IV and V were less likely than others to use ophthalmic, dental and chiropody services, a finding in line with previous studies on preventive services (Richie *et al.*, 1981). Analysis of the 1982 General Household Survey provided evidence that lack of car transport was an inhibiting factor for the sick in rural areas (Haynes, 1991). Economic access also has to be considered. Examination of service use between 1979 and 1985 showed increased prescription charges leading to a decrease in service use (Ryan and Birch, 1991).

Quality of care

The quality of services is also important – the standard of premises and qualifications of staff, the treatment of patients with the same degree of professional commitment and time, whatever their social background. In this context, there is evidence that the resources invested in general practice vary by type of area. Innovative practices (employing practice nurses, improving premises with cost-rent schemes, providing training) had more partners and were often located in rural or affluent suburban areas. Practices which did not take part in schemes to improve premises and employ specialized staff had fewer partners and were more common in urban and working-class areas. Innovative practices were judged to be in the best position to increase their services, thereby increasing their income, in response to the government's primary care reforms. Practices in more deprived areas had been less able to respond to existing incentives and had a smaller margin available for developing their services in future (Bosanquet and Leese, 1988).

On further analysis of high- and low-income practices, it was found that high-income practices were more likely to be larger, have younger partners and to be located in affluent areas. Low-income practices were smaller, located in more urban areas, and more likely to have Asian partners. The high-income practices had higher costs per patient and more staff resources. Low-income practices had fewer practice resources and faced greater disincentives to investment. These practices were concentrated in less affluent areas where the need for improvement was greatest (Leese and Bosanquet, 1989).

Further studies on GP consultations have shown differences in GP responses to different social groups. For example, one study found that higher social class patients received more explanations voluntarily than did lower social class patients (Pendleton and Bochner, 1980). This is despite the evidence that demand for information and advice is widespread among all social classes and is not restricted to middle-class patients (Coulter, 1987; Cartwright, 1979).

A study of home-visiting in a large inner-London general practice found that there was a steady increase in the proportion of home-visits from class II to class V, but the proportion of home-visits was highest of all in occupational class I. When distance was also taken into consideration, class I patients living close to the health centre had by far the highest proportion of home-visits – more than double that of any other occupational class. Of the patients living farthest away from the health centre, occupational class I again had the highest proportion of visits and class V the lowest (Bucquet *et al.*, 1985).

There is also evidence that classes I and II patients are more likely to be referred to specialist services by their GP than classes IV and V patients particularly in the case of older women (Blaxter, 1984). A study in Glasgow found that clinical investigations for heart disease (coronary angiography) were performed more frequently on patients from more affluent neighbourhoods. The men with the lowest level of deprivation had only half the expected death rates from heart disease, but one and a half times their predicated rate of angiographies. In contrast, men in the most deprived areas had death rates one-third higher than average, with only three-quarters of the predicted rate of investigation. A similar pattern emerged for women and raised the question of whether doctors fail to refer or investigate these patients sufficiently (Findlay, 1991).

This leads to the more general question about whether higher social classes receive more effective treatment and whether that is a contributing factor in the differential in survival chances of people from different social classes. There is certainly evidence that higher social groups have better survival chances once disease has been diagnosed; for example, after cancer and coronary heart disease have been confirmed (Leon and Wilkinson, 1989; Kogevinas *et al.*, 1991). While Kogevinas and colleagues concluded that the survival differences for cancers of good prognosis could, in part, be due to differences in treatment, they judged that the delay in seeking treatment was one of the major contributing causes. Another study, looking at cervical cancer, which has a strong social class gradient, could find no differential in survival (Murphy *et al.*, 1990).

On a larger scale, an attempt was made in 1983 to examine the quality of health care delivery in the ninety-eight Area Health Authorities in England and Wales (Charlton *et al.*, 1983). This study chose the eleven diseases regarded as most amenable to medical intervention (excluding conditions controlled mainly by prevention). Mortality for these diseases in the different Area Health Authorities was found to vary considerably, even after adjusting for socio-economic differences between areas. Could differences in quality of health services in these areas account for the variation in death rates? The study raised this question and suggested that the findings warranted further investigation.

Treatment received by ethnic minorities, particularly for mental illnesses, has been called into question. For example, one study of psychiatric hospital patients found that black patients tended to receive harsher forms of treatment (such as electroconvulsive therapy) than their white counterparts with similar ailments (Littlewood and Cross, 1980). Although there are few studies in this area and the extent of differential treatment in the NHS is not known, it is a topic which has been heightening the concern of ethnic minority groups.

The acceptability of hospital services for 'Asian' patients has recently been investigated. The main differences between groups were that 7 per cent of Asians but 100 per cent of non-Asians received written information in their first language; 40 per cent had difficulty in communicating due to lack of English and 90 per cent of them were not satisfied with informal interpreting arrangements. Fifty-four per cent of Asian women did not like to be examined by a male doctor, but half of these did have a male doctor. Ninety per cent of Asians required a special diet, but only 19 per cent received one. This compared with 27 per cent of non-Asians requiring a special diet, most of whom received one. Despite these findings, Asian patients seldom complained (Madhok *et al.*, 1992).

Does uptake match need?

There is plenty of evidence that members of lower occupational classes make less use of preventive services for themselves and their children. Analysis of the second national morbidity survey of general practice confirmed the occupational class gradient in uptake of preventive services (Blaxter, 1984; Crombie, 1984). Differential use of services has also been recorded for screening and health promotion services (Nutbeam *et al.*, 1987; Waller *et al.*, 1990; Pill *et al.*, 1988; Thompson, 1990; Huntington and Killoran, 1991; Gillam, 1992); attendance at local authority developmental assessment clinics for pre-school children (Fisher *et al.*, 1983); frequency of attendance for dental services (Todd and Dodd, 1985; Eddie and Davies, 1985); attendance at well-woman, well-man and cervical cytology clinics (Marsh and Channing, 1986); and use of orthodontic services (Jenkins *et al.*, 1984). This raises the question of *why* these services are used less frequently by the lower socio-economic groups. Is it because of difficulties encountered in using the services or different perceptions of the need for preventive care? Possible explanations are discussed further in Chapter 6.

When the full range of primary care services (preventive and curative) is considered, the problem of assessing 'need' arises. Fig. 7 on p. 274 indicated the *potential demand* for health care and suggested that manual groups would have greater need for health services than non-manual groups. Fig. 8 shows use of GP services by the two groups and indicates that manual groups do indeed use GP services more than non-manual groups. But does their use of services completely match their increased need? This is a key question and one which has proved difficult to answer, particularly when sex and age differences in use are also taken into consideration.

In 1980 newly available data from the 1974 General Household Survey were examined (Collins and Klein, 1980). In 1974 (but not in other years) people who reported both illness and GP consultation were asked whether their consultations had been about the reported illness, thus allowing a more direct comparison of the link between use and need. They found that among men who reported no illness the professional group had higher

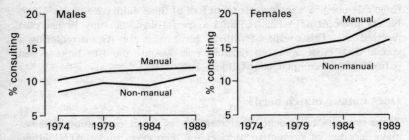

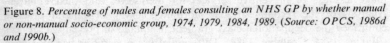

Figure 8. *Percentage of males and females consulting an NHS GP by whether manual or non-manual socio-economic group, 1974, 1979, 1984, 1989. (Source: OPCS, 1986d and 1990b.)*

consultation rates than the rest of the population. Among men who reported acute sickness or chronic sickness without limitation manual groups had higher consultation rates than non-manual groups. For men with chronic limiting illness and for women in all categories consultation rates were not systematically related to socio-economic group. From these results it was concluded that 'the NHS had achieved equity in terms of access to primary health care'. This study has been widely criticized for drawing such sweeping conclusions from the limited data and from the restricted aspect of the system studied (Scott-Samuel, 1981). For example, critics have pointed to the fact that the study was based on figures for only one year, that it was based on numbers of users of primary care and not on frequency of use, and that it took no account of the higher numbers of partly skilled and unskilled workers in the chronic sick category. As it did not cover children's access, severity of need, or nature of conditions, it was premature to suggest that equity of access throughout the NHS had been achieved (Townsend and Davidson, 1982).

OPCS subsequently re-analysed the 1974 data, with some refinements on the technique used by Collins and Klein and with the inclusion of data on children. The study found that for given rates of sickness those in the manual socio-economic groups were more likely to consult a GP than those in the non-manual groups. The result was clearer for acute than for chronic sickness and more marked for men than for women. The conclusion was that, from 1974 data, 'for the aspect studied there was no evidence of bias' (OPCS, 1986d). As similar information was collected in the 1986 GHS, an updated analysis is planned when the data become available.

Looking at the issue from a different perspective, 1980 GHS data were examined to see if the health and social services discriminated in favour of the poor and disabled. Of the elderly, 56 per cent were found to be living in poverty (defined as having income up to 40 per cent above the supplementary pension scale rate). There was no significant difference in service use between the 'poor' and the 'not poor'. When their degree of disability was taken into consideration, no substantial difference in contact rates was observed between the 'poor' and 'not poor' for *health* services (except the district nursing service for the severely disabled). But for the *social* services, especially home-helps, the highest usage rates were found in the 'not poor'. The authors concluded that neither health nor social service departments, for a given level of disability, discriminate in favour of the poor (Victor and Vetter, 1986).

In 1984 two studies using the same data source came to very different conclusions about use of services. One inferred from the results that doctors were discriminating in favour of occupational class V patients. The other study put a completely different interpretation on the findings. Using the national morbidity survey of general practice, Crombie (1984) investigated consultation rates by dividing them into two groups: first-time consultations initiated by the patient, and repeat appointments initiated by the doctor. In the ones initiated by patients, lower occupational classes had fewer consultations for preventive services than higher classes but more consultations for acute episodes like accidents and violence, so that overall there was little difference in consultation rates between the classes. However, for repeat consultations initiated by the doctor, Crombie noted that occupational class V patients had more consultations for a given episode of illness. He reasoned that doctors were compensating for lack of coping skills in class V patients by giving them more return appointments. Blaxter (1984) looked at the conditions for which patients were consulting their doctors. She also found higher consultation rates for occupational classes IV and V, but concluded that these higher rates were justified by the more severe nature of the illness they experienced. The lower occupational classes had more illness which was life-threatening and more painful in nature than higher classes. These two studies illustrate clearly the difficulty of interpreting research in the health service field.

In a community survey of three London boroughs the Nottingham Health Profile was used to compare self-reported morbidity with service use by manual and non-manual classes. The study also aimed to identify which types of morbidity were likely to trigger a consultation and which were not. There were substantial differences in the prevalence of ill-health between social groups. The manual groups were particularly susceptible to tiredness, sleep disturbance, pain and emotional distress. However, their higher levels of morbidity were not matched by higher consultation rates for these conditions (Bucquet and Curtis, 1986).

A detailed local study in general practice has tackled the issue of deprivation and health in one practice serving 15,500 patients (Marsh and Channing, 1986). They selected a sample of 587 'deprived' patients from their register and these were paired with matched controls from a 'more endowed' area. Data on patients for the previous three to five years were abstracted for analysis. Deprived patients were found to have 60 per cent more hospital admissions, 75 per cent more casualty attendances, and almost three times as much mental illness as the control group. Comparisons of serious physical illness, consultant referrals and GP consultations all showed the same trend. There was significantly more non-attendance for appointments and much poorer immunization rates and other preventive care in the deprived group. In total, the deprived patients had provided a 50 per cent higher morbidity load to the health services than their matched controls. The authors go on to describe what a practice can do, in practical terms, to try to improve the health of its deprived patients.

Allocating resources fairly

Before the NHS was set up, resources available for health care varied greatly from one region to another (Whitehead, 1988b). The NHS inherited this unequal distribution, but since 1976, when the Resource Allocation Working Party (RAWP) reported, the service has been committed to the principle of allocating resources more fairly across the country. At that time the expenditure/head of population in the wealthiest regions was approximately 30 per cent higher than that of the poorest regions. The RAWP formula for calculating budget allocation was applied to try to solve the problem.

A decade later, at the regional level at least, there had been a reduction in inequality, with the gap in expenditure/head between the richest and poorest reduced to less than 10 per cent (Holland, 1986). In this particular respect the formula worked well, though it has not been achieved without penalty. In a period of growth, the NHS might have achieved the redistribution relatively painlessly by keeping current expenditure levels fairly steady in some sectors while giving more to others. As it has turned out, there have been severe financial restrictions on the service, and under such circumstances almost the only way of giving more to one region is to cut resources and services in another. This produced its own brand of unfairness, which the RAWP formula was incapable of solving – it is more a political question of deciding the size of the cake to be shared out (Holland, 1986).

It is also important to understand that RAWP only dealt with geographical inequalities of resources in the health service at regional level. It was not designed to tackle inequalities between different social groups in their access to health care, or inequality in resources provided for different services, in particular the lesser priority given to preventive and community health care services compared with the high technology hospital sector.

Following much agitation about underfunding, particularly of the health services in London, a review of the resource allocation system was set up in the mid 1980s. There was debate about the effect of using a mortality measure (SMR) in the allocation formula. Some criticized its use on the grounds that mortality may not be a good guide to need for health services. In fact, SMRs were found to be highly correlated at regional and district level with permanent and temporary sickness rates (Mays and Chin, 1989).

There was also criticism because no weighting was given to extra need for care due to the level of deprivation in an area. Again, it was found that SMR was highly correlated with deprivation indicators that have high values in more northern parts of the country, but it was not closely correlated with indicators which have high values in some parts of London, such as living in rented accommodation or a high immigrant population (Townsend, 1990). The net effect of the RAWP formula was to channel relatively more resources to the higher mortality and historically under-resourced parts of Britain, as intended, but to leave southern regions with too little to manage effectively.

The solution to the resource allocation problem chosen by the government is weighted capitation, to be introduced over a transitional period from 1992 to 1995. This new formula funds regions per head of population, with a reduced weighting given to the level of mortality in each region. No weighting is given for deprivation. The effect of this is to channel more resources back towards the southern regions and away from the north, reversing the effect of the RAWP formula. Problems arise with this at the subregional level if districts are funded on the same weighted capitation basis. Then some deprived health districts with high mortality and morbidity are relatively worse-off than under the RAWP system, and more prosperous districts with better health profiles are relatively better-off. This effect is already being noted and is causing concern in some deprived districts.

To deal with the argument that some account should be taken of level of deprivation over and above that indicated by SMR, a new deprived area allowance was introduced into the new GP contract from April 1990. This is based on the Jarman deprivation index, which also favours areas in London and the West Midlands because one of its components is the percentage of people from ethnic minority groups and these are highly concentrated in London and selected urban areas. There is also a problem highlighted by Jarman himself. The current cut-off point used to define deprived wards includes only 5 per cent of all wards (containing 9 per cent of the population). He feels that this does not give a good measure of deprivation in a family health services authority area: '... a lower cut-off point covering roughly twice this population would be much more equitable' (Jarman, 1991).

Obviously, all these developments need to be monitored carefully and modifications made as discussed further in Chapter 9.

Conclusion

It is difficult to get a comprehensive overview of how the position has changed in the health services over the past decade, and the latest reforms of the NHS add to the uncertainty. Although some recent studies could find no evidence of bias in favour of any social group in relation to GP consultation rates, there is no room for complacency. Other studies have highlighted examples of poorer provision of services in more deprived areas; physical access difficulties for a small proportion of the population – notably among the elderly and manual groups; differences in the quality of care which appeared to favour higher occupational classes; and much lower uptake of preventive services by lower social groups. What is not known is the extent of such inequalities. Concern has been expressed in this chapter about the danger of increases in inequalities in health care with some of the NHS reforms, for example on the provision of primary health care services in prosperous and deprived areas and the effect of new resource allocation arrangements on geographic access to care. On the other hand, there are certainly examples of health and social service workers making strenuous efforts to reduce the inequalities they have identified, and these important initiatives are outlined in Chapter 9, along with a discussion of policy for the future.

Chapter 5

A European Perspective

How does Britain's health record compare with those of other countries in Europe? Do they all experience inequalities in health between their various population groups, and if so, is the size and scale of the inequality the same in each country? Can we learn anything from other countries' attempts to reduce their inequalities? Answering such questions would be of value in developing health policy for the future, but it is no easy task.

The problem is that each country has different methods of collecting information, different definitions of each social group, and covers different time-spans and topics. Only rarely can direct comparisons be made on the type of social factors which are of particular interest here. The difficulties in making international comparisons on inequalities have been reviewed in detail for perinatal and infant mortality (Macfarlane and Mugford, 1984); for chronic illness (Blaxter, 1989); for health services (Macintyre, 1989); and for mortality differentials in general (Lynge, 1984; Wagstaff et al., 1991). In what can only be a brief overview, this chapter looks at inequalities in health *between* and *within* countries in the European Region, noting some promising policy developments.

International comparisons

One way of forming a general picture of how Britain's health record compares with that of other countries is to look at infant mortality and life expectancy at various ages, before going on to consider the health of different social groups. Table 13 shows mortality rates for 1988/89 and illustrates:

1. In all developed countries female life expectancy is greater than that of males by between five to seven years, though in Poland the gap between men and women has grown to nine years for life expectancy at birth.

2. The UK still compares unfavourably with several European countries on infant mortality, being in ninth place in the table, behind the Nordic countries, the Netherlands, France and the former West Germany. We are at

Table 13: *Infant mortality and life expectancy in selected European countries around 1988*

	Infant mortality deaths / 1,000 live births		Life expectancy at birth (years)		Life expectancy at age 45 (years)	
	Male	Female	Male	Female	Male	Female
Finland	6.6	5.5	70.7	78.8	28.9	35.4
Sweden *	6.7	5.5	74.2	80.4	31.5	36.9
Norway	9.2	7.3	73.1	79.7	30.7	36.3
Iceland	7.0	5.4	73.2	80.2	33.1	36.8
Denmark	8.2	6.9	72.2	77.9	29.9	34.7
Netherlands	8.0	5.6	73.7	80.5	30.9	37.0
West Germany	8.7	6.2	72.6	79.2	30.2	35.8
France	8.9	6.7	72.9	81.3	31.2	38.2
UK	10.2	7.7	72.7	78.2	30.1	34.9
Greece	12.2	9.8	74.3	79.4	32.2	36.2
Spain †	10.2	8.1	73.4	79.9	31.4	36.7
Israel*	12.4	9.7	73.6	77.3	29.0	33.8
Italy	10.2	8.2	73.3	79.9	30.8	36.5
Portugal	14.0	12.1	71.1	78.2	30.2	35.6
Poland	18.4	13.9	66.7	75.5	26.2	33.0
Hungary	17.3	14.3	65.5	73.9	25.0	31.8

* 1987. † 1986.

Source: WHO Health For All Statistical Database, September 1991 edition, WHO European Region.

roughly the same level – about eleventh – in relation to life expectancy at birth and at age 45, though the order for some of the other countries changes.

3. The pattern differs markedly for some countries. Finland, for example, has had an excellent record on infant mortality for many years, but a poor record with respect to middle-aged and older men in the population. Greece has a relatively high infant mortality but the highest life expectancy at birth for men in Europe.

League tables like this give only a superficial snapshot of what is going on in different countries. In addition, there needs to be some discussion of trends over time and other significant developments to put the figures in context.

The previous section touched on the position of Britain in relation to other developed countries, but there are wider issues of inequalities between

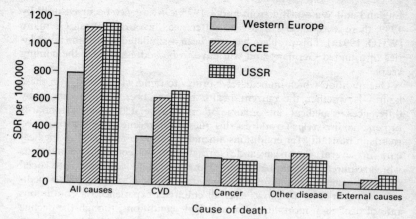

Figure 9. *Differences in mortality between countries of central and eastern Europe and western Europe around 1988–9. (Source: HFA Statistical Database, ESR Unit, WHO/Euro.)*

countries to be considered, in particular the emergence of an east–west health divide. Fig. 9 shows the differentials in mortality between countries in the central and eastern parts of Europe and those in the west. In 1988–9, all-cause mortality in central and eastern Europe was at a level experienced by western Europe in the late 1950s, and long since surpassed.

This difference has not always been so pronounced, but has developed in the past thirty years. An analysis of time-trends for the 1950s to 1987 for ages 50–64 showed that central and eastern European countries such as Hungary, Czechoslovakia and Poland experienced reductions in mortality until the mid 1960s. The decline in mortality then slowed down and, in the case of Hungary and Poland, began to rise in the 1970s and 1980s. Western countries such as England and Wales and West Germany showed a steady improvement in mortality which accelerated in the 1970s (Boys *et al.*, 1991). The picture for the over-65 age-group shows that eastern and western European countries started from a similar position in the 1950s, but over the next forty years large reductions in mortality rates in the west were not matched in the east.

The health gap between East and West Germany seems to have been an even more recent phenomenon. In the early 1970s, life expectancies at birth and at age 45 were similar for the two countries. In fact, at age 45, it was slightly higher in East Germany than in West (and higher than in

England and Wales). But from about 1975 a divergence occurred until by 1989 there was almost a 3-year difference, favouring West Germany (WHO, 1991a). This problem has now been assimilated within the boundaries of a united Germany and will have to be addressed over the coming years.

One question which immediately springs to mind when faced with these figures is whether the current health gap has been brought about by differences in medical care or some other factor related to living standards or personal life-style. To address this question, a recent study has examined trends in mortality for conditions amenable and non-amenable to medical care in several European and North American countries. Conditions which required personal behaviour change or which were related to social or environmental conditions were considered to be non-amenable to medical treatment. Fig. 10 shows that all countries experienced a continuous rate of decline in mortality from amenable conditions, though the decline was more rapid in the western countries. For the non-amenable conditions there was little improvement in the western countries until the early 1970s, when some decline took place. For central and eastern European countries, rates were static until 1970, when each country experienced a worsening of the rates. Ischaemic heart disease acted like a non-amenable condition in the European countries, but followed the pattern of amenable conditions in North America. The authors conclude that the main source of the current east–west divide is connected to the non-amenable deaths rather than a major deficiency in treatment services. However, they point out that the results indicate that there is still some room for improvement in medical care in the east, as deaths from treatable conditions have declined less rapidly than in the west (Boys *et al.*, 1991).

This east–west divide is a matter of concern for the whole of Europe. In September 1990, all the member states of the WHO European Region, including Britain, passed a resolution that all WHO programmes should have a special emphasis on helping the countries of central and eastern Europe through this transitional period, and the European Community is also seeing this as a major responsibility.

Inequalities within countries

Comparisons of this nature do not say anything about the extent of the inequalities in health *within* each country. The Black Report stimulated many other countries to examine the situation in their populations and a body of literature has been building up. Different countries use different social variables to measure inequalities: occupation; income; education;

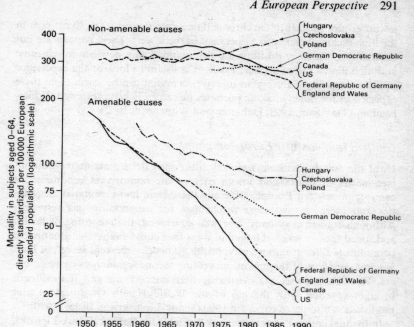

Figure 10. *Trends in age-standardized mortality from amenable and non-amenable causes, various countries in Europe and North America.* (*Source:* Boys et al., *1991. Copyright* British Medical Journal).

social circumstances; rural/urban residence, and so on. But however inequality is measured, every country is found to have disadvantaged and advantaged groups which differ in their experience of health (Blaxter, 1983).

Inequalities between social groups show up in most countries when chronic disease and limiting long-standing illness are measured, with middle-aged men commonly showing rates of chronic disease 40 per cent to 50 per cent higher in the lowest compared with the highest social group (Blaxter, 1989).

Low income is also commonly associated with poorer health, particularly for chronic illness and disability in middle age. In one survey in Finland, for example, the proportion of middle-aged people with chronic illness ranged from 18 per cent in the highest income group to 42 per cent in the lowest group. In France the chronic illness rate ranged from 30 per cent in the high income bracket to 57 per cent in the lowest. These surveys are not comparable, but they do illustrate the common link between low income and high illness rates (Blaxter, 1989). It is useful to look at the experience of different parts of Europe in this respect. What can be learnt from these experiences for policy-making purposes has recently been reviewed (Whitehead and Dahlgren, 1991; Dahlgren and Whitehead, 1992).

Central and eastern European countries

Until the late 1980s there was very little open debate about the issue of inequalities in health and health care in the non-market economies of central and eastern Europe. Officially the system had eliminated inequalities and there was no clear mechanism for questioning this response. Although statistical systems were well developed, the recording of health and social factors was not linked in ways that could enable the situation to be monitored. Most importantly, health statistics were kept secret, at least in some countries in the region, preventing secondary analysis by researchers. Now an analysis has eventually been carried out and the evidence brought together with the aid of the World Health Organization and published in a series of papers in 1990 (Wnuk-Lipinski and Illsley, 1990).

Individual country papers are now available for Poland (Wnuk-Lipinski, 1990), Bulgaria (Minev *et al.*, 1990), Hungary (Orosz, 1990), and the former USSR (Mezentseva and Rimachevskaya, 1990). Several general points have been made from these analyses. Firstly, the social structure cannot be measured in the same way as in western democracies, as income, occupation and so on are not sufficient guides to social position. New class structures have developed in which a person's position in the centrally controlled power structure and political affiliations influence their access to scarce goods and services, health care included. This privileged access is just as important as money in determining standard of living and status, but difficult to capture in official statistics.

Secondly, all countries in this group have experienced intensive development of heavy industry, resulting in serious damage to the environment and pollution which has had an added impact on the health of whole populations and certain regions in particular. Heavy pollution in parts of Poland, for example, has been linked to increases in lung cancer, and deterioration in infant and child health in the affected areas (Jedrychowski *et al.*, 1990; Norska-Borowka, 1990).

Thirdly, the state of economic and social crisis that these countries have been in means that there has been a general deterioration in living stand-

Table 14: *Percentage on 50 per cent or less of average income in Poland*

	1982	1988
Professionals	1	11
Skilled non-manual	4	15
Skilled manual	9	24
Unskilled	10	32
Private farmer	13	40
Self-employed	2	10

Source: Adapted from Wnuk-Lipinski, 1990.

ards. However, the effects are not evenly spread across the population. Some sections of society have experienced much more profound deterioration in living and working conditions. Taking Poland as an example, the increase in poverty has been particularly marked among the private farmers and manual workers. Table 14 shows the proportions living on 50 per cent or less of average income in 1982 and 1988. It can be seen that although the percentage of professionals in poverty increased from 1 per cent to 11 per cent in the 1980s, the percentage of private farmers in this category increased from 13 per cent to 40 per cent and unskilled workers from 10 per cent to 32 per cent (Wnuk-Lipinski, 1990).

At the same time there has been an increase in the proportion of the population in the highest income group – a widening of inequalities in income. This period of increasing poverty also saw high mortality rates, increasing accident rates at work, food shortages and a scarcity of essential drugs.

The health care system became less efficient at a time when it was most needed and inequalities in the provision of care increased as people in higher classes usually had easier access to care. For example, one study in Poland found that the higher the occupational class, the higher was the percentage of patients who personally knew a doctor and the more likely they were to use this acquaintance to get into hospital (Ostrowska, 1980).

The comparative analysis of the four countries by Wnuk-Lipinski and Illsley (1990) came to the following conclusions. On infant mortality, Hungary and Poland have data for educational grade. There is a clear gradient in both countries, with mortality declining with each additional educational grade. The evidence from Hungary shows that these mortality differences between educational grades increased from 1960 to 1987, especially since 1970. There was a sharp social gradient in stillbirth rates in Poland, with the highest rates in manual workers employed in agriculture, followed by non-agricultural manual workers, then non-manual workers, and the lowest rates in the self-employed.

Data on inequalities in adult health comes from Bulgaria and Hungary. In Bulgaria the proportion of people with poor self-reported health increases with declining educational level, except for the highest social category, which has an unexplained high level of reported poor health. In contrast, there was no correlation between poor health and low income, except for the lowest income category.

The trends in Hungary over the past fifty years show that in the pre-war period there were large differentials in mortality rising from non-manual to manual occupations and highest in manual agricultural workers. These differences decreased under the new system after the war, until by 1960 they had virtually disappeared. This lack of inequalities was relatively short-lived, and an increase was noted again for men up until 1983. This resulted from an increase in mortality in both groups of manual workers, with mortality of non-manual men remaining unchanged over the period. For women, inequalities in mortality were also reduced in the immediate post-war period, and when they increased again, this increase was smaller than that found in men.

When causes of death are investigated the greatest differentials in health between educational and occupational groups occur in infant mortality, respiratory disease, infectious and parasitic diseases.

When regional differences are examined, great diversity is seen, especially for the different republics of the former Soviet Union. The Asiatic republics where fertility is high have a correspondingly high infant mortality, whereas the European republics with lower fertility have lower infant mortality, more in line with their western neighbours. In Hungary, regional differences in mortality have widened over time, unlike Bulgaria, where a sharp fall in infant mortality since 1970 has been accompanied by a narrowing of the gap in rates between the twenty-nine regions. In 1984, though, there was still a considerable gap ranging from 12 to 18 deaths per 1,000 live births.

On the issue of health care resources, very great regional differences can be seen in each country. For example, in Hungary in 1985, Budapest had 19 per cent of the population but 36 per cent of the physicians and 30 per cent of the hospital beds, with great concentration of the more specialized services. The inverse care law was evident in the rest of the country, with the poorest provision in the countries with the highest mortality. In Poland and the former Soviet Union, regional variations in health status were found to be partly related to differences in health services between regions, especially for deaths around birth. However, there were stronger associations between mortality and standard of living in a region and between mortality and personal behaviour.

On the policy front, there was a general drive to reduce inequalities in resource allocation in the early post-war period, but this was not sustained after the 1960s. This dying away of interest in creating equitable health care services has been attributed partly to the centrally controlled bureaucratic mechanisms that developed, which were distant from the regions and not flexible enough to respond to local needs. Another important factor was the system of priorities that grew up in these countries, in which high priority was given to the so-called 'productive' sectors of the economy, and low priority to health-related work in general and to health professionals, who were seen as part of a non-productive sector of society. One indication of this is that health workers' salaries were way below the national average in most of these countries.

The Hungarian profile suggests that it was the loss of concern for equity and the overriding emphasis on efficiency that led to a crisis of values. In the restructuring of society the author suggests that there needs to be a return to basic principles such as equity (Orosz, 1990).

With such an upheaval going on in all the major structures in the countries of central and eastern Europe, the challenge will be to build new systems which cut out the inequalities of the old system while avoiding the introduction of defects found in western systems, including those found in health care. In addition to the growing poverty, these countries face levels of unemployment unknown in this part of Europe since the war. Again, there may be lessons to be learnt from the bitter experience of unemployment of the western countries over the last decade. A Europe-wide perspective also needs to be given to the urgently required pollution control in this region.

Southern Europe

Some of the most impressive improvements in health have been made in this part of Europe from about 1950 onwards. Reductions in infant mortality have been most striking for Greece, Spain and Italy, though not so much for Portugal. Life expectancy at birth improved much faster than in the north and west of Europe, and by 1988 Greece had overtaken Sweden and the Netherlands to take top place in life expectancy at birth for men in Europe, with Israel, Spain and Italy not far behind. Life expectancy also increased rapidly for women, though not as fast as for men, with Spain and Greece in fifth and eighth places respectively.

Even so, there are still marked inequalities in health within the countries of the south. Reviews on the issue are available for Spain (Rodriguez and

Lemkow, 1990), Italy (Piperno and Orio, 1990), Malta (Agius, 1990), and Israel (Shuval, 1990).

Looking at Spain and Italy more closely, the familiar pattern of worse health in poorer groups, neighbourhoods and regions within the countries are seen (Rodriguez and Lemkow, 1990; Piperno and Orio, 1990). In Spain there is little association between perinatal mortality and income but a much closer association with the distribution of health services. For post-neonatal mortality and deaths at older ages there is a stronger association with socio-economic status, particularly poverty. Despite economic growth, over 60 per cent of the over-65s in Spain still live below the poverty line and life expectancy and mortality from liver cirrhosis and lung cancer are worse among the poor.

Spain has a distinctive pattern of HIV infection and AIDS cases, which adds a new dimension to the evidence on inequality. Heroin addiction is more prevalent in lower socio-economic groups and, as 50 per cent of people with AIDS in Spain are heroin addicts, AIDS has a socio-economic profile not observed in many other European countries.

As in Britain, Spain has experienced a welcome reduction in inequalities in post-neonatal mortality, particularly from 1975 to 1981, when mortality fell dramatically among manual workers, especially agricultural workers, compared with a moderate fall among professionals.

In contrast, Italy has been experiencing widening differentials in infant health between the more developed north and central regions and the less developed regions in the south of the country. For example, neonatal mortality decreased by 20 per cent between 1980 and 1985 for the country as a whole, but by only 16 per cent in the south and by 22 per cent in the central and northern regions. For infant mortality, some regions recorded a reduction, while others showed no improvement and in some of the poorer districts death rates increased. For example, infant mortality increased in Molise from 9.3 to 14.2 per 1,000 live births from 1980–85 (Piperno and Orio, 1990).

The dramatic improvements in the overall health of the population in Spain and Italy during the 1960s and 1970s have been attributed in part to socio-economic development, leading to improvements in the standard of living for a wide spectrum of the population. At the same time, coverage of essential health services has been growing, promoted in both countries by the introduction of national health systems. These have the potential to influence deaths around the time of birth in particular. In the late 1980s, following the implementation of cost-containment measures in the health services, increased differentials in access to services are emerging. For example, in Italy there has been a decline in diagnostic investigations, particularly in lower socio-economic groups, coinciding with the introduction of co-payments for these services. There are also differentials between professionals and less educated groups in the use of specialist services and admission to the top-quality hospitals. Piperno and Orio concluded that the ability of lower social groups to gain access to the highest-quality services had declined in the late 1980s in Italy, and that it is now generally accepted that the reduction of health inequalities should be a priority for the health services.

The developments in health care policy in Spain show a desire to build more equitable health services. The new constitution of 1978 recognized the right of every citizen to health and free access to health care, and the right for each region to have more control over policies that effect them. In 1986, the Public Health Law created a National Health System (NHS), which combined the efforts of the government and regional health services. Mechanisms were also set up to co-ordinate policy between the centre and the regions and to integrate long-term planning, so that it was easier to pursue a national health policy on a decentralized basis. Equity was one of the national criteria to be taken into account in planning. Other aspects of the reforms have been:

- increasing coverage of the population;
- shift from social security funding to tax-based funding;
- regulation by planning, not market forces, with increasing control over the private sector;
- management improvements, including innovative experiments in audit and other quality assurance measures;
- strengthening of information systems. (Dekker, 1992.)

A national health strategy in line with the WHO Health For All programme has been developed and several of the autonomous regions have also developed plans. In 1990, a commission set up by Congress started a major analysis of the NHS, looking at quality, equity and efficiency (Dekker, 1992). There is a very evident concern in Spain to provide an equitable service. Portugal is also trying to devise equitable resource allocation arrangements for primary care (Giraldes, 1988).

In Italy many experiments have taken place to improve the health and safety of workplaces through joint research between academics and factory-floor workers. In these, workers examine their own working conditions and health problems and put forward suggestions for improvements, based on their experience of the job. Although this approach is not without its problems, it has inspired new ways of doing research to give people the confidence to take action themselves (Reich and Goldman, 1984; Lundberg and Starrin, 1990).

North-western countries

A diverse set of countries could loosely be grouped under this heading, including the Netherlands, France, the former West Germany, Belgium, Britain, Switzerland and Ireland. They are characterized by having above-average health profiles for their populations as a whole, with rising life expectancy in recent decades. Some have shown exceptional progress in specific areas, for example, life expectancy at birth and age 45 for women in France is the highest in Europe; infant mortality in the Netherlands is particularly low, especially for females, and in Britain death rates in young adults are low mainly due to an exceptionally good record on road accidents.

These countries are also characterized by having substantial black or ethnic minority populations, some as permanent citizens and others as migrant workers who are often very low-paid and poorly housed. Whether migrant workers are included in the health statistics of a country can make a big difference to the apparent existence of inequalities. For example in Switzerland, analysis of statistics excludes migrant workers and shows an irregular decline in health, with a higher rate of mortality in the skilled manual group rather than in classes IV and V (Lehmann *et al.*, 1990). However, the statistics only cover 60 per cent of social classes IV and V. The other 40 per cent are foreign nationals employed as seasonal workers in the poorest jobs and it is likely that if they were included the mortality rate of classes IV and V would be much higher (Egger *et al.*, 1990).

Interest in the debate on inequalities in health appears to be low in France, Germany and Switzerland but high in the Netherlands and Britain. Reviews are available for the Netherlands (Mackenbach, 1992), France (Mizrahi and Mizrahi, 1992), Germany (Mielck, 1992), Switzerland (Lehmann *et al.*, 1990), Belgium (Lagasse *et al.*, 1990), and Ireland (Cook, 1990).

A notable trend is that several countries in this group have reported an increase in inequalities in health. For example, in France the results of a longitudinal study linked to the 1975 census have become available to look at adult mortality. For the years 1975 to 1980 the usual occupational class gradient was observed in this study, with a wide differential between top and bottom grades of the order of 2.8:1 for men and 2:1 for women. The health gap between non-manual and manual classes of working age widened between the late 1950s and the late 1970s as mortality declined more rapidly in the non-manual sector (Desplanques, 1984).

The Netherlands also reports a widening gap, for adult mortality at least. It is useful to take the Netherlands as a more detailed example as the literature on the issue is extensive; thirty to forty studies a year are published in this field. These show that lower socio-economic status is associated with higher rates of a wide spectrum of health problems ranging from low birth-weight and adult height to disability, chronic conditions, self-perceived health and mortality. On the other hand there is no consistent pattern for perinatal mortality, children's height, accidents and some short-term and chronic conditions (Mackenbach, 1992).

Small-area studies have also been conducted in cities such as The Hague, Amsterdam and Rotterdam. In Amsterdam, a four- to five-year difference in life expectancy was found between the most deprived and the most affluent areas. For the Netherlands as a whole, there was a strong correlation between socio-economic indicators and mortality for 1980–84. Analysis by cause found higher rates in lower social groups for coronary heart disease, cerebrovascular disease, diabetes, cancer and traffic accidents. The gradient was reversed, with higher rates in higher social groups, for cancer of the breast, lung and prostate and for arterial disease (Kunst, 1990).

Evidence on inequalities in health care systems is sparser, but some studies have indicated restricted access to health care in times of financial cutbacks. For example, during a shortage of hospital beds due to financial cuts, the higher social classes had a disproportionate number of admissions, the reverse being true when there was surplus capacity – more in line with morbidity patterns. In Amsterdam, a study of 55–79-year-olds found that virtually all chronic conditions showed a higher prevalence in the lower social groups, with a correspondingly higher use of nearly all services. However, for chronic sickness the highest social group made more frequent use of specialist services and of physiotherapy services (van den Bos and Lenoir, 1992). Whether quality or effectiveness of services also varied by social status was not known.

The policy debate in the Netherlands has been growing rapidly in the 1980s. The publication of the Black Report and WHO strategy are said to have been the impetus for the Dutch Ministry of Welfare, Public Health and Culture to include a paragraph on inequalities in health in a major policy document in 1986 (Mackenbach, 1992), and a deliberate strategy of raising awareness of the issue on a wide basis was initiated (Gunning-Schepers, 1989). Key policy-makers, including politicians from all parties, trade unions, employers' organizations and medical associations were brought together by the government for a two-day conference in 1987. At this, the evidence on the subject was presented and stimulated these organizations to think about what they could do to address the issue. After the conference, the Ministry commissioned a five-year research programme to inform policy-making; regular reports from this were issued to politicians and were available when major health service reforms were being proposed. The effects of the reforms on equity were taken into consideration. Several small-scale demonstration projects were also commissioned by the government to illustrate at a local level how inequalities in health might be tackled. These included patient advocacy schemes and intensive health education provision in disadvantaged schools.

In November 1991, a second conference on the theme was called by the Dutch secretary of state and the chairman of the advisory council on government policy, to reach agreement on policy opportunities in the field. The consensus from the conference was:

• that socio-economic health differentials had been increasing again since 1960 in the Netherlands;
• that reducing these differentials required an integrated and inter-disciplinary approach by Parliament, various government departments and a wide range of non-government organizations;
• through such an integrated approach, an assessment must be made of the impact policy decisions have on the health status of the lowest social groups, and these effects should play a more important role in future policy decisions (WRR, 1991).

At the conference the responsibilities of a wide range of bodies were set out, including the government ministries concerned with social affairs, employment, education, housing, environment and finance, as well as national and local business and voluntary organizations. A five-year programme (1993–7) of policy development and research was adopted.

The Nordic countries

The Nordic countries of Europe include Denmark, Finland, Norway, Iceland and Sweden. They have had a reputation for a very high standard of health throughout the 1970s and 1980s with exceptionally low infant and maternal mortality. Sweden and Iceland in particular have some of the highest life expectancies in Europe and indeed in the world. The Nordic countries also had some of the highest rates of coronary heart disease in Europe at the beginning of the 1970s, but these showed a sharp reduction during the 1980s. Although deaths from cancers have been relatively low, and are declining further, there are certain exceptions. Lung cancer in women, for example, has risen very rapidly from below the average for the European Community in 1970 to way above it by 1989.

Despite this good record, there is great concern in the Nordic countries

Table 15: *Denmark: neonatal mortality/1,000 live births*

Parent's occupation	1974	1977
Self-employed	5.7	6.6
White-collar	7.5	5.3
Skilled worker	8.1	5.6
Unskilled worker	9.0	5.6
Other/unknown	8.8	6.1
Average	8.0	5.7

Source: Holstein (1985).

about inequalities in health within each country. The evidence has been reviewed for the Nordic countries in general (Kohler and Martin, 1985), for Norway (Dahl, 1990), Denmark (Holstein, 1985), Finland (Valkonen *et al.*, 1991) and Sweden (Diderichsen, 1990).

For a time, it was assumed that inequalities in health did not exist in this group of countries, following reports of a reduction in the differences between social groups in infant mortality and children's height. But more recent studies and re-analyses have shown that although such inequalities may be relatively small they do exist at different stages of life and for both men and women.

Infant mortality (deaths under one year) in Denmark is very low compared with many countries, including England and Wales. Comparisons between occupational groups in the country show that throughout the 1970s initial differences in neonatal mortality declined so that by 1977 the differences had been almost eliminated. The figures given on p. 89 of the Black Report can now be updated in Table 15 to illustrate the point. This shows negligible differences between the five occupational groups by 1977.

Furthermore, the infant mortality rate does not differ between married and unmarried women as it did in the 1960s. Of these reductions in inequality, Holstein comments: 'This result is, in my view, a very important one. It demonstrates that inequalities in health should not be interpreted as an unavoidable "natural law" but as open to change by public health intervention' (Holstein, 1985).

For adults of working age, however, there are still obvious inequalities in health in Denmark. For example, a longitudinal study, examining deaths from 1975 to 1980 in men, found that mortality in the lowest, unskilled group was 37 per cent higher than that of the highest professional group. For women, mortality was 20 per cent higher in the equivalent groups (Andersen, 1985). From studies quoted later in this chapter it seems that occupational differences in Denmark are smaller than in several other European countries. Morbidity studies have found the familiar pattern of increasing disease rates with decreasing social class, except in the 20–29 age range, where professional classes have poorer health.

Although regional differences in infant mortality have been noted, these change from year to year without showing a stable pattern of regions with high and low rates, so the differences appear to be the result of random fluctuations (Holstein, 1985).

On the other hand, the regional differences in dental health in Denmark seem to be more systematic. Comparing the Copenhagen area with Western Jutland in the 1980s the ratio of children with decayed teeth was 1:2 – a difference which reflects the variations in preventive programmes and regular dental examinations in these areas. The Danish municipalities with public dental care for children have 10 per cent less caries than those without public dental care.

In relation to health services, no major differences in use of services are apparent, and use of free primary health care varies only slightly with income. However, use of dental care, which is not always free for adults, varies considerably with social class and income (Holstein, 1985).

Fresh evidence concerning inequalities in women's health in Norway has recently emerged. Traditionally, analysis has been by a woman's own social class and this has shown much smaller differences in mortality between women of different social groups. Analysis of the same data by husband's social class (as is often the case in Britain) reveals larger differentials which have been attracting more concern.

In Finland, there is a regional pattern of mortality with north-eastern Finland considered less healthy than the south-western parts. Over the decade from 1970 to 1980 mortality declined in all four provinces but the differential in mortality between them remained the same. However, over the same period the differences between cities and rural areas in mortality rates for men aged 35–75 disappeared. Among women there were no obvious urban/rural differences.

Interesting changes have occurred in relation to the health services. In 1964 there were noticeable regional differences in consultation rates with doctors in the state-subsidized health care system. Residents in the 'healthier' south of the country made more use of doctors' services than those in the 'less healthy' east and north. However, between then and 1976 these regional differences had diminished, especially among those who were chronically sick, and the relative differences are now said to be negligible in the rural areas and much reduced in the urban areas.

What has still to be tackled in Finland, though, is the inequality in the use of health services by different income groups. Consultation rates with doctors increased with increasing income, when adjustments were made for the variation in the number of days sick. Hospital use also varied with income, and large regional differences still persist in the use of the private dental services (Koskinen *et al.*, 1985).

On trends in Finland, a study looking at differences in mortality between 1971 and 1985 used occupational class and education as social indicators. The findings on education agreed with earlier studies that there was a marked difference in mortality of middle-aged men between educational groups. In 1971 at the start of the period under study, a 35-year-old man with basic education had a 50 per cent greater chance of dying before the age of 65 than a man with a higher education. The gaps between the mortality of educational groups narrowed slightly in the mid 1970s, but increased again in the 1980s (Valkonen *et al.*, 1991). For occupational class the gap in mortality between the upper white-collar employees and other groups widened in the late 1970s and early 1980s, as the relative position of unskilled workers worsened. Only slight differences were observed in women by occupational and educational group (Valkonen, *et al.* 1991).

Extensive studies have now been carried out in Sweden on the issue. During the first years of life differentials in mortality are bigger than in the rest of childhood, and are particularly noticeable for boys. Children in families of non-manual workers had significantly lower mortality than children of manual workers or the self-employed. This difference grew smaller as the boys grew older. From this study of 1.5 million children, it was calculated that the proportion of deaths attributable to a child's socio-economic group was 20 per cent among boys and 8 per cent among girls. If mortality among children aged 1–19 in general could be reduced to that of children in families of non-manual workers, an estimated 150 deaths out of 1,000 deaths occurring each year in Sweden could be prevented (Vågerö and Östberg, 1989).

In the early adult years (20–23), differentials in mortality also exist (Östberg and Vågerö, 1990) and they persist throughout working life, though the gap decreases with age. After retirement, differentials are smaller for men, but larger for women classified by their own occupational class (Olausson, 1991). Morbidity differentials have also been observed in men and women aged 16–74 (Vågerö and Lundberg, 1989). It has been pointed out that heavy smoking was more common in older non-manual men who had higher mortality from coronary heart disease. On the other hand non-manual women smoked more but had a lower mortality from coronary heart disease than manual workers, so smoking habits are not a sufficient explanation for this pattern (Vågerö and Norell, 1989).

Much interest in Sweden is focused on working conditions as a possible key determinant of the inequalities in health in Swedish society. One analysis concluded that a large part of the class differences in mental and physical health seemed to be a result of systematic differences between classes in their living conditions, especially their working environment (Lundberg, 1991b). Further evidence is focused on the widening inequalities in cardiovascular diseases for middle-aged men from 1961–86. There was a decreasing mortality among professionals, but for manual workers in industry mortality increased from 1961 to 1980, then remained static. As mortality for professionals continued to decrease after 1980, the gap continued to widen. The increase in mortality was highly concentrated in manufacturing industries, not in manual occupations or lower educational groups in general, pointing to the importance of working conditions and the labour market. The widening of inequalities in health in this respect corresponded to a period in the 1960s and 1970s of intense rationalization of Swedish industry, creating stressful, monotonous working conditions (Diderichsen, 1991).

Because of this concern for working conditions, several initiatives in Sweden have focused on the workplace. There is very strict safety regulation, and Sweden has one of the lowest levels of industrial injury in Europe. At the national level, the government set up the 'Swedish Working Life Fund' which raised a large amount of money from a short-term levy on business from September to December 1990. Over a five-year period this money is being distributed to companies – initially the ones with the most hazardous jobs – that put forward sound proposals for improving the conditions in their workplaces, provided the companies concerned match the government grant.

The demonstration of inequalities in health was also the trigger for initiatives by the unions in Sweden. For instance, the Labour Organization (LO) – the national confederation for manual workers – realized that its two million members included most of the groups in employment with high risks of poor health compared with the rest of the population. The debate within the LO about this led to the setting-up of a five-year health programme in 1987, in cooperation with the National Health and Welfare Board, and the umbrella organizations for the local authorities and community groups. Although advice, information and training were provided centrally, the local union branches were left to choose their own priorities for action. The result was that by 1990 all branches had devised workplace schemes, but these differed greatly in content depending on local views. In one company near Stockholm the focus was on heart disease, leading to negotiations for improvements in the factory canteen, changes in working hours, better provision for shift-workers, and more appropriate first-aid training for safety delegates, in addition to education on personal behaviour change. In the less populated areas of the country, the Transport Workers Union identified a particular problem for long-distance lorry drivers in obtaining regular, nutritious meals. The priority chosen in this case, therefore, was to establish contact with hotels and cafés along the main routes to gain agreements on a more healthy choice of menu, available at convenient times for the drivers (Lundberg, 1991a).

Finland has initiated policies to tackle inequalities in health care between different regions of the country. It was recognized that there was an unfair geographical distribution of medical personnel, and an Act of 1972 enforced a two-pronged strategy:

1. Health resources were preferentially allocated to northern and eastern parts of the country. Cities which had hospitals and health centres were deliberately left lagging behind. Subsidies were offered to set up new medical posts in priority areas. Higher salaries were offered in community health centres than in the hospital sector.

2. Building expenditure was switched from hospital to health centre buildings. By 1981 the community and hospital sectors were taking equal shares of the building budget (formerly the hospital sector took the major share).

The policy seems to have been successful because the health centres in rural areas in Lapland and eastern Finland 'are today better manned than those in the big cities'. There has been a corresponding improvement in the number of nurses and dentists in the priority areas, too. In effect, primary health care has become the centrepiece of the national health service rather than playing a subordinate role. Unfortunately, in recent years there has been some slippage in this policy, with rural health centres becoming less attractive and a deterioration in access to services in some large urban areas, indicating a need for constant vigilance.

In Norway, the national food and nutrition policy takes in aspects of equity in trying to ensure a supply of cheap nutritious food, and improvements to the distribution networks to all parts of the country. In 1976 the Norwegian parliament passed a national nutrition and food policy – the first of its kind in the world. It had four main goals:

1. to encourage healthy dietary habits, by pricing policies and improvement in the food distribution networks;

2. to help stabilize the world food supply by contributing to emergency food reserves and decreasing reliance on imported food;

3. to promote consumption of domestically produced food;

4. to strengthen and stabilize the rural economy, stopping the decline in the number of small farms by making farming more profitable and attractive.

National dietary goals were set and, uniquely, the policy focused on structural changes to encourage the desired dietary changes, rather than emphasize the individual's responsibility alone. Differential food pricing and incentives for production of healthy food were proposed, with the whole policy co-ordinated across the nine government departments which could have an influence on the issue. The aim was to provide reasonably priced, nutritious food accessible to all.

After ten years of the policy, evaluations show mixed progress. On the positive side, it has been noted that the policy has survived three different governments; all the goals and objectives are still valid and indeed have been strengthened by subsequent research findings; all the major political parties still support it, and there have been great efforts at cooperation at national and local level. In addition, the proportion of the gross national product given in aid to developing countries has also increased over the decade, reaching 1.15 per cent in 1984. The level of farming incomes and the area of cultivated land has also increased (Klepp and Forster, 1985).

On the negative side, it has proved very difficult to change existing farming and pricing policies in the face of a strong lobby from the agricultural sector, in effect protecting the producers rather than the consumers. Even the interdepartmental government committee is reported to be dominated by the Ministry of Agriculture. Against this background the policy has made most progress in a wide variety of health education programmes, and much less on the pricing and food-production fronts (Winkler, 1987). The strategy, however, has not been abandoned but is entering a second phase, supplemented by more intensive research on how to change pricing policy and build on the successes so far.

All the Nordic countries have made extensive efforts with policies to improve maternal and child health, and in the case of Sweden this was specifically triggered by concern about social inequalities in infant mortality in the 1930s. The threefold difference between the most favoured group and the rest of the population was reduced to about 10 per cent, with the aid of policies on universal coverage of health care, welfare benefit, employment and housing improvements (Dahlgren and Diderichsen, 1986; Diderichsen, 1990). The gap has not entirely disappeared, as detailed in the next section.

In Denmark the reduction in neonatal mortality has been attributed in part to an intensive preventive public health effort, coupled with social changes concerned, for example, with freer access to abortion services (Holstein, 1985).

In relation to the Finnish record on low birth-weight and infant mortality the Black Report has already outlined the rapid development of primary health care services in Finland which aim to cover a large proportion of the population with outreach programmes (p. 98). Since then, further improvements have been made. To advance the target set on low birth-weight, new social maternity benefits for all pregnant and nursing mothers were introduced in the 1970s. By 1982 all women were entitled to 258 days of paid maternity leave (compared with 72 days in 1971), and men were entitled to 6 to 12 days of leave around the time of birth, and between 25 and 100 days' paternity leave in exchange for some of the maternity leave (compared with nil in 1971). Twenty per cent of men take advantage of this benefit.

The Nordic countries have also been among the most active in taking up the WHO Health For All strategy. Finland and the Netherlands volunteered to be the first two countries to test out models of policy development under the Health For All banner, and as a result a national health strategy was produced in Finland as early as 1985. It contained equity goals in relation to the distribution of health care and on other aspects such as homelessness and housing conditions. By the time England produced its first draft strategy in 1991, Finland had just undergone a detailed review of the first five years of operation of its strategy (WHO, 1991b). Norway and Iceland also have national strategies. Although Sweden has only recently developed such a strategy, it has introduced important policy bills in Parliament. For example, in June 1991 a bill was adopted requiring all national public agencies to report to Parliament on specific goals to reduce social and occupational inequalities in health. It also required them to do health impact assessments on all national policies. In effect this put into place formal mechanisms for monitoring and planning action on inequalities in health across a range of departments and agencies.

Comparative studies

A number of recent studies have tried to compare the size of the differentials in health.

Valkonen (1989), for example, compared mortality by level of education in Denmark, England and Wales, Finland, Hungary and Norway in the 1970s and 1980s for the age range 35–54. Among men, mortality rates were highest in Hungary and Finland, and among women, in Hungary and Denmark. Death rates were found to decline with increasing years of education with a remarkably similar pattern in all six countries. Changes in inequalities over the decade were also analysed. The gap in mortality between groups with different levels of education had increased in England and Wales in the 1970s. In men there was no change in mortality in the lowest educational category, whereas there was a decline of between 10 per cent and 20 per cent in the other categories. In women there had been a large increase in the health gap due to a decline of more than 40 per cent in the death rates for the higher educational category. No significant increases in inequality were noted for the Nordic countries over the same period (Valkonen, 1989).

Occupational mortality in the four Nordic countries has been compared for 1971–80, making use of compatible census-linked longitudinal studies. Standardized Mortality Ratios were based on the *whole* Nordic population who were economically active (Andersen *et al.*, 1987). Clear differentials in mortality in men could be seen between occupational groups. Finnish men had the highest mortality in almost every occupational group, followed by Denmark, then Norway and Sweden. It was noticeable that the same groups were advantaged and disadvantaged in each of the four countries. Thus non-manual groups (especially teachers, nurses and doctors) had relatively low mortality, while manual groups had high mortality (particularly those in heavy industrial jobs, and in hotel and domestic work). When causes of death were investigated in the study it was found that groups with high mortality overall had high mortality for almost all causes of death, not just for a few specific occupational hazards (Andersen *et al.*, 1987). Valkonen (1987) has used the results from the above study to compare the gap in mortality between white-collar and blue-collar occupations in the four Nordic countries. Mortality was between 9 per cent and 14 per cent higher for blue-collar occupations than for white-collar occupations in Denmark, Norway and Sweden, while in Finland the difference was 25 per cent. This suggested that inequalities in mortality were greater in Finland than in the other three countries, which had roughly equivalent levels of inequality (Valkonen, 1987).

In a detailed review of these and other comparative studies in 1987, Valkonen came to the following conclusions:

For working age adults,
- inequality in mortality is greatest in France, somewhat less marked in

England and Wales, Hungary and Finland, and smallest in Denmark, Norway and Sweden;

- inequality in mortality among men in different occupational classes had increased during the last two decades in France, Hungary, and England and Wales, but has remained constant in Norway, Denmark and Finland;
- there are smaller gradients in mortality among married women than among men but changes in inequality reflect those seen in men, with increased inequality in England and Wales and Hungary but not in the Nordic countries.

For babies,

- in Denmark and Sweden socio-economic differences in infant mortality throughout the first year of life have all but disappeared. In most of the other countries discussed above the differences are still marked, though they have decreased somewhat in England and Wales. (Valkonen, 1987.)

To allow a closer comparison between Sweden and England and Wales, data on mortality and chronic sickness rates in men and women of working age in Sweden have been coded to the British Registrar General's social class schema. Differentials in mortality were observed in all three countries, but the differences were greater in England and Wales than in Sweden, whether measured by the ratio of manual to non-manual classes or the ratio of IV + V to I + II. For chronic sickness, class differences were also present in the three countries and greater in England and Wales, measured by the ratio between classes V and I (Vågerö and Lundberg, 1989). The data from this study have recently been re-analysed to provide additional information about the pattern. This showed that in England and Wales the class gradient declines fairly gradually throughout the social scale. In Sweden, in contrast, there was relatively little inequality among the manual classes and class IIIN, but a substantial gap between the top two classes and the rest (Wagstaff *et al.*, 1991).

Using the same classification techniques, the latest evidence shows the existence of social class differences in all three countries in infant mortality. Within Sweden, there was a difference of 20 per cent between the neonatal mortality rate of the non-manual and manual classes. For post-neonatal mortality the difference was 38 per cent. Within England and Wales, there was a somewhat larger differential of 27 per cent between non-manual and manual classes for neonatal mortality, and of 43 per cent for post-neonatal mortality. There was also a big difference between the overall death rates in each country, with neonatal mortality rates one and a half times higher in England and Wales than in Sweden, and post-neonatal rates twice as high. The authors calculate that if all Swedish infants had the same level of mortality as the non-manual classes in Sweden, then 10 per cent of neonatal and 29 per cent of post-neonatal deaths would be avoided. If English and Welsh babies had the same level of mortality as the Swedish non-manual classes, then 40 per cent of neonatal deaths and 63 per cent of post-neonatal deaths in England and Wales would be avoided (Leon *et al.*, 1992).

Conclusions

So what conclusions can be drawn from these international comparisons? Certainly Britain is not alone in experiencing inequalities in health. Every country to a greater or lesser extent experiences differences in health between regional, social or income groups. The question of whether some countries have less inequality in health than others is very difficult to answer. The comparative studies quoted lend support to the suggestion that the Nordic countries, particularly Denmark, Sweden and Norway, experience less social inequality in health than other European countries, including England and Wales.

What is instructive in these comparisons is the commitment shown in several countries to addressing the issue of inequalities in health, even if it is acknowledged to be a slow and difficult process.

Chapter 6

Explaining Health Inequalities

Of crucial importance for policy-making is the question of how health inequalities are generated and maintained. The Black Working Group examined the evidence on causes of occupational class differences in health under four main headings: artefact, health selection, cultural/behavioural and materialist/structuralist explanations. Material and structural factors were judged to be the main contributors to inequalities, though the other explanations were not mutually exclusive and could be seen to play some part at varying stages of life.

This chapter looks at fresh evidence published from 1980–92 which has taken the discussion further forward. A number of useful reviews are available (Macintyre, 1986b; Wilkinson, 1986a; Davey Smith *et al.*, 1990b and 1992).

The artefact explanation

This approach, espoused by Illsley (1986) and Bloor *et al.* (1987), suggests that the method of measuring occupational class – by the Registrar General's social class classification – is unreliable and may artificially inflate the size and importance of health differences. The authors maintain that the Registrar General's classification and the nature of occupations open to the labour force have changed so much in recent decades that any comparisons with earlier decades this century are meaningless, using this classification as a tool. The arguments and evidence concerning this explanation have already been outlined in greater detail on pp. 265–75. Briefly, the recent evidence continues to point to very real differences in health between social groups which cannot convincingly be explained away as artefact.

Firstly, important new evidence has come from the OPCS Longitudinal Study showing the existence of a clear occupational class gradient in mortality, free from one of the statistical problems – numerator/denominator bias, as outlined on p. 229 (Fox *et al.*, 1986). Secondly, Chapter 3 has already given examples of recent studies which have made serious attempts to control for some of the measurement problems related to time-trends to control for some of the measurement problems related to time-trends and occupational class, and none of the results alters the picture to any great extent (Pamuk 1985 and 1988; Goldblatt, 1989, 1990a and 1990b; Marmot and McDowall, 1986). Thirdly, the last ten years have seen an upsurge in studies (quoted in Chapter 2) which have used other indicators of social circumstances to examine their relationship with health. Whether social position is measured by income, housing tenure, household posses-sions or education, a similar pattern emerges on inequalities in health between the top and the bottom of the social scale, consistent with that found by using occupational class. Fourthly, analysis has been extended to people beyond retirement age and to women in different social circum-stances, showing the same general conclusions (Fox *et al.*, 1986; Moser *et al.*, 1990). Finally, results from major longitudinal studies have provided fresh evidence of a social gradient in mortality when alternative measures are used, with a differential *greater* than that found when occupational class alone is used as a measure (Goldblatt, 1990b; Marmot *et al.*, 1984b). This and other studies suggest that the Registrar General's classification might be under-estimating the size of the health gap rather than over-estimating it (see p. 232). There can be no doubt that these inequalities exist, however imperfect the measuring tool.

The argument that we could do with a better measure of social class than one based on occupation is widely accepted not least in relation to women, and new studies are developing such approaches. Occupation is just one of the many interrelated factors which contribute to the concept of social class. It has been pointed out that there is a tendency for some social groups to be relatively privileged in almost every respect – power, status, income, education, etc. – and for other groups to be relatively disadvantaged in almost every respect, and one measure cannot hope to capture all these factors.

Theories of natural and social selection

Explanations in terms of selection accept that social inequalities in health exist, but suggest that the differences are caused by a health selection process. According to this explanation, people in poor health would tend to move down the occupational scale and concentrate in the lower social classes, while people in good health would tend to move up into higher classes. The gap between the health of the higher and lower classes would therefore be kept open indefinitely and would be inevitable whatever overall improvements in health occur over the entire population. The same sort of explanation has been discussed on p. 254 in relation to unemploy-ment – the possibility that ill-health may lead to subsequent unemployment rather than unemployment leading to ill-health. This explanation has been reviewed by Blane *et al.* (1993) and West (1991).

Has any new evidence shed more light on this explanation? A distinction has been drawn between inter-generational and intra-generational selection. Inter-generational selection would operate when people move into a different social class from their parents, as they move from childhood into adulthood. Intra-generational selection would operate when there is movement from one social class to another in adult life.

On inter-generational selection, a theoretical model has been constructed showing that it would be possible to create the observed occupational class differential in health through social mobility, provided that selection for health was a *major* determinant of social mobility (Stern, 1983). However, evidence from social mobility studies suggests that the main factors in social mobility are education and the material and cultural background of the family, rather than health (Goldthorpe, 1980; Halsey *et al.*, 1980).

Further data have been presented for the three decades from 1951 to 1980 which confirm early studies on first-time mothers in Aberdeen and the outcome of their pregnancies. There was a gradient in perinatal mortality, birth-weight of babies and height of mothers between the occupational classes. It was noted that taller women tended to move up the occupational classes at marriage, while shorter women tended to move down at marriage. As height can be taken as an indicator of health before marriage, this evidence shows that some sort of health selection was taking place at marriage and contributing to the class differential (Illsley, 1986). It has been pointed out, however, that most of the social mobility at marriage in this study took place between social classes III and IV plus V. This mobility was associated with very small differences in maternal height yet large differences in prematurity and obstetric death rates (Blane *et al.*, 1993).

The 1980 OPCS survey of heights and weights in Great Britain confirmed that the 'shortest women were least likely to raise their social class through marriage and that, to a lesser extent, the tallest were most likely to raise their social class in this way'. However, OPCS were less certain about what interpretation to put on these findings (Knight, 1984).

Data from the National Survey of Health and Development cohort study have shown that *serious* illness in childhood can affect social mobility. Whatever their class of origin, seriously ill boys were more likely than others to experience a fall in occupational class by the time they were twenty-six (Wadsworth, 1986). This kind of evidence suggests that unhealthy people are more likely to move down the social scale, but estimates suggest that this effect would not make more than a small difference in the overall figures. For example, an estimate of the effect of serious childhood illness suggests that only about 1.5 per cent of those seriously ill in their early twenties had suffered a drop in occupational class as a result of previous childhood illness (Wilkinson, 1986a).

Additionally, the National Child Development Study, which has been following a cohort of children born in 1958, has been used to check this explanation. Results confirm that some social mobility in childhood was related to health, but again this mobility did not account for the social class gradient in health observed (Power *et al.*, 1986). A second study from this project has used housing tenure as well as occupational class to check the results. It compared not only the health of young adults who were upwardly or downwardly mobile, but also the health of those who had stayed in stable socio-economic circumstances from birth to the age of twenty-three. Significantly, the health of those young people whose circumstances were stable differed between socio-economic groups as much as, if not more than, that of those who were mobile; this difference in health could not be explained by social mobility because there had been no movement between classes in this group of people (Fogelman *et al.*, 1987).

A completely new argument has been put forward in recent years to support the idea that inter-generational health selection takes place. The concept of 'indirect health selection' is introduced in which socio-economic factors experienced in childhood influence the ability of children to attain their full health potential in adulthood. Empirical evidence from Sweden shows that young adults who claimed to have experienced economic hardship in childhood stand a greater chance of downward mobility and a reduced chance of upward mobility than those who do not experience hardship (Lundberg, 1991b). In addition, evidence from a longitudinal study, the National Child Development Study, found that low social class, living in rented accommodation, overcrowding, large family size and receipt of free school meals in childhood were all closely associated with social class differences in health at age 23 (Power, 1991). Several other studies have also found an association between growing up in a deprived area with high infant mortality and poor health in middle age (Barker *et al.*, 1989; Barker, 1990). However, there are two fundamental problems in interpreting these findings. Firstly, it is difficult to disentangle the effects of childhood deprivation on adult health from the influence of more recent deprivation. For example, in the National Child Development Study noted above, both childhood deprivation factors and recent experiences such as unemployment and early parenthood were associated with the social class differences in health at age 23 (Power, 1991). Secondly, and most importantly, evidence that socio-economic conditions in childhood influence adult health cannot really be classed as a form of health selection. The definition of health selection is that prior health influences subsequent social position, not the other way round.

In relation to intra-generational selection, there is a possibility that as people become sick in adult life, they could move down into a lower social class, and conversely, that healthy people could move up because of their better health. There is no doubt that people who are chronically sick do tend to become poor, but there are several reasons why such an explanation cannot account for the bulk of the differentials in health observed.

Firstly, some of the major diseases of today, such as lung cancer, have a short period between onset and death – too short a time for downward mobility. Yet just as steep gradients are seen in lung cancer mortality as in chronic bronchitis, which usually does have a long period between onset of disease and death.

Secondly, the OPCS Longitudinal Study has been able to track the social position of the same individuals from 1971 to 1981 and monitor their mortality rates from 1981 to 1985. In men aged 45–64, no consistent relationship has been found between those who move to a higher or lower social class and their mortality. From the Longitudinal Study there was no evidence that downward mobility maintained or increased social class differences in mortality in middle age (Goldblatt, 1989).

Thirdly, the Longitudinal Study has been able to examine deaths from 1976 to 1981 in men over retirement age at the 1971 census. A substantial social class gradient in mortality was found even in men aged 75 and over. These men would have retired ten or more years before death and their social class would be fixed at what it was before retirement. Therefore, by the nature of the way they were recorded by the census, they could not change class even when they became ill. Whatever caused the social class gradient in the over-75s, it could not have been downward or upward social mobility in the ten years or more before their death (Fox *et al.*, 1986).

In the Whitehall study the men were given a rigorous medical examination on entry to the study. Among those with no detectable disease at the beginning of the study, there were still much greater death rates in lower than higher grades. Recruitment of sicker men into lower grades in the Civil Service would not explain the gradient in this case (Marmot *et al.*, 1984b).

To sum up, there is some evidence that health selection operates at younger ages, and new evidence for men over fifty that no such selection effect is evident after this age. Estimates of the size of the selection effect suggest that it accounts for only a small proportion of the overall differential between the social classes.

Cultural/behavioural and materialist/structuralist explanations

The health selection explanation suggests that health can determine subsequent social position. The third and fourth explanations both take the view that social circumstances can affect subsequent health, but differ in where they put the emphasis.

The cultural/behavioural explanation stresses differences in the way individuals in different social groups choose to lead their lives: the behaviour and voluntary life-styles they adopt. In this explanation inequalities in health evolve because lower social groups have adopted more dangerous and health-damaging behaviour than the higher social groups, and may have less interest in protecting their health for the future.

The structuralist/materialist explanation emphasizes the role of the external environment: the *conditions* under which people live and work and the pressures on them to consume unhealthy products. Inequalities in health in this context would come about because lower social groups are exposed to a more unhealthy environment. They do more dangerous work, have poorer housing, and have fewer resources available to secure the necessities for health and to use the available health services. At a more general level, the whole structure of society is implicated.

But several commentators are beginning to question whether the distinction between the two approaches is artificial, as behaviour cannot be separated from its social context (Blane, 1985; Blaxter, 1983). The classic example of childhood accidents has been quoted to illustrate the point. The observation that children from lower social groups have more accidents than children from higher groups may be explained by the behavioural view as due to more reckless, risk-taking behaviour in this group and inadequate care by parents. The materialist view would highlight the unsafe play areas, the lack of fenced-off gardens and the greater difficulty of supervising children's play from high-rise housing. In the latter view, the environment is dictating the behaviour of both mother and child.

The following new evidence supports the behavioural and the structural/materialist explanations but shows that the two are interrelated rather than mutually exclusive.

Evidence on cultural/behavioural differences

Latest evidence confirms previous observations that there are life-style differences between the social classes which are related to health. Cigarette-smoking would be a prominent example.

Smoking habits

Table 16 gives the percentages of cigarette-smokers in each socio-economic group over the period 1972–88. It is clear that in almost every year the percentage of smokers increased steadily from the professional group through to the unskilled manual group. For example, in 1988 16 per cent of professional group men and 17 per cent of professional group women were smokers compared with 43 per cent of men in the unskilled manual category and 39 per cent of women in that category.

The table also shows that there has been a decline in the prevalence of smoking in most socio-economic groups, but the decline has been more rapid in some groups than in others. For example, prevalence in women in the manual groups has shown only a small reduction since 1972, whereas that in the professional group has halved.

Smoking habits varied with economic status, too. For example, in 1988 33 per cent of men in work were smokers, compared with 56 per cent of unemployed men. The corresponding figures for women were 33 per cent and 44 per cent. Smoking prevalence by region also shows higher levels in Scotland and the North than in the rest of the country.

Class trends in mortality from lung cancer and coronary heart disease show some similarity to the smoking trends. Thus there is a social class gradient in mortality for both diseases, with lower rates in the professional classes to highest in the unskilled manual class. In addition, mortality over the decade has been declining faster in non-manual groups than in manual groups, as Fig. 6 on p. 271 has illustrated (Marmot and McDowall, 1986).

Mortality from lung cancer and coronary heart disease is higher in the unemployed than in the employed population, and regional variations in mortality from the diseases mirror the smoking variations to a certain extent.

In the case of coronary heart disease, there are further similarities. Before 1950 mortality from the disease in men was marginally higher in classes I and II than in IV and V, but during the 1950s the gradient reversed and mortality became higher in classes IV and V than in I and II (Marmot *et al.*, 1981; Morris, 1981).

Alcohol

Drinking habits also vary between the social groups but in a much more complex way, as shown in Fig. 11.

The association between alcohol consumption and socio-economic group is stronger for women than for men, and shows a *reverse* gradient, with the

Table 16: *Prevalence of cigarette-smoking in Great Britain, 1972–88, by sex and socio-economic group[1] (persons aged 16 and over[2]): percentage smoking cigarettes*

	Professional	Employers and managers	Intermediate and junior non-manual	Skilled manual and own account non-professional	Semi-skilled manual and personal service	Unskilled manual	All aged 16 and over
Men							
1972	33	44	45	57	57	64	52
1974	29	46	45	56	56	61	51
1976	25	38	40	51	53	58	46
1978	25	37	38	49	53	60	45
1980	21	35	35	48	49	57	42
1982	20	29	30	42	47	49	38
1984	17	29	30	40	45	49	36
1986	18	28	28	40	43	43	35
1988	16	26	25	39	40	43	30
Women							
1972	33	38	38	47	42	42	42
1974	25	38	38	46	43	43	41
1976	28	35	36	42	41	38	38
1978	23	33	33	42	41	41	37
1980	21	33	34	43	39	41	37
1982	21	29	30	39	36	41	33
1984	15	29	28	37	37	36	32
1986	19	27	27	36	35	33	31
1988	17	26	27	35	37	39	30

[1] Members of the Armed Forces, persons in inadequately described occupations, and all persons who have never worked have not been shown as separate categories. They are, however, included in the figures for all persons.

[2] Aged 15 and over in 1972.

Source: OPCS (1990b).

proportion of heavy drinkers higher among non-manual than manual groups. For example, 14 per cent of professional women consumed more than the recommended sensible limit compared with 8 per cent of women from semi-skilled and unskilled groups. Among men, employers and managers and skilled manual groups were more likely than others to be heavy drinkers. Moreover, men and women in the manual groups were more likely than those in the non-manual groups to be classified as non-drinkers or to have very low consumption. Among women, this trend was most marked, with 46 per cent of semi-skilled groups and 56 per cent of unskilled groups being non-drinkers or having low consumption compared

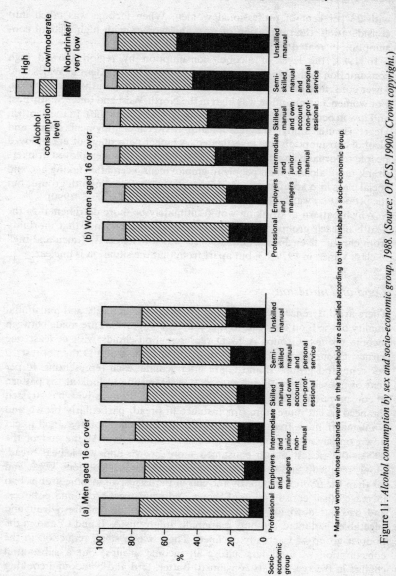

* Married women whose husbands were in the household are classified according to their husband's socio-economic group.

Figure 11. *Alcohol consumption by sex and socio-economic group, 1988. (Source: OPCS, 1990b. Crown copyright.)*

with 23 per cent of professional women. When income was taken into consideration, the proportion of men and women with high alcohol consumption increased with higher household income.

In 1988, the level of alcohol consumption by region showed high consumption in the North, North-West and to a lesser extent in Wales, and lower consumption in Scotland, East Anglia and the South-West for men. For women, consumption was high in the North-West and outer South-East and low in Scotland, Wales and East Anglia (OPCS, 1990b). In the Scottish Heart Health Study, the relationship between employment status and alcohol consumption was investigated. A higher percentage of unemployed people reported being non-drinkers. Nevertheless, the unemployed drinkers drank more alcohol than people in employment, even after taking age and social class into account. 'Binge drinking' was common in both groups, but the proportion was higher among the unemployed (Lee *et al.*, 1990).

Which pattern of drinking would ultimately be more detrimental to the health of each group is debatable. There is some evidence that mortality from chronic liver disease and cirrhosis was lower in class I men and high in class V men in 1979–83, but apart from that the situation is unclear.

Food and nutrition

There are differences between social groups in the quantity and nutritional quality of the food they eat. In this context comparisons are made between income groups. Groups A to D represent households with at least one earner. Group A contains the richest 10 per cent, group D the poorest 10 per cent, and groups B and C are intermediate, each representing 40 per cent of households with one earner. It is interesting to look at the pattern of consumption, bearing in mind that recent nutritional advice has stressed the need to eat more fibre (for instance in bread, particularly brown and wholemeal), more fresh fruit and vegetables including potatoes, and to cut down on sugar, salt and fat, particularly animal fat. At the end of the 1970s, the richest group consumed more brown and wholemeal bread, more fresh fruit and vegetables, and less white bread, potatoes, sugar and fat than the poorest group. By the end of the 1980s, all income groups had increased their consumption of brown and wholemeal bread and potatoes, and had cut down on sugar. However, consumption of fresh fruit and vegetables had increased only marginally in groups A, B and C, and in the poorest group had actually declined. There was a small reduction in the consumption of total fats across all income groups, but a substantial change in the *type* of fats consumed. Butter, lard and compound cooking fat consumption declined markedly, and there was a corresponding increase in margarine and 'all other fats' consumption in all income groups (MAFF, 1991). Thus in terms of the foodstuffs listed the richest income group continues to have a healthier diet than the poorest group. However, there are signs that, within the limits of their income, the poorest group may have responded to nutritional advice to the same extent as other groups, for example in wholemeal bread consumption. How much the poorest group's choice of food is restricted by low income is discussed in greater detail on pp. 331–4.

In relation to diet and heart disease, poorer families and residents of the North and Scotland have been accused of eating too many fatty foods, unlike their more health-conscious counterparts in the South. The evidence does not support this view. What is evident is that intake of vitamin C shows great variation between different groups and regions because consumption of most of the main sources of the vitamin is lower in Scotland and the north of England, and in larger and poorer families. Table 17 shows the nutrient value of the diets of different household types. Vitamin C intakes ranged from 40mg to 62mg per day, with intakes highest in the south of England, in richer households and in smaller families. In contrast, there is very little variation in the proportion of energy derived from fat – between 40 and 42 per cent in all categories of household, except in very large families where it is lower. The ratio of polyunsaturated to saturated fatty acids (P/S ratio) showed only small variation. What variations there were in the proportion and type of fat did not match the variations in heart disease observed in Britain (MAFF, 1991).

Given that the recommendation is for no more than 30–35 per cent of energy to be derived from fat, *all* groups in the table appear to be consuming too much. These findings on fats were confirmed in a study of the diets of middle-aged men and women living in three English towns. Consumption of fat and the other main nutrients was lowest in the northern industrial town which had the highest death rates from heart disease and from all causes combined (Cade *et al.*, 1988).

There is also evidence of higher consumption of sweets by children in lower social groups (Charles and Kerr, 1985).

The links between nutrition and health are many and varied, ranging from effects on growth, to links with specific diseases like coronary heart disease and obesity, to general resistance to infections, and all of these show higher rates in lower social groups.

Exercise in leisure-time

Data on leisure-time activities by socio-economic group were available in

Table 17: *Nutritional value of diet by region, income group and in households with two adults and different numbers of children in 1990*

				Regions of England							
	Scotland	Wales	England	North	Yorkshire/ Humberside	North-West	East Midlands	West Midlands	South-West	South-East/ East Anglia
P/S ratio	0.39	0.40	0.40	0.39	0.40	0.38	0.42	0.40	0.40	0.41
% energy from fat	40.5	42.1	41.6	40.3	41.3	41.1	42.3	41.3	42.2	42.0
Vitamin C (mg)	50	47	53	53	52	45	52	47	57	57

	Numbers of children					Income group			
	0	1	2	3	4 or more	A	B	C	D
P/S ratio	0.40	0.41	0.40	0.40	0.41	0.40	0.41	0.40	0.38
% energy from fat	42.4	41.7	40.6	40.3	38.5	42.1	42.0	41.3	40.8
Vitamin C (mg)	62	55	46	42	40	62	53	48	44

Source: Adapted from MAFF (1991).

Table 18: *Exercise in leisure-time in Great Britain by socio-economic group. Persons aged 16 and over (1977 and 1986). % participating.*

Socio-economic group	Walking (over 2 miles)		Indoor swimming	
	1977	1986	1977	1986
Professional	29	30	9	16
Employers and managers	23	24	6	11
Intermediate – non-manual	27 ⎫		7 ⎫	
Junior – non-manual	20 ⎰	22	5 ⎰	12
Skilled manual	15	17	4	7
Semi-skilled manual	12	15	1	7
Unskilled manual	10	12	2	3

Source: OPCS *General Household Survey* for 1977 and 1986.

the 1973, 1977, 1983 and 1986 General Household Surveys. Table 18 shows two of the most popular activities: walking and swimming. In both, the professional group had the highest participation rates and the unskilled manual group the lowest. There was an increase in participation from 1977 to 1986 for all groups, but the social gradient remained.

When considering strenuous activity at work, the gradient is reversed, with higher activity in manual occupations in Scotland for both men and women (Crombie *et al.*, 1990). In Wales, a similar increase in exercise at work with decreasing social class was seen for men, but no gradient was evident for women (Nutbeam *et al.*, 1987). It is difficult to say from these results whether any social class has a 'healthier' pattern of physical activity than another, especially as levels of vigorous activity are so low in all social classes that those who take adequate exercise are in a minority in every group.

Exercise may be linked to health in several ways, including a possible protective effect against coronary heart disease mortality, which is, of course, class-related (Morris, 1981).

Poorer take-up of preventive services by lower social classes has already been noted; it is clearly a possibility that this is due to cultural norms and voluntary behaviour choices rather than to material barriers to take-up, such as limited access. More detailed studies have to be carried out to find out which explanation is correct.

How much of the differential does life-style explain?

The evidence outlined above suggests that differences in life-style could indeed account for some of the class differential in health, but how much of it do the

Table 19: *Relative risk* of CHD death in ten years controlling for (a) age, and (b) age, smoking, systolic blood pressure, plasma cholesterol concentration, height and blood sugar*

	Administrators	Professional/ executive	Clerical	Other
(a) Controlling for age	1.0	1.6	2.2	2.7
(b) Controlling for other risk factors	1.0	1.5	1.7	2.1

* Calculated by multiple logistic regression.

Source: Marmot *et al.* (1984b).

life-style factors account for? A more systematic investigation of coronary heart disease risk factors was carried out in the Whitehall study (Marmot *et al.*, 1984b). The two major smoking-related diseases, coronary heart disease and lung cancer, were related both to smoking and employment grade. Of the top grade, 29 per cent were smokers, compared with 61 per cent of the lowest grade. However, it was found that even for non-smokers coronary heart disease was strongly associated with grade, with higher rates in lower grades. Table 19 shows what happened to the class gradient for coronary heart disease when controlled for age, smoking, systolic blood pressure, plasma cholesterol, height and blood sugar. The risk associated with employment grade reduced by less than 25 per cent. Likewise, controlling for exercise in leisure-time had little effect on the differential. In addition, steep gradients were found for diseases thought not to be related to smoking.

In the United States similar results have been found from an important longitudinal study, the Alameda County Study in California (Berkman and Breslow, 1983; Kaplan, 1985). The study has been assessing levels of health in the sample and trying to determine factors associated with health since 1965. When family income was studied, those with 'inadequate' income had much poorer survival chances over eighteen years of follow-up. For example, compared with the richest group, the poorest group had more than double the risk of death over that period. The study went on to analyse whether harmful behaviour patterns accounted for the increased risk. Even when the data were adjusted to take account of thirteen known risk factors including smoking, drinking, exercise and race, there was still a substantial gradient of risk associated with income. For example, the poorest group still had one and a half times the risk of death as the richest group. They concluded that behaviour patterns were not the major factors related to the increased risk of death, and suggested that factors related to the general living conditions and environment of the poor were more likely to be implicated. This line of enquiry is continuing.

Likewise, in the study of unemployed and employed groups reported on p. 254, excess mortality in the unemployed group was still evident when the study controlled for smoking and drinking (Cook *et al.*, 1982).

Evidence from other European countries also raises questions about the role of smoking in the class gradients. For example, in Sweden the pattern of smoking cannot explain the higher coronary heart disease rates in manual class women. In the age group 50–69, there was a higher proportion of heavy smokers among self-employed people and non-manual workers for both men and women. The proportion of people who had been smoking for over twenty years was also highest among non-manual workers. While the pattern of heart disease mortality in men was consistent with these smoking trends – with higher mortality in non-manual and self-employed men – the reverse pattern was evident in women, with lower mortality in non-manual groups (Vågerö and Norell, 1989). Anomalies also exist in other countries, suggesting that for coronary heart disease in particular, the differential in mortality observed cannot be attributed solely to smoking habits. In some cases none of the differential can be attributed to smoking.

Analysis of the Health and Life-style Survey has also produced results which introduce new possibilities. In a complex analysis, the study looked at various aspects of the health of individuals in relation to their material living conditions, their social support networks, and their 'healthy' and 'unhealthy' habits related to smoking, exercise, diet and alcohol. One important finding was that few people had life-styles that could be described as totally healthy or unhealthy as far as their personal habits were concerned. For example, only 15 per cent had 'healthy' habits on all four areas of personal behaviour, and only 5 per cent had totally 'unhealthy' lives on these four counts. Most people adopted a mixture of 'good' and 'bad' habits (Blaxter, 1990).

A new finding from the study was that people who had adopted two or more 'healthy' habits and who lived in a favourable environment with good social support, had better health than people with 'unhealthy' habits living in similar circumstances. However, there was much less contrast in the health of people with 'healthy' and 'unhealthy' habits living in less favourable circumstances with fewer social supports. The implication of this finding is that, relatively speaking, personal behaviour makes more difference to the health of groups living in good circumstances than in bad. As yet the finding is only suggestive, but it is an important line of inquiry to follow up with further research.

As the studies on diet in the previous section showed, the small variation in fat consumption between regions and income groups does not explain the large difference in heart disease rates between these groups. All these studies suggest that the differences in life-style between social groups account for some, but not all, of the observed health gap. Indeed in some cases *most* of the difference in health is not explained by these factors.

Several new studies have touched on the cultural aspect of this explanation – the suggestion that beliefs about health and health care may differ among social groups. The 'culture of poverty' idea – that poorer groups have more negative concepts of health and a lack of orientation towards the future which inhibits preventive health action – has been re-examined. For example, Calnan and Johnson (1985) compared the health beliefs of women from social classes I and II with those of social classes IV and V on two issues: concepts of health and perception of vulnerability to disease. Both of these issues are claimed to be related to decisions to take action on health. Findings showed that there was no social class difference in theories about vulnerability, or in concepts of health when defined in relation to personal health. Only when health was defined in the *abstract* were there marked social class differences and this may have been because middle-class women found it easier to express abstract ideas.

Similarly, Blaxter and Paterson (1982), in a study of disadvantaged mothers and daughters in Scotland, found no evidence that would fit a simple 'culture of poverty' model in either generation. Problems in health service use in the younger generation seemed to stem more from a lack of skill in dealing with the system rather than from adverse cultural beliefs. These and other studies (Pill and Stott, 1985a, 1985b) suggest that the importance of the 'culture of poverty' model as an explanation of poor service use and health-damaging behaviour may have been over-estimated in the past, and new appraisals of health behaviour are needed. This applies also to studies of middle-class families, where conflicting views about health and barriers to the adoption of healthier behaviour, also exist and suggest that behaviour change is not easy even in the best of circumstances (Backett 1990; Backett and Alexander, 1991).

Evidence that material factors affect health or health-related behaviour

Several studies published recently have investigated how material and structural factors affect health. Others have looked at how such factors influence behaviour or limit choice about health. The evidence for a clear causal link between unemployment and mental ill-health has already been presented on p. 256, together with evidence of higher mortality in the unemployed which cannot easily be explained away other than by some direct or indirect effect of unemployment. The strong association with aspects of material deprivation and ill-health in small-area studies has also been discussed on p. 251. This section therefore concentrates on a number of additional factors, such as housing and income, to add to the evidence in previous chapters.

Housing conditions and health

Housing as a health issue came to prominence in the mid 1880s in England, highlighted by reports from Edwin Chadwick. Many of the nineteenth-century public health reforms were concerned with improving these living conditions, but for much of the twentieth century the subject has been neglected. In recent years the issue has been regaining attention, although the problems encountered have changed:

Nowadays, the relation between housing and health is mediated in subtler ways than in Chadwick's time. Illness is brought about by factors such as faulty design (which contributes to falls and fires in the home), inadequate heating and lighting (which is also linked to falls), damp (which is related to the growth of moulds and mites and thus linked to chest diseases including asthma), and lack of safe amenities for recreation. Houses with multiple occupancy (bedsits, converted flats and bed-and-breakfast hotels) may be particularly hazardous especially when the supporting services such as sanitation and fire escapes are overburdened and families have to share washing, toilet, food storage, and cooking facilities. (Acheson, 1990)

Some of the more recent studies look at aspects of poor housing, like damp and mould, in relation to physical health. Others are concerned more with the stress and safety aspects imposed on people by poor design. For example, a study in Gateshead was carried out in 1983 on eight council housing areas, from the very best to the very worst in the district. Controlling for age, there were marked and consistent differences in self-reported health between individuals from different areas. People from 'bad' housing areas reported poorer health, more long-standing illness, more recent illness and more symptoms of depression than those living in 'good' housing areas. The position was reversed for the over-65s because of a local authority letting policy which gave priority to the less-fit elderly. Nearly a third of households reported defects in houses which they thought affected health, and these came disproportionately from the three 'bad' areas, especially in connection with respiratory conditions. 'Bad' council housing areas did not necessarily conform to the stereotype of non-traditional construction and high-rise flats. Location, poor environment and low quality of construction were the important factors (Keithley *et al.*, 1984).

A further paper by the same team looked in greater detail at respiratory conditions in council house tenants. It was found that smoking, an unhealthy working environment and age were the most important determinants of respiratory problems. When these were held constant, people in areas of 'bad' housing reported more respiratory conditions than those in 'good' housing areas. The problems were associated with flats rather than houses, and with older accommodation (McCarthy *et al.*, 1985).

A large-scale study investigated whether the design of buildings could lead to social malaise among the inhabitants. It covered over 4,000 blocks of flats and 4,000 houses in London, with additional information from around the country and abroad. Fifteen design variables in blocks of flats were identified which affected the behaviour of at least some of the residents, especially children. The degree of social malaise was indicated by the extent of litter, graffiti, vandalism, children taken into care, and urine and faecal pollution. Circumstances worsened with larger buildings and grounds, as the number of interconnecting walkways increased, and also where residents could not see or control the approach to their dwellings. The study concluded that such badly designed blocks 'made it difficult for normal people to cope', and thus contributed to social malaise (Coleman, 1985).

Also of relevance is the growing problem of infestation of housing estates, with the associated health risks. It has been pointed out that the design of high-rise buildings, with their interconnecting ducts and heating systems, allows rapid spread of vermin over which the individual tenants have very little – if any – control (Young, 1980).

An analysis of 'difficult to let' council housing in Liverpool concluded that the unsatisfactory housing conditions on one estate were contributing to high rates of infectious diseases, respiratory disease and mental illness. One source of infection was traced to unhygienic mobile food vans which residents used because no shops had been provided on the estate. Respiratory illnesses were aggravated by ducted warm-air heating and the practice of drying clothes indoors because of inadequate facilities (Department of the Environment, 1981a). Another study of families living in flats found that serious accidents among children were linked to the design of the building (Department of the Environment, 1981b).

The Housing and Environmental Health Departments of the Wirral, Merseyside, identified serious design and construction faults in their high-density housing. Water penetration, ventilation, heating and insulation problems, inadequate under-floor electric heating, deck access and high child-densities 'combined to produce disaster'. These faults resulted in dangerous and severely limiting conditions for the tenants, including lack of privacy and play facilities, noise, lack of clothes drying facilities, dependence on lifts, inadequate refuse disposal, and the obvious safety aspects of the height of buildings (Darley, 1981).

On the subject of damp, a study in South Wales suggested that respiratory symptoms may be aggravated by damp housing and by open coal fires which were thought to cause some pollution of the air inside the house (Burr *et al.*, 1981). Another found clear effects of damp housing on the health of children in a deprived area of Edinburgh in 1986. In particular, respiratory/bronchial symptoms, headaches and diarrhoea were much more common among children living in damp housing. The effect of damp was independent of the effect of low income or smoking in the household (Martin *et al.*, 1987). This study was repeated on a larger scale in England and Scotland and the original findings were confirmed (Platt *et al.*, 1989). A study in Edinburgh in 1984 had also found an association between respiratory problems in children, reported by their parents, and damp or mouldy housing. However, such environmental factors were not linked to GP consultation rates for these illnesses. This highlights the dilemma of which measure of morbidity to use in community studies (Strachan and Elton, 1986).

Evidence that some reporting bias may be occurring comes from a later study relating to asthma, in which a significant association was found between reports of mould in the home and reports of wheeze in children, but when objective measurements of bronchial reactivity were taken there was no association between the reports of mould and the degree of bronchospasm (Strachan, 1988). Strachan suggested that parents aware of damp in homes may be more likely to report symptoms in their children than parents living in houses without damp or mould, and this certainly has to be taken into consideration in the design of studies.

Cold conditions in houses are also a risk in countries like Britain. A review of the evidence on temperature and health concludes that for each degree Celsius by which the winter is colder than average, there are about 8,000 extra deaths. Each year about 40,000 more people (mainly very elderly) die in Britain in winter than in summer. Some deaths are due to hypothermia but most are due to respiratory and cardiovascular diseases. At a room temperature of 12 degrees Celsius, changes occur in the heart and blood vessels which increase the risk of heart attack and stroke (Lowry, 1989). The poor spend twice as much on heating as a percentage of their total income as the rest of the population, yet still struggle to keep their homes warm if living in poorly constructed dwellings.

Income

There have been few studies in this country of the direct effect of income on health, partly because of the enormous difficulties encountered and partly because of political sensitivity. To be meaningful, all sources of income would have to be assessed, including the value of fringe benefits, property, etc., and such statistics are not readily available in this country. A preliminary analysis has been carried out on occupational incomes and mortality in twenty-two occupations, comparing 1951 and 1971. Over twenty years those occupations which had increased their income relative to average earnings tended to experience a relative decrease in mortality rates. In occupations where income had gone down relative to the mean, mortality rates tended to go up relative to the mean. The death rates of old people also seemed to vary in a similar way with changes in the real value of state pensions over the years from 1965 to 1982 (Wilkinson, 1986c).

Using cross-sectional data, a series of calculations has been carried out to investigate the relationship between income and mortality at the macro-economic level. First, the relation between average income and life expectancy was assessed using gross national product per head in the twenty-three countries in OECD. There was virtually no correlation between the increases in GNP per head and increases in life expectancy in the developed countries in the sixteen years from 1970–71 to 1986–7. In contrast, the relation between income distribution and life expectancy showed a strong correlation in developed countries. Those countries with a shallower gradient from the richest to the poorest sections of the population (more equal income distribution) had the higher life expectancies. In addition, when changes in relative poverty in the EC countries were investigated at different periods of time, a fall in relative poverty was significantly related to a more rapid improvement in life expectancy. Furthermore, in the countries of OECD, changes of disposable income showed that increases in the share of income going to the least well-off were associated with faster increases in life expectancy. This is an interesting line of investigation and should be extended with further studies, as the implications for public health are considerable. For example, the calculations suggest that if Britain adopted a more equal income distribution similar to that found in some European countries, then about two years might be added to the population's life expectancy (Wilkinson, 1992).

Another study has looked at the effect of income, but this time on children's height. A study of families in poor areas in London in 1973–6 found that a low amount of money spent on food/person/week in a household was highly correlated with poor growth in children. Among these children protein intake was 92 per cent of the recommended daily intake, iron 80 per cent and vitamin D 40 per cent of that recommended. Of the children in the survey 11 per cent were mildly or moderately malnourished (Nelson and Naismith, 1979).

The *indirect* effect of income on health, for example on choice of diet and eating habits, has been more widely investigated. As outlined on p. 321, people from low-income households tend to eat less fruit, vegetables and high-fibre foods, and more sugar, than people from high-income households.

Studies of why this should be so have found lack of money to be a major factor, restricting food choice as well as limiting the quantity of food consumed. For example, a study of sixty-five families living on supplementary benefit in 1980 found that some parents went without food to provide enough for their children, and lack of money was frequently cited as the reason for lack of fruit and vegetables in the diet (Burghes, 1980). In a study of 1,000 low-income people in the North of England in 1984, approximately a quarter of respondents reported that they did not have a main meal every day. One-third of these said this was because of cost. Four out of ten unemployed people went without a main meal because of lack of money (Lang *et al.*, 1984). An in-depth study of 107 women living with pre-school children in Milton Keynes in 1984 found that 51 per cent of single parents and 30 per cent of low-income mothers in two-parent families were cutting down on food consumption for financial reasons. Of low-income women, 67 per cent found it difficult to afford what they considered to be a healthy diet for their children (Graham, 1986). When over 350 families living on low incomes were studied in 1991, a similar pattern was seen. One in five parents said they had gone hungry in the last month because they did not have enough money to buy food. Nearly half of the parents had gone hungry in the past year in order to make sure other family members had enough. One in ten children under 5 had gone without food in the previous month, and two-thirds of children and over half of parents were eating poor diets (National Children's Homes, 1991). The study also found that a 'healthy' shopping basket was £5 a week more for low-income families than an 'unhealthy' basket. That represented 20 per cent of the total weekly food expenditure for these families (National Children's Homes, 1991).

It is commonly found in such studies that food is treated as a flexible item in the household budget (unlike rent and rates); when money is short, spending on food tends to be cut back. Unfortunately the cheaper foods are often higher in fat and sugar.

A number of 'desk-top calculations' have been carried out to estimate the cost of following advice on a 'healthy diet', to see whether recommendations are realistic for people on low incomes. One, looking at the cost of an 'adequate' diet in pregnancy, concluded that the cost may be beyond the means of families dependent on low wages or benefits. For example, an average couple living on supplementary benefit in 1984 spent 9 per cent to 10 per cent of their income (excluding housing) on one person's food. However, it was estimated an 'adequate' diet for a pregnant woman would have taken up 28 per cent of the couple's income (Durward, 1984). The British Dietetic Association has considered the dietary problems of special groups at risk of malnutrition – children, pregnant women, ethnic minorities, the handicapped and elderly – and concluded that existing benefits for some members of these groups were insufficient for their dietary needs (Haines and de Looy, 1986). One recent study, basing the 'healthy diet' on the advice of the National Advisory Committee on Nutrition Education, calculated that the recommended diet could cost up to 35 per cent more than the typical diet of a low-income family (Cole-Hamilton and Lang, 1986). Some would dispute the figure of 35 per cent and suggest that community studies are now needed to check how valid these calculations are in real-life settings.

In recent years an increasing number of studies have gone out into the community to do just that: to document how people in different circumstances live and how they cope with aspects of health. In the field of family health care, Graham (1984) has collected and reviewed over 250 studies relevant to the question: 'How do parents meet their responsibility to family health?' This provides a valuable insight into the literature. It becomes obvious from such studies that all household resources have the potential to influence health – income, housing, fuel, food and transport. The pattern of spending on these basics varies between rich and poor families. For example, in 1990 poor households spent 56 per cent of income on necessities (food, fuel, housing), whereas rich households spent 35 per cent of their income on these products (Central Statistical Office, 1991). While 96 per cent of professional households have at least one car available, only 57 per cent of unskilled manual households have one (CSO, 1992). It is found that the poorest families may have little choice of fuel, and often have to rely on the most expensive kind (Boardman, 1986). Families who are economizing on fuel risk making their homes cold, damp and prone to condensation. Even within families, there is evidence of resources not being shared out equally. For example, parents may go without food to provide for the children, and the adult breadwinner may be given more food than those who stay at home. If a family has a car it cannot be assumed that women and children have access to it for food shopping and health appointments during the day. Frequently it is found that the male breadwinner in a household has priority over use of the car for work. The issue of transport has been growing in importance as food outlets and medical services become centralized. The time and money spent on travelling becomes a factor to be considered in health service use. One study of pregnant women found that women going to the hospital antenatal clinic spent twice as long travelling and waiting than mothers going to local GP clinics. They also experienced great problems in travelling with young children (Graham, 1979).

Several studies examine how mothers cope with the stress of caring for the family on a low income, which often involves a juggling act of keeping within a very limited budget while at the same time seeing that the children are well and relatively contented. There is evidence that mothers find a variety of ways of relieving stress in the short term without leaving the child alone. Graham (1984) points out that this often leads to parents going against medical advice. Sweets tend to be used as a quick and easy way of keeping children quiet on shopping trips and on other stressful occasions (Charles and Kerr, 1985), breast-feeding may be abandoned to allow more time for other members of the family (Graham, 1980), and babies' milk may be mixed with cereal to help cope with crying and sleep problems (Graham and McKee, 1980). Cigarette-smoking was used by some mothers as a way of easing tension without leaving the room (Graham, 1976). Another review has also recently highlighted the use of smoking by women to help them survive their stressful workload (Jacobson, 1988).

Graham (1984) points out that such actions, which would be labelled irresponsible by some professionals, may be the only way in which mothers can stay sane and act responsibly towards their family. Poor attendance for preventive health services is also examined in terms of costs and benefits. Graham concludes: 'For poor families in particular a *rational* decision may be one which rejects professional care. The mother may choose instead to invest her limited resources of time, money, and energy in other areas of family health' – in food for the family for example, or in keeping her children warm (Graham, 1984).

These studies on family health, in particular, indicate a complex relationship between individual behaviour and structural and material factors. When researchers start to ask why behaviour differs between classes, it becomes clear that socio-economic circumstances do play an important part. It is far too simple an explanation to put it all down to ignorance or laziness.

Explaining sex differences in health

Parallels can be drawn between the explanations of social class inequalities and those of sex inequalities in health. The artefact, natural selection, behavioural/cultural and materialist/structuralist explanations have all been applied to sex differentials.

For instance, some of the sex differences in morbidity (with high rates for women) have been attributed to artefact, though the exact extent of this is unknown. Morbidity may be under-estimated for men relative to women due to more proxy reporting for men in surveys; or women may have a greater predisposition to report illness. Additionally, women may be more inclined to take care of their health, resulting in increased consultation rates or days of restricted activity for the same amount of illness (Waldron, 1983). All these points need further investigation and, of course, none of them can explain away the sex differential in mortality.

The natural selection or genetic explanation suggests that women's greater longevity and low mortality rate is an intrinsic feature of the human species. This view is supported by the fact that even before birth female foetuses have better survival rates than male foetuses (Hart, 1991). Whatever the merits of the genetic explanation, evidence that the sex differential in mortality is reversed in less developed countries (like Nepal and Bangladesh), and that even the morbidity differential is not a fixed phenomenon in the same country, suggests that the social and cultural environment and health services can play a powerful part in modifying the differential. If that is so, then there should be scope for improvement in health for both sexes.

Very little work has been published on the causes of the sex differential in Britain, though studies in the United States and Europe attempt to answer the question: 'Why do women live longer than men?' Male mortality exceeds female mortality by 100 per cent for seven of the major causes of death in the United States: coronary heart disease, lung cancer, emphysema, motor-vehicle and other accidents, cirrhosis of the liver and suicide. These causes account for 75 per cent of the sex differential in mortality in the United States. Reasons for the differential have been analysed at the behavioural/cultural level. It was estimated, for example, that well over half the difference between male and female death rates could be accounted for by differences in behaviour, for example cigarette-smoking, alcohol consumption and occupational hazard. The study concluded that sex differences in behaviour are more important causes of higher male mortality than genetic factors (Waldron, 1976).

A comparison of sex differentials in health and illness in Sweden, Denmark, Finland and Norway found great variation in the morbidity differential. For example, the sex differential in symptoms of anxiety was much smaller in Finland and Sweden than in Denmark and Norway. Type of employment also had an effect on the differential. There was excess female morbidity in agricultural and manual workers. In white-collar groups, students and pensioners, however, men and women had similar standards of health. In some countries, like Finland and Norway, white-collar women were healthier than their male counterparts. Overall, the excess female morbidity rate was mainly due to higher rates for female manual workers and full-time housewives (Haavio-Mannila, 1986). In general it was concluded that in countries where many women work outside the home, rates of illness and hospitalization for women are lower than those for men. In countries, and at certain periods of time in the same country, when women mostly stay at home, women's illness rates are higher than for men (Haavio-Mannila, 1986). In Britain there is debate about the differential effect on health of employment outside the home for groups of women living in different social circumstances, as explained on p. 247 (Arber *et al.*, 1985; Moser *et al.*, 1990b).

Another study in 1985 was interested in the causes of the difference in life expectancy between men and women. The authors argued that if much of the difference between males and females was due to environmental factors, then there may be situations where the difference could be reduced. They hypothesized that kibbutz life might be capable of narrowing the gender gap in life expectancy by providing a closely matched environment for men and women with less difference in gender roles than in other developed countries. Calculating the expected gap in life expectancy from international data, they found that in the kibbutz the observed gap was much smaller – at birth the gap was 4.5 years instead of the expected 7.1 years, and at age fifty the gap was 2.7 years instead of the expected 5.1 years. The gap had been reduced by improvements in male life expectancy rather than by a reduction in female life expectancy (Leviatan and Cohen, 1985).

These recent studies open up intriguing possibilities for improvements in the sex differentials in health, though investigations are only at a preliminary stage. They certainly illustrate the potential importance of social and environmental factors on the health of both men and women.

Conclusions

The four explanations of inequalities in health put forward by the Black Working Group have been reviewed in the light of new evidence. From the evidence, the inequalities between social groups are genuine and cannot be explained away as artefact. Further evidence has confirmed the existence of a health selection effect – in particular, showing that serious illness in childhood is linked to a fall in occupational class later on. There is also renewed evidence of selection for height at marriage. Estimates suggest that the selection effect is small and does not account for the much larger differentials in health observed.

The weight of evidence continues to point to explanations which suggest that socio-economic circumstances play the major part in subsequent health differences. For example, the evidence that health-damaging behaviour is more common in lower social groups continues to accumulate, especially concerning smoking and diet. But can such life-style factors account for all the observed differential in health between different social groups? The short answer is: no. When studies are able to control for factors like smoking and drinking, a sizeable proportion of the health gap remains and factors related to the general living conditions and environment of the poor are indicated. In this context there is also a growing body of evidence that material and structural factors, such as housing and income, can affect health. Most importantly, several studies have shown how adverse social conditions can limit the choice of life-style and it is this set of studies which illustrates most clearly that behaviour cannot be separated from its social context. Certain living and working conditions appear to impose severe restrictions on an individual's ability to choose a healthy life-style.

The evidence suggests that policies to reduce inequalities which focused entirely on the individual would be misguided. The importance of social and material factors highlighted by the research suggests that broader policies incorporating structural improvements in living and working conditions would be required in addition.

Chapter 7

Action on Inequalities: A Framework for Policy-making

From the evidence reviewed in the previous chapters, it is clear that inequality in health and health care cannot be dismissed as a marginal issue. It is a substantial problem for Britain, and for many other countries. Tens of thousands of excess deaths, and extra suffering and disability each year, point to a massive waste of potential across the population as a whole – potential to live a healthy, productive, satisfying life. Whether an economic point of view is taken, or a public health or a humanitarian stance, it does not make sense to ignore the problem and make no attempt to address it.

However, it is one thing to highlight a problem, but another to say what, if anything, can be done about it. In comparison with the hundreds of reports adding to our knowledge of the extent and nature of inequalities in health, there have been little more than a handful analysing the broad policy issues involved. Nevertheless there have been pockets of intensive activity to draw upon, not only in this country but in Europe and North America.

The rest of the report will concentrate on practical action to tackle inequalities. This chapter details the emergence of a consensus on broad policy aims and outlines a framework for thinking about policy development. Subsequent chapters look at research and information needs, policy in the caring services, and the wider involvement of other sectors.

A consensus on policy emerges

The publication of the Black Report rekindled debate in many countries about the seriousness of the problem and what could be done about it. It was one of the first government-sponsored reports to draw conclusions from the evidence for policy-making purposes. It is instructive to look at the Black Report's analysis, and how the debate has developed since then, towards strategies for action.

1. The Black recommendations

Inspection of pp. 198–208 in this volume will reveal the Black Report's plan of action, based on research, health and social service initiatives, and a wider strategy to raise living standards among the most disadvantaged in society.

It is noteworthy that at least seventeen of the thirty-seven recommendations of the Black Report relate directly to policy-making within the caring professions. Although the evidence presented in that report – and confirmed by the latest research – suggests that health and social services cannot be expected to solve the problem of inequalities in health singlehanded, the Working Group was convinced that there was a vital role for these services to play. The improvement in the quality of life which health care can bring about, particularly for the most disadvantaged groups, was considered to be of substantial importance.

The policy outlined on pp. 133–64 has three main thrusts: priority for children, for disabled or elderly people, and for preventive and educational action.

In addition, as material living standards and social circumstances were seen to play a major role in maintaining inequalities in health, a broad social policy was proposed by the Black Working Group through the three main strategies outlined on pp. 165–97. First and foremost the abolition of child poverty was proposed as a national goal for the 1980s, achieved through various means involving

- increases in child benefit and maternity grants;
- the introduction of an infant care allowance;
- attention to nutrition of children, particularly in school meals, which should be free for all;
- increased pre-school education and action on child accidents involving planners, engineers and architects.

Secondly, the Working Group recommended improvements in housing and working conditions, together with a fairer deal for disabled people through a comprehensive disability allowance and special funding for housing adaptations and services (recommendations 29–35).

Thirdly, a co-ordinated government policy was envisaged, involving national and local government and an overseeing Health Development Council responsible for planning and monitoring progress of the policy (recommendations 36, 37).

Although these proposals were not welcomed with open arms by the government of the day, there is no doubt that they attracted widespread interest on an international scale, and they coincided with discussions taking place in the World Health Organization on a European health policy level.

2. The World Health Organization strategy

In 1984 the European Region of the WHO drew up a strategy for attaining 'Health for All by the Year 2000' and in 1985 issued detailed targets to which the UK has agreed. Firstly, it acknowledged that there are certain fundamental conditions which have to be met before any real improvements can be made – the prerequisites for health:

- freedom from the fear of war;
- equal opportunities for all;
- satisfaction of the basic needs for food, basic education, clean water and sanitation, decent housing, secure work and a useful role in society;
- political will and public support to launch the necessary action.

'Without peace and social justice, without enough food and water, without education and decent housing, and without providing each and all with a useful role in society and adequate income, there can be no health for the people, no real growth and no social development' (WHO, 1985).

Secondly, it recognized that the region would have to come to grips with two major issues if the European goal is to be reached by the year 2000: the reduction of health inequalities among countries and among groups within countries, and the placing of just as much emphasis on strengthening health as on reducing disease and its consequences.

Not surprisingly, therefore, the first of the thirty-eight detailed targets which followed this statement was concerned with 'equity in health'; 'By the year 2000, the actual difference in health status between countries and between groups within countries should be reduced by at least 25 per cent by improving the level of health of disadvantaged nations and groups' (WHO, 1985). The WHO considered that this target could be achieved 'if the basic prerequisites for health were provided for all; if the risks related to life-styles were reduced; if the health aspects of living and working conditions were improved; and if good primary health care were made accessible to all'. It emphasized that the main determinants of present health differences were living and working conditions; that the struggle against poverty and social deprivation was an integral part of any policy for better health; and that approaches to changing life-styles should be supportive rather than victim-blaming and should recognize the limits placed on the choice of a healthy life by social and economic conditions. It also stressed the need for responsive, outreach health services. What the WHO strategy goes on to do is to carry the theme of 'equity in health' right through the rest of the targets to form a broad, long-term policy touching on many aspects of health.

These points and the finer details of the strategy were in complete agreement with the policies advocated by the Black Working Group. The two analyses agree on the main problem, the underlying causes and the most likely solutions. The documents can be read and considered together as outlining a way forward for the future.

3. Professional proposals

It is obvious that this is precisely what is happening already in some local government and health authorities, and also in the discussions taking place in the professional bodies. For example, the Faculty of Community Medicine issued a Charter for Action in 1986 to identify the specific actions that would be required in the UK to pursue the WHO targets successfully (Faculty of Community Medicine, 1986). This spelt out in detail what the targets would mean for central and local government, for health authorities and health professions, for training institutions, for all organizations and for individuals.

The British Medical Association, in direct response to its members' concern about findings of the Black Report, set up a working group to consider the evidence on deprivation and ill-health and came up with recommendations from a medical perspective (BMA, 1987). There are two strands to the action proposed in the BMA discussion document: short-term health service initiatives which could lessen the incidence of specific illness in deprived groups, and long-term structural changes in social policy.

The long-term suggestions on structural changes included:

- action on unemployment;
- financial support for vulnerable groups;
- school meals;
- an enlightened approach to inner-city building and the safety of children;
- a review of legal control of workplace health and safety;
- a new generation of public health laws to combat present-day problems of housing design, damp and disrepair.

The report does emphasize, however, that the problem cannot be solved by juggling existing resources between different health and social services. There would need to be a national commitment to take action and to provide the necessary resources to do so.

Adding a further dimension to the debate, the Archbishop of Canterbury set up a Commission in 1983 to examine social and economic conditions in the urban priority areas. When it was published in 1985 the Commission's report, entitled 'Faith in the City', was influential in forcefully focusing public attention on the plight of the inner cities. In graphic detail it set out the structure of inequality within the cities; the economic and physical decline and social disintegration experienced in the outer housing estates as well as in the central urban areas. It concluded:

Chapter after chapter of our Report tells the same story: that a growing number of people are excluded by poverty or powerlessness from sharing in the common life of our nation. A substantial minority are forced to live on the margins of poverty or below the threshold of an acceptable standard of living. The critical issue to be faced is whether there is any serious political will to set in motion a process which will enable those who are at present in poverty and powerlessness to rejoin the life of the nation. (Archbishop of Canterbury's Commission, 1985)

The recommendations for the nation stemming from the study were very much in tune with those of the Black Report, with radical proposals for concerted action on poverty, unemployment, housing conditions, homelessness, community care, public safety and national policies on health. Prominent researchers in the field, although differing in where they put most emphasis, came out in favour of similar action.

4. The Chief Medical Officer's analysis

Throughout most of the 1980s there was a conspicuous silence from both government and civil servants on the subject of inequalities in health. There seemed to be almost a taboo about even mentioning the phrase in official documents.

This silence lasted until 1990, when it was gradually broken, first in Wales and then most notably by the Chief Medical Officer for England. For example, in a lecture in October 1990, he said:

We can now turn to two recent reports – the Black Report and Margaret Whitehead's 'The Health Divide'. I believe that, on the epidemiological data presented, the major conclusion of their authors is inescapable. This conclusion is that, despite the continuing general decline in mortality and improvement in health, the forty years since the introduction of the NHS have seen little progress in the reduction of inequalities in health among the various social groups. Indeed, for some variables the differences have grown. (Acheson, 1990)

He went on in that lecture, and in his final annual report as Chief Medical Officer, to put forward his analysis of the problem and the possible solutions. The clearest links with the excess burden of ill-health were seen as low income, unhealthy behaviour, and poor housing and environmental amenities. Success in reducing observed inequalities required a wide strategy to reduce deprivation and improve the physical environment, in addition to the most obvious points of initial attack such as health promotion initiatives on personal risk factors (Acheson, 1991).

These illustrate the emerging consensus that something should be done and the direction in which policy should be developing. The debate has obviously moved on since the Black Report made recommendations, but it is remarkable how salient those recommendations were and how similar are the conclusions of a variety of bodies up to the present day.

A framework for policy-making

Over the past three years, WHO has been engaged in clarifying the concepts of equity in health (Whitehead, 1990), and looking at policies and strategies to promote greater equity (Dahlgren and Whitehead, 1992); the following section draws on this work.

It is potentially a vast area and the approach advocated in the WHO discussion papers is to concentrate on the soluble – to sort out which health differences are both avoidable and considered unacceptable. Four main determinants of inequalities in health are widely considered to be at least partially preventable and at the same time unfair. First, the substandard or dangerous living and working conditions to which people in disadvantaged groups are more often exposed are clearly inequitable. Secondly, there are risk factors associated with personal behaviour – smoking, inadequate nutrition – which are more common in lower social groups and would be considered unfair if choice of personal life-style is restricted by socio-economic conditions. Thirdly, there are factors associated with health care – poorer provision, uptake and quality of essential services in communities at greatest need of such care. Fourthly, there is the tendency for sick people to become poor. This is a special category, because the original ill-health may not have been preventable. However, the low income of disabled people could be considered both preventable and unjust.

Most of these factors would be singled out in a general policy to improve the public health, but the point is that all these factors are at a higher concentration in more disadvantaged sections of society and any improvement in them would benefit these groups especially.

What are we trying to do?

It is important to sort out what policies are trying to do. A policy to tackle any of these risk factors or health hazards could have one of three quite distinct aims:

1. To tackle some of the main determinants of inequalities directly – housing problems, unemployment, barriers to healthier life-styles, and so on.

2. To minimize the health damage from these root causes so that people are less liable to fall ill when they experience them. For example, counselling and support of people when they become unemployed will not prevent unemployment but may help them avoid the psychological damage caused by the experience of unemployment.

3. To match the volume and quality of health services to the increased volume and complexity of ill-health found in communities facing these excess risks. This third goal is an attempt to cope fairly with the increased need that inequalities create, rather than a direct attack on inequalities. However, the end result may well be a reduction in inequalities in access to care.

It is clear that the activities going on in health and social service fields are often directed at goals 2 and 3, though there is scope for action on goal 1 as well, as some of the illustrations in Chapter 9 make clear. For example, the job creation schemes and welfare rights campaigns (pp. 366 and 367) can make a small but valuable contribution to alleviating the experience of unemployment and poverty. This fact is often overlooked when people perceive that only massive structural changes on a national or international scale can have any effect on the problem.

To achieve any of these policy goals, strategies are needed which consider information needs, the possible points of intervention, organizational arrangements, and monitoring. These will be examined in the following chapters.

Chapter 8

Action on Inequalities: Information Needs and Research

For policy to be soundly based, improvements need to be made in the collection of routine information and in developing better measurement tools through research. This chapter discusses information needs and the gaps identified in existing data, before going on to outline some current developments in this area.

Information needs and gaps

Several recent reviews have outlined the kind of information needed for the planning and evaluating of policies to reduce inequalities in health and health care (Thunhurst, 1989; Dahlgren and Whitehead, 1992; Thunhurst and Macfarlane, 1992).

In general, there is a need for increased recording of socio-economic factors in routinely collected health statistics and, conversely, an injection of health information into routine economic and social statistics. A pragmatic approach has been advocated by such organizations as the Core Indicators Group of the Healthy Cities network. The group takes the view that it is better to take practical steps to improve and use existing data, even if inadequate, rather than waiting for the production of an idealistic set of indicators that may never materialize (Thunhurst, 1989).

Existing health information systems could be adapted to include more social data if the commitment was there. The Hospital Episode System, for example, originally contained no information on socio-economic circumstances of patients, but through pressure from statisticians, from 1992 ethnic origin will be recorded and consideration is being given to including social class. Records will be aggregated by district of residence rather than hospital of treatment, which will allow better planning for local populations, and patients' NHS numbers will be added to records to increase the potential to link records together (Thunhurst and Macfarlane, 1992). Adaptations such as these help with the monitoring of inequalities and related policies. Other new information systems currently coming into operation need to be examined for their potential to include social factors – for example, the NHS District Information Support Systems and computerized record-keeping in general practice. Child health computer systems have been used to monitor inequalities in children's health (Reading *et al.*, 1990) and it has been suggested that this computer system could form the basis of a total community register, forming links with primary care and recording events into adulthood (Ross and Begg, 1991).

The Black Working Group considered that it would be easier to trace and assess continuing inequalities

- if school health statistics routinely recorded the height, weight, hearing and other health indicators of school children in relation to occupational class;

- if statistics on accidents to children routinely recorded the circumstances of the accident, and the age and occupational class of the parents;

- if the National Food Survey were adapted to be a more effective measure of nutritional status, and be able to identify 'at risk' groups in the population;

- if the General Household Survey developed a more comprehensive measure of income and command over resources, so that the influence of poverty/affluence could be related to self-reported illness in the Survey.

None of these four recommendations on data collection has been adopted in the intervening twelve years so policy-makers still have to rely on special surveys carried out from time to time at national or local level.

The idea that routine economic and social statistics should include data related to health has been taken up in the 1991 census. For the first time since 1911 it did contain two important new questions, one asking about chronic illness and the other about ethnic origin. Although the wording of the health question was not ideal, the response to these questions will be of enormous help in linking health and social factors together once the data become available for secondary analysis.

There is still an urgent need for more data on all dimensions of health that can be disaggregated below regional level, to give information at the district, city and town level. Many national surveys related to health or personal risk factors do not give reliable information at these levels.

In the longer term, development work is needed to produce:

- better indicators of social inequality;

- improved measures of health, especially morbidity;

● resource allocation formulae sensitive to inequalities in health;

● ways of auditing inequalities in the outcome of health care.

Many of the gaps in information and research needs identified by the Black Working Group still remain, including the recommendations on a major research programme co-ordinated by the research councils and the Department of Health.

Furthermore, for much of the 1980s it has become even more difficult to obtain information on social class and health even from the traditionally available sources. The Black Working Group drew heavily on detailed analyses from the occupational mortality supplements of the Registrar General's Office produced for the years around each census. However, the latest supplement, published in 1986, did not carry out such analysis of the data, and several researchers have expressed their frustration at this latest obstacle to research (Townsend *et al.*, 1988; Morris, 1986).

There was an even stronger reaction from the *British Medical Journal* in a leader entitled 'Lies, damned lies and suppressed statistics'. It commented:

The latest [supplement] has just been published, and something strange has happened – reference to the social class differences in mortality have almost slipped out. Why is this? Could it be because somebody in the government or in the Registrar General's office is anxious to play down the widening gap in mortality between rich and poor ... it would seem that yet again the government is exerting its influence and suppressing potentially adverse information. (*British Medical Journal*, 1986)

This implication was flatly denied by the chief medical statistician responsible for producing the supplement. He argued that the information on occupational class in the supplement was less reliable than in previous decades and was also no longer suitable for studying the very deprived groups in society, and that was why the customary analysis had not been carried out. Because in the months that followed there was still much disquiet about the affair, the Medical Research Council called a meeting in May 1987 to consider the collection of information on inequalities in health. Several researchers pointed out that the information on occupational class collected by the Registrar General was still valuable if used properly. Indeed it was considered one of the best sources for investigating deaths by different causes or in a variety of subgroups because of the large number of deaths it covered. There were plenty of suggestions for improving the reliability of data, including more field surveys, more longitudinal studies following people over a period of time, and the use of 'marker' occupations representing each occupational class. Many ideas for further research were put forward, including greater understanding of the ways in which unemployment, psychosocial differences and nutrition could bring about inequalities in health. However, the *British Medical Journal* commented that the government's chief medical statistician 'did almost too good a job at demolishing the value of the data that he is responsible for collating, and other researchers at the meeting had to reassure him that they were still valuable' (Smith, 1987b).

Despite this rather negative picture at national level and the difficulties encountered, there have been positive developments in the field of official statistics. Following the criticism of the last Decennial Supplement for not including analysis of the social class data, the next one, due to be published in 1995, promises to be a much improved document. It will have extended analyses not only on social class, but also on several alternative classifications based, for example, on tenure and car ownership. Also promising are developments at the OPCS Longitudinal Study. This was not originally set up with health studies in mind, though it has already proved invaluable for examining questions on inequalities in health. Now the Longitudinal Study Unit has had a team of research officers attached to it by OPCS, to look directly at health issues and extend the analyses still further.

There have also been notable responses from various organizations and individual researchers around the country on developing tools for monitoring inequalities in health, as the following examples illustrate.

Post-coding

Social indicators from the census small-area statistics are now readily available on tape from OPCS, down to the level of wards. From this, over 250 variables are available for analysis, including housing and overcrowding factors, consumer-durable ownership, employment status, family composition and so on. Since 1981 (1974 in Scotland) OPCS has provided post-coded death records, and also post-coded birth records. Since 1982 birth-weight has been recorded almost universally on birth and perinatal death certificates. In Scotland all in-patient statistics and cancer registrations have been post-coded since 1975.

This opens up much wider opportunities for analysing small areas below the level of local authority or health district. For instance, it makes it much easier to pinpoint areas of poor health and to explore which social and other factors in those areas are implicated. In this context, the Black Report called for further research 'on the development of area social conditions and health indicators for use in resource allocation' and 'the study of the interaction of the social factors implicated in ill-health over time, and within small areas'. Numerous studies of this kind have been undertaken by health and local authorities in direct response to the Black Report, making use of these newly available data. These studies have already been outlined in Chapter 2, but in the following section some of the technical considerations will be discussed.

Developing measures of social inequality

Small-area analysis does have some unique problems which have been reviewed by Carstairs (1981a). In particular, small areas produce small numbers of events, for example only a handful of deaths in a year. To compensate for small numbers, results have sometimes been aggregated over several years. Alternatively, results for areas with similar social profiles have been combined. OPCS sponsored a series of studies in the 1970s to find ways of identifying and grouping together wards with similar socio-economic composition irrespective of where they were in the country. For example, in the resulting Craig–Webber classification forty variables from the census data have been employed to group census wards together to form thirty-six socially distinct 'clusters'. Clusters range from 'high-status suburban areas' to 'poor-quality housing in areas of economic decline', and this classification has been used in other studies – for example in the OPCS Longitudinal Study described on p. 250. A Classification of Residential Neighbourhoods (ACORN) is a similar approach which has been developed commercially, based on the age structure of an area together with its employment level, family composition, type of housing, car ownership and social status. Only the post-code is required to identify the social profile of a neighbourhood. The value of using the ACORN system in health studies is being investigated (Morgan, 1983; Morgan and Chinn, 1983).

Other studies have combined several indicators of social and material deprivation into a composite deprivation index. Areas can then be ranked by their degree of disadvantage or affluence according to their score on the index. The question of which social indicators to include in the index is crucial and has been thoroughly discussed in three papers (Thunhurst, 1985b; Townsend, *et al.*, 1986b; Morris and Carstairs, 1991). The points made there warrant closer inspection. Table 20 shows the social indicators used to define deprivation in four well-known indices.

Note that some indices combine direct indicators of deprivation, like overcrowding and unemployment, with indirect measures of the number of people *at risk of deprivation*, for instance the proportion of one-parent families, elderly people or ethnic minorities in an area. The problem is that

Table 20: *A comparison of the social indicators used in four well-known indices*

	Proportion of:
Department of the Environment (1983) Indicators of urban deprivation	unemployed persons; overcrowded households; single-parent households; households lacking exclusive use of basic amenities; pensioners living alone; population change; residents living in households where head of household was born in the New Commonwealth or Pakistan. Standardized Mortality Ratio.
Jarman (1983, 1984) Underprivileged Area Score	children aged under 5; ethnic minorities; single-parent households; elderly living alone; lower social classes; highly mobile people; non-married-couple families (indicating less stable family groups). Overcrowding-factor. Poor housing factor. Unemployment.
Carstairs Index (Carstairs and Morris, 1989)	overcrowding; unemployment among men; low social class; not having a car; –combined into single score for each post-code sector.
Townsend Index (Townsend et al., 1988)	economically active residents aged 16–59/64 who are unemployed; private households lacking a car; private households which are not owner-occupied; private households with more than one person per room.

not all people in such groups are deprived. Mixing material conditions and 'at risk' groups like this can result in certain pitfalls. For example, Townsend points out that the Department of the Environment's score finds that the ten most deprived local authority areas in England are all in London, with none in the North. Similarly the Jarman index finds seven of the ten most deprived health districts are in London and none in the Northern Region: figures which fly in the face of other observations. Thunhurst (1985b) points out that such results are obtained when an index is dominated by certain highly skewed variables such as ethnic minority and one-parent family households which are more highly concentrated in the inner London boroughs than elsewhere. If no correction is made for this skewed distribution, then high-scoring areas on the index may simply be high-scoring areas for ethnic minority or single-parent households.

Ways of overcoming this problem have been put forward, for example by the use of more sophisticated statistical techniques and by using 'grass-roots' surveys to check and extend the statistical results (Thunhurst, 1985b). Townsend and his colleagues solve the problem by choosing only indicators of material deprivation, such as the proportion of households with no car, or with electricity disconnected, or with an unemployed head. Likewise social class is not included in the composite index, but is analysed separately so that the interrelationship between health, deprivation and social class can be investigated.

Several comparisons of the various indices have now been carried out. In one study five common indices were examined to measure their relative performance in explaining the variations observed in health indicators, using data from post-code sectors in Scotland. The Carstairs Index (Scottish Deprivation Score) and the Townsend Index were found to explain most variations, and to adhere most closely to the concept of material deprivation. The Jarman Index, on the other hand, was less effective because it included some individual variables which correlated very weakly, or even negatively, with the health indicators (Morris and Carstairs, 1991). ·

Other studies have compared the use of unemployment rates with the common indices, to judge their relative usefulness to district health authorities for indicating need at a small-area level. One study concluded that unemployment rates merited further consideration and that the Jarman Index was the least appropriate of several other indices for health authority use (Campbell *et al.*, 1991). A new index for measuring the impact of relative deprivation on general practitioners' workload has also been developed, claiming to overcome some of the shortcomings of the Jarman Index (Balarajan *et al.*, 1992). There is heated debate about the relative merits of each index at present, as a search is on for the best one to use for resource allocation under the NHS reforms. The Jarman Index is already used to allocate deprivation supplements to general practices, though some question the wisdom of this (Carr-Hill and Sheldon, 1991; Davey-Smith,

1991). The authors of the three best-known indices have jointly pointed out that it is important in the debate about which is best not to lose sight of the common message coming out of all these indices – the strong link between deprivation and ill-health, however measured (Jarman *et al.*, 1991).

Beyond occupational class

Although occupational class has traditionally been used to measure social class it is not without its problems, particularly in relation to women (McDowall, 1983). In mortality statistics and studies on morbidity (in the General Household Survey, for instance) married women have often been classified by their husband's occupational class and single women by their own occupation. At least three major problems arise:

1. Fifty-two per cent of married women now work outside the home either full-time or part-time. Classifying them by their husband's occupation may conceal health hazards linked to their own employment.

2. Such classification may also conceal differences in health between married women who are housewives, those who are unemployed and those who are in paid employment.

3. The earnings of working women may well influence the standard of living and material resources of the household, but this is not taken into account if the husband's occupation alone is used.

Difficulties also arise with the unemployed, the elderly and children. For these groups, occupational class may not fully encapsulate the circumstances in which they live.

Several alternative approaches have been put forward and are being investigated. For instance, Arber (1989) suggests that the most appropriate measure would be *household class*, rather than individual class, based on the occupation of the spouse who is economically dominant. Groups with very poor health can also be differentiated by a combination of household characteristics and area-based indicators, and the OPCS Longitudinal Study has done extensive work on this as detailed on p. 244. Promising measures are emerging from this study in relation to the social circumstances of women.

In relation to children, one alternative measure is the Social Index developed for use in the Child Health and Education Cohort Study and intended to be more in tune with the home environment of the child than occupational class alone. This incorporates seven socio-economic variables associated with the child's environment:

occupational status of head of household;
parents' education;
social rating of neighbourhood;
tenure;
crowding index (persons/room);
bathroom availability;
type of accommodation.

If any one variable, such as occupational class, is not available, a score can still be obtained for the family by adjusting the index accordingly. The Social Index provides a continuous scale running from the most disadvantaged to the most advantaged social groups, and appears to be more sensitive to social inequalities in childhood than the Registrar General's social class scale. For example, it has identified disadvantaged groups experiencing difficulties in health service use which were not detected by the use of occupational class (Osborn and Morris, 1979).

Developing measures of health

The Black Report also recommended that policy decisions on, for example, resource allocation at district level should not be based on area mortality data alone. Further indicators of health care and social need were required.

There were calls for the use in area studies of morbidity data and measures of positive health, in addition to mortality rates. With the advent of post-coded birth records containing birth-weights, the incidence of low birth-weight in small areas can now be used as a health indicator in such studies. For example, it has been used in the study of health inequalities in the Northern Region (Townsend *et al.*, 1986b), and the Greater Glasgow Health Board used a range of birth-related information (for example low birthweight, breastfeeding and immunization status) to compile health profiles of general practice populations (Forwell, 1991).

Another promising tool for surveying health problems is the Nottingham Health Profile (Hunt and McEwen, 1980). It defines, much more specifically than, say, the General Household Survey, the *nature* of health problems in the population and the impact of those problems on everyday activities. The profile is in two parts. Part I assesses health in six problem areas considered to be important by the lay population, i.e. pain, energy, physical mobility, sleep, social isolation and emotional reaction. Part II measures the effect of these health problems on paid employment, ability to perform jobs around the house, and the effect on relationships, sexuality and so on. Each section carries a score of 100 – the higher the score, the greater the number of problems experienced. The profile has been shown to relate well to more traditional measures such as the presence of chronic illness and the seeking of medical care, but it provides an added insight for policy-making. Studies using this profile were described in Chapter 2. For unemployed and re-employed men, a comparison with the General Health Questionnaire (GHQ) found that the Nottingham Health Profile provided a broader assessment of perceived health, giving additional information on pain and physical mobility problems (McKenna and Payne, 1989).

Blaxter has reviewed the many different measures commonly used as health indicators in inequality studies and has been experimenting with five measures of health to assess their usefulness for future large-scale surveys. The five dimensions are disease, functional disability, 'illness' or frequent symptoms, 'malaise' (lack of psychological well-being) and fitness. The problems of measuring health are considered in depth in this study (Blaxter, 1985).

The Health and Life-style Survey, a national sample study of 9,000 people, has provided data on a whole range of health factors which have not been available on a national scale before. As well as collecting data on illness symptoms and conditions in the sample, the Survey has taken physiological measurements and collected information on life-style factors, self-assessment of health and orientation towards healthy behaviour, and can relate these to a variety of socio-economic parameters including income (Cox *et al.*, 1987; Blaxter 1990).

The Welsh Heart Health Survey of 1985 (and 1990) is also providing valuable data in the realm of positive health. In the nine health authorities in Wales 20,000 people were interviewed to provide a baseline of health indicator and life-style factors against which to assess health promotion activities (Nutbeam *et al.*, 1987). A similar survey was piloted in 1991 in England, and will be sampling 17,000 people per year from 1993.

One of the issues highlighted for further research by the Black Working Group was in the field of disability and handicap. The Working Group called for prevalence studies of disability in the community which made assessments of the severity of disablement, for example by self-care criteria. They also wanted studies on the *interaction* of processes leading to physical and mental handicap and disadvantage, and on how some children escape the effects of disadvantaged conditions p. 137. The Child Health and Education Study, based on a cohort of children born in 1970, has been engaged in studies of this nature. One of its aims has been to investigate the extent of disability and learning difficulties in the national sample of ten-year-old children. To do this, it has been developing a measure of disability based on an inventory of skills and behaviour. With the inventory the parents of each child in the sample can make an assessment of the child's ability, and norms for the population can be derived. Results from groups of disabled children can then be compared with the norms. In addition it is making assessments of educational achievement, undertaking medical examinations to assess physical health, and collecting information on a range of social and environmental factors associated with each child. From the data it may be possible to map the development of disability and learning difficulties and to assess the importance of the factors involved (Butler *et al.*, 1982).

Conclusions

The Black Working Group highlighted major deficiencies in data collection, and twelve years later these deficiencies have still not been fully remedied. In addition, some statistics which were previously available have become less accessible and gaps in new information systems for the NHS have now been identified. Improvements have been made in some fields, for example in the production of statistics for use on a small-area basis, but the inherent problem spreads far beyond research on inequalities in health to encompass public health research in general.

Above all, there needs to be increased recording of socio-economic factors in routinely collected health statistics as well as a parallel injection of health information into routine economic and social statistics.

Despite the shortcomings in data collection there has been some progress and upsurge in research on social inequalities in health, as the numerous studies reported in earlier chapters testify. It is significant that many of these studies were directly stimulated by the publication of the Black Report in 1980. Furthermore, there is intense activity to develop better tools for monitoring the situation and for allocating resources more equitably.

Chapter 9

Action on Inequalities: Policy in the Caring Services

A policy for the caring services should be seen as a complement to a wider strategy, rather than a substitute for action on a broader front. Nevertheless, there is still a valuable contribution to be made by the health and social services, even though it is recognized that the determinants of health in general, and inequalities in health in particular, mainly lie outside this sector.

Indeed, in a cold political climate when no lead is being taken at a national level, this may be one of the few sectors where progress can still be made. Action could be aimed at one of four goals:

1. Efforts can be made to reduce those inequalities in health *care* that result directly in inequalities in *health*. Inadequate access to preventive services may contribute to the increased infectious disease and death rates seen in lower social groups. Restricted access to contraception, maternal and child health care may contribute to the higher prevalence of risk factors such as early and unwanted childbearing, insufficient spacing between births, and high parity, which in turn influence infant mortality rates and many aspects of the health and well-being of mothers. For the conditions amenable to medical care, being offered poorer quality and less effective investigation, treatment and follow-up may lead to a greater incidence of death and disability in less favoured social groups. Given that procedures such as hip replacement and cataract surgery can have an immense impact on the quality of life experienced by older people, inequalities in this dimension of health may result if one social group is consistently selected for such operations in preference to others. The same is true for rehabilitation services. With vigilance and audit, the caring services can put their own house in order so that such inequalities in health care are minimized.

2. To a lesser extent, but still of value, is the impact the caring services can have on wider determinants of health: on improving working conditions; on reducing poverty; on influencing personal behaviour.

3. Another major task is to alleviate the health damage caused by these other determinants of inequalities in health. For example, when people working in hazardous conditions or children in unsafe housing experience higher accident rates, it is the speed and quality of response of the health service that can make all the difference to whether the injury is fatal, or whether it results in permanent or only temporary disability. Lack of services in high-risk localities can compound the damage done by the environmental factors. When unemployment strikes, sensitive services can help to prevent that experience causing lasting psychological harm. Health services may not be able to provide housing for homeless people, but they can ensure ease of access to essential services for the homeless when they need them. The provision of additional child care facilities in disadvantaged areas can help to compensate children for the effects of that disadvantaged environment. The role of the caring services in this respect should not be under-estimated.

4. Matching service provision to increased need in disadvantaged areas can also make a contribution. Assessing the health needs of the population, which planners of services are now supposed to do, should automatically lead to greater weight being given to the needs of disadvantaged sections of the community, even if reducing inequalities in health care was not an explicit aim of the planning process.

This chapter looks at some of the practical details relating to these aims. In particular, it discusses resource allocation, which is central to all four aims; improving access and quality of care; and what can be done on issues such as unemployment, poverty, housing and encouraging healthier personal life-styles. These are considered at different policy levels within the limits of the health and social service sectors.

Resource allocation

For the fair and equitable distribution of resources, there must be an awareness at all levels that there is an added burden of ill-health in disadvantaged areas and communities, and that historically there has been a tendency for poorer-quality services to exist in those same areas. It can be seen from Chapter 4 that there is still a problem in this respect, and current resource allocation policy may be making the situation worse.

When considering the national allocation to regional health authority level, for example, the formula as it stands–with weighted capitation–pays less attention to social inequalities in health than the RAWP formula. In relative terms, it shifts funds away from high mortality, high-deprivation regions of the country towards lower mortality, lower-deprivation regions, in the south and east. A revised formula needs to be devised which takes these two key factors into account. One problem seems to be that whichever of the existing formulae is used, some districts of London seem to be in an anomalous position with respect to the rest of the country. The 1991–2 review of London's health care needs, it is hoped, will come up with a solution for London that is adequately funded and does not damage allocation to the rest of the country.

Allocation from region to district is currently a problem in those regions where the national weighted capitation formula has been applied, without modification. This would result in loss of revenue in some relatively deprived districts, even in southern regions. Bearing in mind that deprived areas tend to have less adequate services anyway, this would lead to a decrease in access to and quality of services for people in need in such areas. Health authorities need to be aware of this potential problem and monitor the effects of funding arrangements on provision. This problem has been tackled in the four Thames regions. In City and Hackney Health Authority – one of the most deprived districts in the country on the DoE index – the funding predicament was highlighted in the 1990 public health report. A change to weighted capitation would have led to a £2 million loss in revenue from the district over the period 1992–5. Instead, representations from City and Hackney and other deprived districts led to a re-evaluation by the North-East Thames Region, which has now been persuaded to alter its formula to introduce a deprivation weighting. The three other Thames regions have agreed to the same formula. The index chosen is one devised by the University of Surrey, incorporating factors for social class and housing tenure. As a result, instead of losing £2 million, City and Hackney is now estimated to gain in the order of £10 million over the next four years. Mersey Regional Health Authority has also recognized the problem and introduced a weighting based on unemployment rates for allocations to all its districts.

At the family health services authority level, it has already been noted that there was a quality divide in general practice set to widen under the terms of the 1990 GP contract (Pringle, 1989). Some FHSAs have analysed the situation in their areas and have criteria for the allocation of development funds for staff, premises and computer technology in underdeveloped practices.

There are other aspects of resource allocation, of course, that are not directly dealt with by such mechanisms, such as the imbalance between primary and secondary care, and between resources going into prevention and promotion on the one hand, and treatment services on the other.

Improving access and quality of care

To improve access and quality of care, policy-makers and practitioners at all levels first need to be aware of the potential barriers to access, and second, to have a mechanism in place for monitoring services so that problems can be recognized if they materialize. It is not only geographic access that needs attention, but also economic and cultural access (Dahlgren and Whitehead, 1992).

Economic access is concerned with equal access to good-quality services regardless of the ability to pay. Even in a system like the NHS, barriers can arise, for example, if charges are introduced for certain services at a level which causes a serious decline in uptake.

The introduction of the 'internal market' into the NHS also raises potential dangers from an equity point of view. Problems arise because patients from disadvantaged groups are often more costly to treat and care for than the average, as they tend to suffer more illness of a chronic nature, for longer periods of their lives. They may also take longer to recover because of less nutritious diet, poor living conditions or lack of social support. Disadvantaged neighbourhoods tend to have a higher prevalence of illness than more affluent areas. Therefore a contract calculated on *average* costs of a specific treatment or average cost per head of population may fail to cover the *actual* cost for these patients. Without regulation there is a danger that providers will avoid bidding for contracts for 'unprofitable' deprived communities, preferring to compete for business to serve more 'profitable' affluent populations. Alternatively, the quality of services in deprived areas may have to be lowered to keep within the fixed price contract. When services are being rationed there is also the question of who gets chosen from the queue. Is one section of society always losing out?

Geographical access is concerned with the fair distribution of services around the country in different localities and relies in part on resource allocation discussed in the previous section. There are also local difficulties, for example with transport, to be taken into consideration.

Cultural access is concerned with the relationship between patients and health workers: whether differences in education, culture or religion cause barriers to communication and effective use of services.

Attention can be paid to these three types of access and to quality issues by:

● monitoring the effect of funding arrangements, changes in policy, and rationing processes, on provision of services for different sections of the population;

- monitoring uptake rates and patterns of service use and acceptability;
- monitoring quality of premises, staff numbers and their training, and the distribution of services in different localities;
- including equity considerations in the setting and monitoring arrangements for contracts;
- auditing referral and treatment patterns by social group.

There are examples of policy-makers who are already taking equity into consideration in their service planning. East Anglia Regional Health Authority, for instance, is developing ways of setting contracts with equity as one of the basic principles. A survey of district health authority contracts on health services for children in 1991 found that although most did not contain any acknowledgement of the link between poor child health and social deprivation, some did. One, for example, required providers to 'enable disadvantaged children to have equal access to health services'. Another required clinical audit in policies to develop provision for vulnerable groups such as travellers and the homeless. As the survey was undertaken at an early stage in the contracting process, the fact that some contained a consideration for inequalities in health was thought to be encouraging for the future (Benzeval *et al.*, 1992).

How to improve local access and quality of services has been given serious attention in many areas and progress has been made by groups around the country, especially in the maternal and child health field, as recommended in the Black Report. Dowling (1983) and Wood (1991) reviewed new developments in preventive health care in pregnancy and early childhood and documented over sixty schemes operating in England and Wales which have tried to ensure that services reach those who need them. Dowling concludes that, 'when attention is given to the life-styles and needs of the parents, most families can be contacted, often with surprising ease'. How is this done?

For a start, attention has been given to the difficulties of parents with young children trying to reach the clinics. Transport, for instance, is a particular problem for people on low incomes relying on public transport – which can be expensive, time-consuming and fraught with stress if small children have to be taken along too. Both rural areas like the Isle of Wight and urban areas like Hounslow and Edinburgh have been running decentralized antenatal clinics staffed by a consultant and community midwives. Mobile clinics have been used by Southwark to improve immunization in areas with low take-up rates, and by Ormskirk District to take child health services to outlying areas. Other health authorities have organized minibuses and other forms of transport to bring parents and children into central antenatal and child health clinics. Another successful approach has been the timing of clinics to suit parents who work during the day, or mothers with children who need to be collected from school in mid afternoon, or Asian women reluctant to visit the clinic at times when their husbands cannot accompany them. Some hold evening clinics, for example, while others make sure that mothers with school-age children to collect are given early-afternoon appointments. Many now provide play areas for children in clinics and general practitioners' surgeries to relieve the stress of long waits. The point is that sizeable improvements can be made in access and convenience of the services for the patient without necessarily costing large amounts of money.

Then there are projects which have set out to provide opportunistic health care for those who would not usually use preventive services. Shopping centres are obvious choices. Bolton Community Health Council and Health Authority, for example, set up a pregnancy walk-in clinic in the centre of the town, staffed by a midwife. The TUC and the Spastics Society have pioneered workplace antenatal care projects in Scotland and Oldham for pregnant women mainly working on the factory floor (Dowling, 1983).

Some projects have encouraged women to carry and keep their own obstetric notes as a way of improving communication between staff and patients and boosting confidence in women. A recent evaluation of six community-based projects of this nature concluded that such care can result in improved accessibility and uptake, improved communication and consumer satisfaction, without any deterioration in the outcome of pregnancy (Wood 1991).

Services trying to break the link between deprivation and child health have been reviewed by Goodwin (1991). New initiatives are continually being evolved to try to help deprived communities. In Nottingham, for example, an experimental programme has been investigating the organization of a child health clinic serving a deprived population. A community paediatric team approach has been used and has resulted in attracting older, more deprived pre-school children, and the detection of more treatable medical disorders (Nicoll, 1986). In the same city extra health-visiting has been provided for deprived groups. In this case areas of the city suffering from deprivation were first identified by a City Council project. From this, babies at high risk of post-neonatal death could be identified and their families supported with extra health-visiting. As the ratio of health visitors to population was already well below the DoH recommended level, any transfer of staff from one area to another was considered unfair on the community in general. The solution was to obtain joint funding for extra health visitors from City Council and Department of the Environment sources (Madeley, 1982).

A simple screening and educational programme has been developed for inner-city general practices. Pre-school children were screened for iron deficiency, sickle-cell disease and thalassaemia when they attended for immunization. This was found to be acceptable to families in socially deprived areas and the accompanying education may have accounted for some of the observed reduction in the prevalence of iron deficiency in the community (James *et al.*, 1989).

The Health Visitors Association has also recommended that school nurses should extend their role with children into counselling of pupils and support of staff, to develop health-promoting schools (HVA, 1991).

In the primary care setting, a group of GPs in the North-East of England has been exploring ways of improving preventive care for deprived patients, with various outreach programmes and schemes for tracing and responding to missed care through patients' records. Action is based on comprehensive, computerized medical records. The front of each record card shows the missing care for each member of the patient's household. An offer of preventive care can therefore be made whenever the doctor sees the patient for a sickness appointment – and the care is given immediately, to avoid return appointments. In addition, letters go out to each household listing and offering the missing care, with follow-up letters sent to non-responders from time to time. To make use of every opportunity, health visitors are provided with household lists with the missing care for each household member so that the topic can be brought up when visiting (Marsh and Channing, 1986). They succeeded in raising the uptake of preventive care for patients from a deprived area to a higher level than that of a more endowed neighbouring community (Marsh and Channing, 1988).

In another general practice setting in a socially deprived community in Wales, GPs have devised accessible and flexible ways of case finding and audit of the care of chronic disease and risk factors that allow for continuity of care. These methods have been shown to be effective in the control of chronic conditions and reduction of risk factors because they are responsive to the demands of patients living in difficult circumstances (Hart *et al.*, 1991). Bury Community Health Council has shown how community health councils can document inequality in access to health services in a deprived part of town and put practical suggestions to the health authority for making services more accessible (Walsh *et al.*, 1985).

Caring for disabled and elderly people

The situation concerning access and quality of services for disabled and elderly people is in a state of flux at the present time. Recommendations for improvement from the Black Report and other sources have been aimed mainly at improving the care of elderly and disabled people in their own homes. The strategy involved reviewing hospital, residential and domiciliary care for the disabled elderly, reviewing sheltered housing provision, encouraging joint care programmes and increasing community support especially in the form of nursing services for disabled people and home-help services with greatly extended functions.

A most unsatisfactory situation has evolved over the 1980s, and it is unclear whether it will be resolved in the near future. It is useful to look at some of the background to the present situation in order to understand how it came about. In 1986 the government-appointed Audit Commission reported on its study of community care policies. Were policies such as those in the DHSS 'Care in Action' document being adopted in practice? Were funding and organizational policies helping or hindering the desired developments? The Commission concluded:

There are serious grounds for concern about the lack of progress in shifting the balance of services towards community care. Progress has been slow and uneven across the country; and the near-term prospects are not promising. In short the community care policy is in danger of failing to achieve its potential . . . community care is far from a reality for many of the very people it is intended to help. (Audit Commission, 1986)

For the elderly, the Commission found that although there had been a decrease in the numbers accommodated in hospitals, this had been more than offset by an increase in accommodating old people in private residential homes. Apart from an increase in local authority day-care in the late 1970s, home-based services like home-helps, meals-on-wheels and community nursing had not increased in real terms but had been struggling to keep pace with the growing number of elderly in the population.

Furthermore there were great regional differences in the provision of care. For example, home-help provision by local authorities ranged from 7/1,000 people aged over 75 in some authorities, to 44/1,000 in others. The level of private and voluntary residential accommodation for the elderly varied from 7.6/1,000 people aged over 75 in Cleveland to over 70/1,000 in Devon. Indeed, all along the south coast of England there was much greater provision of this kind of service in relation to the relevant population than in the rest of the country. This could have far-reaching effects, as will become apparent shortly. The rapid expansion of private residential and nursing homes began in 1983 when the DHSS for the first time allowed local authority social service departments to make payments to private residential homes to place frail elderly people. Homes have been springing up all over the country and social security payments to them in 1983 totalled £102 million, rising to £200 million in 1984 and over £500 million in 1986 (Audit Commission, 1986). The BMA points out that this large expenditure on private residential homes conflicts with the government's stated policy of redirecting resources to community care. There is also the fear that elderly people may be pressured into accepting places in nursing homes when they could continue in their own homes *if they had adequate support* (BMA, 1986).

Support for this concern came from a 1985 study of elderly people admitted to residential homes in three authorities. About half the residents did not need to be there. They could have been supported in the community if the necessary resources had been available (Audit Commission, 1986).

Because of the perverse way in which the social security system works, it appeared to be easier to obtain state benefit payments for board and lodging in private residential homes than to obtain either Attendance Allowance or Invalid Care Allowance for care in a person's own home. And the amount of the benefit was greater. 'In short the more residential the care, the easier it is for people to obtain benefits and the greater the size of the payment.' Under this system there was, and still is, a further temptation for local authorities to turn some of their council-owned homes over to private management so that eligible residents could claim supplementary benefit to cover their fees. Substantial 'savings' have been made by local authorities by doing just that. The overall effect, however, was a serious undermining of community care initiatives because:

● it was encouraging high-cost residential care while starving some of the low-cost, home-based options;

● it was undermining the efforts of resource allocation policies by channelling public funds to people in the better-off, least deprived areas of the country.

What is more, local authorities which had increased expenditure to fund community care were sometimes penalized by having their grant from central government cut. As a result of this, the Audit Commission made recommendations for immediate action on funding and managerial policies. The Commission warned that if action was not taken, 'the result will be continued waste of scarce resources and, worse still, care and support that is either lacking entirely, or inappropriate to the needs of some of the most disadvantaged members of society and the relatives who seek to care for them' (Audit Commission, 1986).

There is no doubt, however, that the need for community support services is undiminished. The British Medical Association report on the elderly recommends the urgent development of respite care to help the carers of disabled and elderly people, as well as greater provision of home-help services, telephone alarms, laundry services, meals-on-wheels and so on – all services which allow disabled people to remain in their own homes (BMA, 1986).

Partly to deal with these problems, the NHS and Community Care Act is to be brought into force by 1993. This new legislation will give local authorities responsibility for assessing the requirements of each individual in need of care, whether elderly, disabled or mentally ill, and buying an appropriate package of care for that person. Money released from social security budgets, previously paid out for private residential care fees, may be available to councils, but exact funding arrangements are unclear. This could be a key opportunity to expand the sort of domiciliary services preferred by many older people, but to work well there has to be adequate funding designated specifically for community care, rather than going into a general fund. Vigilance will also be needed to ensure that preventive and home-based services are encouraged, rather than too much emphasis being placed on hospital-based or residential care.

Action on unemployment and poverty

Since the Black Report was written there has been a dramatic rise in unemployment in this country, first in the early 1980s, then again in the early 1990s. With it has come rising poverty and growing concern for the possible health consequences, and a questioning of the action the caring services could take on the matter.

A research project explored the issue with three professional groups. Health visitors, health education officers and social workers in London, the Midlands and Scotland were interviewed to discover how unemployment was affecting their work and their response to it. The study found that 80 per cent of the sample of health visitors and social workers and 50 per cent of health education officers, considered that unemployment was affecting their day-to-day practice. It was found that the increase in poverty was the most striking feature, though health visitors and social workers also found added individual and family problems created or exacerbated by unemployment. Most were ignorant of local initiatives and were responding in an *ad hoc* way to the situation. Though well-meaning, very few had stopped to think whether their actions were really suitable for dealing with the problem. The poor response was put down to lack of time and resources, but for some their attitudes were holding them back. For example, some felt that it was not really a task for them, but was for other professions. There was also confusion about what could be done, or a lack of conviction of the effectiveness of their actions – a realization that they would only be ameliorating rather than removing the difficulties. Some were apprehensive that their superiors would not see unemployment and its effects on health as a legitimate issue for health workers to tackle (Popay *et al.*, 1986). In response to this research, training materials for these professionals were produced (Dhooge and Dooris, 1988).

But what response can realistically be given? The Unemployment and Health Study Group (1986) and a series of articles by Smith (1987a) have examined the question in depth and put forward suggestions for action:

Responding to unemployment

District Health Authorities could

1. monitor unemployment and its health effects in the locality;
2. have a clear strategy to deal with the issue;
3. relay the information to staff;
4. take unemployment into account when targeting responses and resources to those most in need;
5. train staff in benefits and facilities available to the unemployed;
6. liaise with local authorities over local community initiatives;
7. create jobs and work.

Source: Adapted from Harris and Smith (1987).

Recommendations from these reviews include the drawing-up by health authorities of clear strategies to deal with unemployment and health; the monitoring of local unemployment and its effects on health using the special expertise of the district public health director, for instance; the training of all health workers on the health effects, the state benefits and local help available to the unemployed; and the setting-up of appropriate counselling services for them. Recognizing that the NHS is a major local employer, it was further suggested that health authorities could create jobs and work opportunities for the unemployed and handicapped people through the various government training and employment schemes, for instance, and ensure that orders for supplies went wherever possible to local firms. An important role for Community Health Councils was also advocated in raising the awareness of both the public and the health authorities of what could and is being done about the problem.

At the end of 1986 a survey of District Health Authorities was carried out to find out what they were doing about unemployment and health. Encouragingly, about half the health authorities in Britain were found to be responding to the problem in some way. For instance, those in areas of high unemployment were more active than those in low unemployment areas. There was great variability in the extent of the action, though, with health education and public health departments leading the way. The monitoring of health and social factors, including unemployment, had been undertaken by many districts, though only a few had passed the information to staff (Harris and Smith, 1987).

Some authorities, like Somerset, had been training staff in the benefits available to the unemployed, and the Greater Glasgow Health Board had produced a comprehensive study pack – originally intended for the unemployed, but which had become popular for professional training purposes (Black and Laughlin, 1985). Resource allocation to areas of high unemployment had proved difficult, though, because of the large proportion of expenditure taken up by hospital services. South Sefton Health Authority had been at the forefront of action in creating work opportunities. At one stage in the 1980s, it employed 250 long-term unemployed people through the Manpower Services Commission Community Programme, covering such topics as dental health education, community surveys and hospital security. Other districts have been following this example. Although this source of funding has now dried up, other government and EC schemes have come into being and could be tapped if people were alert to the opportunities.

Wider strategies are, of course, needed to tackle unemployment. But the point made by these commentators is that local action to ease the situation is possible at a very practical level. The same is true of poverty.

Responding to poverty

While economic policy at national and international level will determine overall levels of poverty in the country, some useful tasks can be carried out within the realm of the caring services. The role of health visitors in responding to poverty has been extensively reviewed recently and a practical guide for the caring professions has been produced (Blackburn, 1991 and 1992). Table 21 summarizes the suggestions for action coming from these reviews. However, the recommendations could just as easily apply to the practice of other health and social service workers, and indeed there are examples of this happening.

Table 21: *Responding to poverty: what can health visitors do?*

Monitoring:

- monitor level and distribution of poverty and related ill-health in neighbour-hoods;
- monitor and evaluate effectiveness of service provision and gaps;
- monitor how specific social policies affect families, e.g. the Social Fund.

Preventing and supporting:

- acknowledge to families that they are not to blame for poverty;
- give realistic advice and have realistic expectations of what families can do in their circumstances;
- make advice easier to follow, e.g. devise safety equipment loan schemes;
- help families to claim welfare benefits;
- negotiate with other services on their behalf;
- provide easy-to-use and flexible services;
- provide opportunities for families in poverty to meet together.

Pressing for policy change:

- raise awareness of issues among local agencies and community;
- encourage development of policies that will help, e.g. child care policies;
- develop community development skills to help local people to participate;
- join local pressure groups and press for policy statements from professional bodies.

Source: Adapted from Blackburn (1991).

For example, in Birmingham family health services authorities are funding welfare rights advice sessions in general practice health centres, funded as part of the health promotion clinic scheme. In Bristol the health authority and social services department are funding a similar project in deprived parts of the city. Tens of thousands of pounds in unclaimed and refused benefits have been gained by health centre users as a result (Richards, 1990).

Action on homelessness and housing

There is no doubt that homeless people face additional health problems which put them in great need of health services, but at the same time they face greater barriers in gaining access to care than the settled population. Among the added health problems for families living in temporary accommodation are high accident rates, food poisoning and nutritional difficulties, infestation, high infection rates, and stress-related illnesses. Because homeless people may be moved on from one hostel to another and one authority to another, there is difficulty in maintaining records and continuity of care from one GP and health visitor; and difficulty in being accepted on to other GPs' lists and in maintaining preventive care such as immunization. Many resort to the use of accident and emergency departments of hospitals, with no proper follow-up care.

Various proposals for positive action to ensure ease of access have been put forward (Lowry, 1990; Wall, 1991; HVA/BMA, 1989; Connelly *et al.*, 1991). These include adapting existing services to make them more accessible, or providing separate services for homeless people. Various schemes have proved successful, including special drop-in clinics where homeless people can get primary care attention without an appointment; sessions held in hostels for the homeless; and assigning responsibility to one or more health workers for monitoring the needs of homeless people and keeping track of their records, and then co-ordinating the care they need. In addition, suggestions have been put forward on how health workers could use existing laws to help improve housing conditions and to press local councils on unfit homes (Battersby, 1991).

Suggestions for directors of public health and planners have also been put forward (Roderick *et al.*, 1991; Connelly *et al.*, 1990). These include:

- conducting epidemiological research on the health problems associated with temporary homelessness, to inform planning;
- cooperation with local authorities and voluntary agencies for the more accurate collection of information on homelessness in the area;
- using the annual public health report to highlight effects of housing on the health of local people;
- withdrawing from the practice of determining medical priority for rehousing as this may be an inefficient and ineffective use of time;
- pressing for more training for doctors on housing policy and for more training for social service and housing staff on health;
- pressing through national channels for the establishment of health standards in house-building. (Roderick *et al.*, 1991.)

Planning services for ethnic minorities

The issue of ethnic minorities and the health and social services has been attracting more attention in recent years, although there have been suggestions that the health professions have been slow to recognize that this client group may have special needs (Johnson, 1984). For example, the

NHS has been criticized for a lack of effective action on two conditions which especially affect ethnic minority groups – sickle-cell anaemia and rickets. People of Afro-Caribbean origin are particularly at risk from sickle-cell anaemia, but although a test for it can be carried out at birth, as yet there is no comprehensive screening programme. With rickets, caused by a deficiency of vitamin D, the Asian population appears to be most at risk. Pressure to have Asian food fortified with vitamin D has, however, failed so far (Radical Statistics Health Group, 1987).

On the other hand, there has been criticism of the health service for a blinkered approach which sees the important health problems of Asians in particular as anaemia and rickets, infant mortality, and infectious diseases such as TB. This is reflected in the priority given to research and in the available health education literature. Major health problems, such as coronary heart disease, are given little or no attention when it comes to adapting services to the needs of different ethnic groups (Bhopal, 1988 and 1991). Bhopal recommends that, where possible, existing services should be adapted if required, with separate projects and services implemented only when these fail.

Donaldson and Odell (1984) list seven areas of concern where cultural differences may have implications for services: uptake of and encounters with services; perceptions of health and presentation of illness; life-style and cultural practices; differing patterns of disease and the use of alternative medicine. It is clear that in order to plan and provide health services with the needs of ethnic minorities in mind, routinely available information is required at the District Health Authority level. But does this information exist?

A survey in 1984 set out to discover what information bases were used at local level, what special services were provided (in this case for the Asian population), and whether health workers were undertaking training and research on transcultural health issues. Only health authorities with Asian populations over 500 were included. The vast majority of these authorities (81 per cent) derived estimates of the size of the Asian population from the census, which indicates country of birth only. Others had incorporated local data into the census data (16 per cent) and still others used data from local surveys only (8 per cent). Only 19 per cent had details of the religious composition of their Asian population. A total of 21 per cent of authorities had further details, such as the language spoken by various groups, but the two latter measures were mostly based on guess-work or general impressions. Authorities did not have morbidity data available by ethnic origin, though a number did have the country of birth recorded on some of their information systems. Despite these deficiencies many District Health Authorities were providing special services – mostly health education and special diets in hospital. Thirty per cent were also providing staff in-service training, and a high proportion were making use of informal interpreters, mainly relatives and volunteers (Donaldson and Odell, 1984). This study highlights the urgent need for sample surveys at a local level and suitable health information collection to provide the necessary data on ethnic minority populations. A plea was made in this study for renewed efforts to devise an acceptable question on ethnic origin for the 1991 census, and this has now been implemented (White, 1990).

Many of the initiatives developed so far have centred on services for mothers and babies. Tower Hamlets, for example, has employed interpreters in antenatal and child health clinics. Some employ health aides who, in addition to interpreting, give information about nutrition, child development, family planning and so on. Others have established new antenatal clinics in Asian communities, staffed by people who can speak the relevant languages (Dowling, 1983).

One of the best-known and respected projects in this area is the Hackney Health Advocacy Scheme in the East End of London, where half of the babies are born to mothers born outside the UK – 33 per cent of the total being from the New Commonwealth and Pakistan. The staff of the maternity hospital there estimated that a quarter of their patients did not speak English. Asking friends and relatives to translate was unsatisfactory because it caused embarrassment to women, especially if the interpreters were male. The Community Health Council initiated the Multi-Ethnic Women's Health Project in 1980 to meet the needs of the non-English-speaking women at the local maternity hospital. Women who worked for the project were called 'health advocates' and not only did they provide an interpreting service, but they also mediated between patients and professionals to make sure that women were offered an informed choice of health care. The advocates 'booked' new patients following a set protocol and presented the history to the midwife or doctor. The advocate then followed each woman through her pregnancy and was present at every antenatal visit. The project had an impact on hospital policy and practice; for example, in hospital food; introducing a protocol for breaking bad news; changes in labour ward protocol; stopping the practice of asking for passports and devising more sensitive ways of asking for post-mortems. An evaluation compared 1,000 women who had been helped by a health advocate with women from a control hospital and with a group from the same hospital before the scheme got under way. There were statistically significant differences between the groups in three areas. The antenatal length of stay was reduced to the level of the control hospital, although initially it had been higher. The proportion of induced labours to non-English-speaking women increased from 14 per cent to 16 per cent at the control hospital but stayed at 9 per cent at the hospital with the health advocates. The Caesarean section rate was less than half that of the control hospital. The study demonstrated that health advocacy can influence clinical practice as well as lead to patient satisfaction (Parsons and Day, 1992). Other link-worker schemes have also shown that hospital policy can be altered by such schemes (Rocheron and Dickinson, 1990).

Such ideas could be developed further if health workers became more aware of the issues. In this context the National Extension College has been developing training materials for the health professions, and the College has also carried out a survey of training needs on health and race, to identify priority topics in this area (National Extension College, 1984, 1986; Pearson, 1985; Larbie and Mares, 1986). A guide on health education for nurses has also been produced (Elliott, 1992).

One way forward in the promotion of health services more sensitive to the needs of ethnic minority groups is that taken by Liverpool Health Authority, which in May 1987 agreed a ten-year race relations strategy. The strategy's four goals are broken down into objectives and action programmes, together with time-scales for achieving them. A staff training programme supports the strategy, and targets will feature in the performance review of senior managers. The goals are notable in covering health care issues as well as employment matters.

Encouraging changes in personal behaviour

Differences in personal life-style between different social groups account for some of the inequalities in health observed, though, as emphasized in Chapter 6, it is not a sufficient explanation without some understanding of the severe restrictions on life-style faced by many living in disadvantaged conditions. There is a place for sensitive education and support by health professionals, but only if two factors are fully taken into account: first, that low-income and other disadvantaged groups have many limitations on personal behaviour, and second, that education rarely works without being linked to complementary social and public policy. Chapter 10 details proposals for the direction that wider policy could take to make it easier to choose a healthier life-style.

The kind of one-to-one personal contact that happens daily between professionals and individual patients can provide an excellent context for education and advice if approached with care. The full potential of such opportunities is often not realized partly because advice given is often totally unrealistic for the situations in which people live and also because attention is not given to choosing methods of education that are the most appropriate for the purpose (Whitehead, 1989a and 1989b; Whitehead and Tones, 1991). The problem of inappropriate advice has been examined in relation to smoking and low-income mothers with young children (Graham, 1989), and nutritional advice to similar families (James *et al.*, 1991). Successes have been achieved when methods have been tailored to suit each situation. For example, controlled studies of GPs giving smoking advice in consultations have shown that practical demonstrations of exhaled carbon monoxide are particularly valuable in influencing less educated patients (Jamrozik *et al.*, 1984). Similarly, a study of health visitors giving home safety education in a deprived area found that specific, practical advice on the particular hazards found in each home was more effective than more generalized advice from impersonal sources (Colver *et al.*, 1982). Sensitive education for ethnic minority women has been found to increase the uptake of cervical smears (McAvoy and Raza, 1991). In Edinburgh, a controlled study found that counselling by health visitors in eight weekly visits was valuable in the management of post-natal depression in socially disadvantaged women (Holden *et al.*, 1989).

Community development approaches have also been used effectively in disadvantaged communities. These put the emphasis on what the local community feels is important rather than what an outsider has decided is good for them. Sometimes people living in difficult circumstances are more responsive to this kind of approach than to more traditional methods. In the Greater Glasgow area the Health Board has been involved in such projects for a number of years. In one initiative a community development health education officer was employed to work in a severely deprived area. The local community identified high food prices (leading to poor nutrition) as a major priority, and the officer helped them to set up and run their own food cooperative providing reasonably priced fresh fruit and vegetables (Black, 1984).

Similarly, the Salford Community Health Project has been funded by the district health authority since 1982, with two community health workers acting as facilitators for residents of two areas of multiple deprivation in the city. Pressing issues identified by the residents included lack of child care facilities, high levels of depression with dependency on tranquillizers, and difficulties in living on a low income. In response to the child care problems, the Salford Crèche Project has grown up, employing twenty local crèche workers so that women can take part in other activities. On the issue of depression, community groups and training have developed not only to tackle stress reduction and tranquillizer withdrawal, but also on the more positive side, to build confidence and assertiveness (Youd and Jane, 1986). There are now over forty long-running community development health projects in this country as well as hundreds of smaller initiatives and individuals endeavouring to incorporate the principles of community development into everyday practice, sometimes under major constraints (see R UHBC, 1989). When reviewing the most effective methods, health and social service authorities could give more encouragement and support to such approaches, where appropriate.

Authorities in this field could also help people to maintain a healthier life-style by providing more smoke-free environments for staff and patients, by adopting food and nutrition policies, and so on. In this respect, there has been much progress already. For instance, by 1989 82 per cent of District Health Authorities and Health Boards had a formally approved policy on food and health (HEA, 1990), and nearly all had developed a smoking policy. Whether these policies work in practice is another matter, which requires close monitoring.

All these aspects of health promotion policy can be incorporated into the planning process in a much more structured way. For example, the ten-year health promotion strategy of Oxford Regional Health Authority illustrates one model of how equity could be taken into consideration in health promotion planning, even though the NHS reforms have now altered the way the authority can operate. The region's original strategy adopted a traditional approach in proposing action on risk factors such as smoking, exercise and diet, undifferentiated by different population groups. Evidence from a regional health and life-style survey, however, revealed great variations by gender and social class in different parts of the region. An untargeted strategy would have increased these differences still further. Refinement of the strategy therefore took place, firstly by setting differential targets by social class and by gender. For example, a target was set of 80 per cent for the proportion of non-smokers belonging to non-manual social class in 1994 (from a baseline of 75 per cent in 1986), and a target of 70 per cent for manual social classes (from a baseline of 58 per cent). Although the target is lower for manual classes, it actually represents a much larger shift in smoking patterns than that for non-manual classes. Secondly, resources were focused on the three most socially deprived districts in the region and then focused within those districts on the most deprived areas so that an impact could be made, rather than spreading the funding thinly over the entire region. Thirdly, disadvantaged groups in the selected areas were targeted. In this way, it was argued, resources would be used most effectively by tackling the problems of those with the worst health and life-styles. Fourthly, the strategy was refocused on to settings rather than diseases. The emphasis was on finding the best opportunities for health promotion available and using the most effective methods for each setting. This led to the adoption of outreach and community development methodologies, as they were considered more effective in the most disadvantaged settings. Three community projects were therefore funded. The issues these projects have tackled include debt counselling; isolation and mental stress; vandalism and safety. The regional team concluded from their experiences that:

A targeted, community-based approach alone will reach social groups which need the most support – any other strategy could waste scarce resources. (Griffiths *et al.*, 1991)

Summary

There is a vital role for the caring professions in taking action on inequalities in health. By attention to resource allocation, access and quality of care issues, people working in the health care sector can help to reduce those aspects of inequality in health caused by inequality in health care. To a lesser degree, they can also take action to help improve living and working conditions, to reduce poverty and to influence personal behaviour. However, all these policies have to be seen as complementary to a wider strategy outside the realm of the health services, rather than a substitute for action on a broader front.

One vital task for the caring services is to help alleviate the health damage caused by other determinants of inequalities in health. In this respect, the contribution good health care can make to the quality of life of a wide range of people should not be under-estimated. A plea is made to introduce a consideration for equity into every aspect of policy-making in the caring services. This is particularly important with the current restructuring of the NHS and the forthcoming changes in community care provision. These have the potential to increase inequalities in health care if they put undue emphasis on profit-making and competition, and great vigilance is needed to avoid this outcome. Sir Douglas Black put into words the concerns of many on this point in a recent letter to the national press:

It is my belief that until . . . we restore a health care system grounded in equity, and not one which allows market forces to dictate a shallow entrepreneurism, health problems will not be tackled in the most economic and efficient way. Good health care cannot be achieved for the rich or the poor, unless there is good health care for all. (Sir Douglas Black, 1992)

Chapter 10

Action on Inequalities: a Wider Strategy

As material living standards, social circumstances and life-styles are seen to play a major role in maintaining inequalities in health, a general consensus has emerged on the areas to be tackled, as outlined in Chapter 7. These go beyond the health services to encompass many different sectors.

Any wider strategy to do something about inequalities in health could move forward on four broad fronts:

- ensuring an adequate income for all, but most urgently, tackling the poverty that still exists in this country, especially in relation to children and disabled people;
- improving living conditions; not just the physical structure of individual dwellings, but improving the wider social environment and the chance to obtain housing in the first place that is safe and affordable;
- improving working conditions and the chance of safe and fulfilling employment;
- removing barriers to the adoption of healthy personal life-styles.

These are very general aims, but there are specific actions that could be taken relating to the British context. This chapter looks at the policy problems and possible ways forward on some of these fronts. As action involves many different sectors and political commitment, consideration is also given to co-ordination of strategy at national and local level.

The poor get poorer

The Black Working Group proposed that we should adopt a national goal for the 1980s of abolishing child poverty. Not only have we failed to make progress towards this goal, but in some respects the situation has grown worse, as more families with young children have fallen into the low-income category.

There are several ways of demonstrating this. For instance, we can look at which groups occupy the bottom 20 per cent of the income range, that is, the poorest fifth of the population. In 1971, over half the families in this category were pensioners and just over a fifth were families with children. By 1988, pensioner families only accounted for a quarter of this poorest section, while the proportion of families with children accounted for nearly a half.

This approach tells us who the poor are but will not, of course, say anything about how widespread poverty is in the population. To answer this question we have to choose a minimum standard of decency and assess the number or proportion of the population falling below that level. Problems arise here because there is no universally agreed poverty line. Some define it in *absolute* terms, assessing a minimum level of income required for basic subsistence and defining anyone with less than that minimum as in poverty. Others believe that poverty is *relative* to the standard of living common in the rest of society. Those who cannot afford to participate in the normal activities of the community and have only enough income to 'exist' are defined as poor in relative terms.

There is no agreement about what the basic necessities are, either. Sir Keith Joseph has been quoted as arguing that 'a family is poor if it cannot afford to eat' (Joseph and Sumption, 1979). On the other hand, MORI polls of the general public in 1983 and 1990 found a broader concept of a minimum standard of living which included damp-free housing with basic amenities; clothing and shoes; money for public transport; adequate heating and carpeting; and toys for the children (Mack and Lansley, 1985; Frayman, 1991). By Joseph's definition there may be very few poor people in Britain today (though we have no way of knowing), while defined by public opinion the number is put at eleven million (Frayman, 1991).

A 'benefit poverty line' can be taken by using the level of Income Support as a guide. This is the amount of money the state provides for those with little or no income. In May 1990 (the latest figures available) 1.82 million children were dependent on Income Support in England and Wales (18 per cent of the under-16 population), and nearly 217,000 children in Scotland (21 per cent of the under-16 population) (Hansard, 1991). In 1979, 9 per cent of children in Britain were dependent on the equivalent benefit, so on this measure there has been a doubling of child poverty over that period. It has to be said that as benefit levels are considered to be inadequate this provides a low estimate of the degree of poverty in Britain. Alternatively, an 'income poverty line' can be used, defining as poor those living on less than half average income after housing costs. As outlined in Table 22, the figures show an increase in poverty from 9.4 per cent of the population in 1979 to 21.6 per cent in 1988. This represents 11.8 million people, 3 million of whom are children (Social Security Committee, 1991).

The drastic rise in unemployment in the early 1980s accounted for most of the observed rise in poverty in children, as families with young children were particularly hit by the recession.

Some have argued that in the 1980s disposable incomes have risen for everyone, including the poor, so that even though over 20 per cent of the population are living on less than half average income, they are still better off in real terms than they were in 1979. This has been termed the 'trickle down effect', in which a general growth in the economy and the creation of wealth at the top of the social scale trickles down to benefit everyone, including those at the bottom of the scale. The government statistics on which this argument rested have now been shown to be incorrect, and revised figures published by the Department of Social Security for 1979–1988/89 show that the poorest tenth of the population had a decrease of 6 per cent in their real disposable incomes, after paying their housing costs,

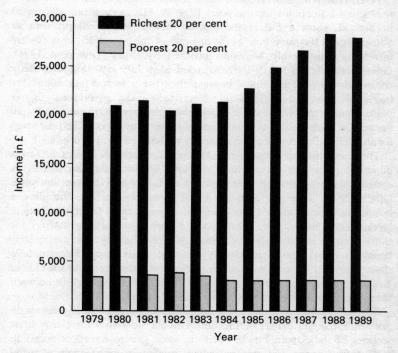

Figure 12. *Trends in the average annual disposable income of poorest and richest UK households, 1989 prices. (Source: Townsend, 1991.)*

Table 22: *Changes in the extent of poverty: the income poverty line*

Numbers and percentages of people living on less than 50% average equivalent income, after housing costs

	Number of people (in millions)	Proportion (%)
1979	4.9	9.4
1983	6.2	11.5
1988	11.8	21.6

Source: Social Security Committee (1991).

while the average had an increase of over 30 per cent (Department of Social Security, 1992).

Peter Townsend has extended the analysis to include the experience of the richest households for the years 1979–89. His calculations, illustrated in Fig. 12, show a fall in the income of the poorest 20 per cent of households at the same time as the incomes of the richest 20 per cent were increasing considerably, widening income inequalities (Townsend, 1991). Government figures for 1979–88/89, released in July 1992, are not strictly comparable with Townsend's because they use a formula to adjust for household size and composition. Nevertheless, the government figures paint a similar picture of static or declining incomes within the poorest 20 per cent of households, with increases of 40 per cent (over £5,000 per year) for the richest 20 per cent (Parliamentary written answer, 16 July 1992).

The widening gap between rich and poor in incomes and other forms of wealth since 1979 is confirmed by Inland Revenue statistics, as the tax system has benefited the rich more than the poor (Central Statistical Office, 1992). This has been attributed to several factors, including a boom in the stock market, the easing of certain capital taxes, and cuts in income taxes linked with substantially bigger increases in gross pay for those on high incomes (Huhne, 1986). All these factors have particularly benefited those who were already wealthy, while doing little to help those who were poor. Consequently a review of social trends in the United Kingdom pointed to a growing social division since the mid 1970s between the prosperous majority and the poor minority (Halsey, 1987).

Townsend has also pointed out that statistics on disposable incomes do not show the full extent of the fall in living standards for the poorest sections of the population. In addition, some groups have lost access to certain free goods and services which previously eased their financial situations. For example, poorer groups have experienced:

- loss of free and subsidized school meals;
- selected increases in rents and associated charges;
- having to repay loans from the Social Fund instead of obtaining grants;
- loss of access to single grants for clothing, diet and heating;
- new obligations to pay water charges and 20 per cent of poll tax.

On a wider scale, during the 1980s social security provision has changed for other vulnerable groups, including the sick and disabled. A large number of benefits were removed or their real value reduced. For example, those that were removed include earnings-related sickness and unemployment benefits, a range of industrial injury benefits, maternity grant and a large part of maternity benefit. Those that were reduced in value include invalidity pension, child benefit, child dependency additions paid with a variety of benefits, and means-tested benefits paid to the under-25s. As unemployment increased in the first half of the 1980s, eligibility for flat-rate and means-tested unemployment benefit was restricted.

The social security reforms of the mid 1980s may have made the situation worse. For example, many older and disabled people lost eligibility for additional weekly allowances. Further cuts were made in disability benefits in 1990, and the earnings-related addition to invalidity pension was phased out in April 1991. The overall assessment is that the reforms have failed to ameliorate the poverty of a substantial number of pensioners and have left some of them worse off (Townsend, 1991).

Responding to low income

It is clear from the evidence that much is wrong with the present system of taxes and benefits. The policies adopted over the 1980s, even if introduced with the best of intentions, have had negative side-effects. For example, ending the indexing of social security benefits to earnings in 1980 has been credited with being one of the key factors in increasing the experience of poverty in the 1980s (Piachaud, 1991).

There is no shortage of proposals for how to improve the situation (Parker, 1989; Hills, 1988; Becker, 1990; Quick and Wilkinson, 1991; Delamothe, 1991). Most agree that in the long term there needs to be a complete review of the tax and benefit system at the national level, so that taxation is progressive and social security benefits more adequate. Some put the emphasis on improving the income of people in poverty; others propose a more even distribution of income across the whole community. Whatever the final choice of policy following a review, it is clear that the present system is unfair and is creating desperate conditions for those in greatest need.

The National Children's Homes, among others, have put forward proposals for more immediate action to improve the lot of children in poverty, including:

- identifying a clear food element in Income Support, based on the 'healthy eating' standards advocated by the Department of Health;
- raising Income Support to a level that will ensure that families can provide an adequate diet;
- raising Family Credit to enable the nutritional needs of families with children to be met;
- making cooking facilities a priority need under the Social Fund and providing grants, rather than the present loans, for essential goods;
- reintroducing quality standards for school meals.
(National Children's Homes, 1991).

Such policies could be adopted in a relatively short space of time, and would make an immediate impact.

While changing the tax and benefit system is a national responsibility, improvements in people's income can be made – even if in a more modest way – at regional and local level. For instance, advice and public awareness campaigns can help to increase take-up of state benefits. Debt counselling services can also be helpful. The provision of free school meals by local education authorities can make a big contribution to the nutrition of children with inadequate diets, provided the meals are of sufficiently good nutritional quality. Encouraging mutual support in poor communities can also have a beneficial effect on mental health and help people gain in confidence. For example, several regional and city councils in Britain have developed anti-poverty strategies. Strathclyde Regional Council's is possibly one of the most comprehensive. It has an eight-pronged strategy involving financial assistance within its powers; welfare rights campaigns; money and debt counselling; the provision of additional Council services in poorer areas; community development initiatives and improvement in employment and training opportunities as a route out of future poverty (Strathclyde Regional Council, 1990).

In Manchester, shortly after the Black Report was published, the City Council sponsored two seminars for health authority, City Council and Community Health Council members, with the aim of publicizing the findings of the report and considering what to do locally. Out of those seminars came a ten-point plan identifying those areas of action which could be implemented fairly swiftly. These included action to improve the take-up of welfare benefits, to improve the statistical information on health available at ward level (for example on accidents to children) and to continue improvements in housing to tackle the problem of damp, as well as the promotion of strategies on cigarette-smoking and nutrition. As part of these developments, an Anti-poverty Sub-committee of the City Council was set up to promote measures to tackle poverty across the city as well as in the most deprived areas. Included in the anti-poverty programme were initiatives to stimulate employment, to tackle low pay and to promote uptake of welfare benefits. In this context twenty welfare rights officers were appointed to work around the city encouraging uptake of benefits and training other Council staff in the help available to low-income groups (Manchester City Council, 1986).

The initiatives taken on poverty in health services have already been mentioned in Chapter 9, involving family health services authorities, district health authorities and individual health workers. At the neighbourhood level, local health authorities have been funding community development workers to help in other ways. For example, in some neighbourhoods where commercial moneylenders have been charging extortionate rates of interest for small loans, residents have devised credit unions. These provide loans at low interest rates and are run by people in the community themselves, with help in setting them up from the community development workers.

At every level, there can be, and has been, complementary action to improve financial situations.

A crisis in housing

Many people consider decent housing to be one of the prime prerequisites for health, and certainly the Black Working Group saw it as such. But there are still sections of the population in this country who have yet to attain that goal. In 1990, 170,000 households were accepted as homeless by local authorities in Great Britain. This was an increase of 15 per cent on 1989 and a 50 per cent increase since 1985. Of these, 156,000 were in a priority need category, and two-thirds of these households contained dependent children (Central Statistical Office, 1992). An additional 85,000 homeless households were given advice only, as the councils did not accept responsibility for them.

To house these families, local authorities are having to rely increasingly on temporary bed-and-breakfast accommodation. In 1990, 48,000 households who had applied to local authorities as homeless were placed in temporary accommodation; more than double the mid 1980s figure. As noted earlier, these mainly represent families with children, and such accommodation is often among the worst as far as children's safety and

health are concerned. In addition, for the first time the census of 1991
counted the number of people sleeping rough on 21 April 1991; 2,700
people were found in England and Wales on that night sleeping in the
open air, nearly half of them in London.

As far as housing standards are concerned, the latest major survey on
housing conditions was carried out in 1986 and showed that 900,000
homes in England were 'unfit for human habitation', while an additional
460,000 lacked one or more basic amenities. Added to this were homes
needing major repairs, to give a total of 2.4 million properties classed as substandard.

Between 1971 and 1986, the number of homes lacking basic amenities
fell by over 80 per cent. Over the same period there was a less dramatic fall
in unfit homes, but an increase in the number in serious disrepair (Department of Environment, 1988). The elderly, unemployed or ethnic minorities
are more likely than other groups to be in poor-condition housing with the
common factor being low income.

There have been real improvements in the matter of overcrowding,
though. Between 1971 and 1989–90, the percentage of households judged
to be overcrowded on a bedroom standard fell from 9 per cent to 3 per
cent. However, ethnic minority households were at greater risk of overcrowding than the rest of the population. For instance, in 1988 10 per cent
of households with a non-white head were overcrowded (less than one
room per person), compared with only 1 per cent of all households. Of
households with a head from a Pakistani or a Bangladeshi ethnic group,
about one-third had less than one room per person (Central Statistical
Office, 1992).

Much of the improvement in housing conditions took place in the 1960s
and the beginning of the 1970s, with little progress made since then. Two
additional factors are now giving concern for the future – the shortage of
houses and the poor state of repair of existing houses. In 1977 it was
estimated that 200,000 new dwellings/year were needed throughout the
1980s. In reality there has been a severe drop in building to the level of
40,000 dwellings/year in the public sector, with the private sector unable to
make up the difference. Shelter has estimated that the public sector has
experienced a 60 per cent cut in investment between 1982 and 1989, so
efforts have had to be concentrated on the repair of existing stock rather
than on new building programmes. However, the housing stock is in a
poor condition. In addition, home improvement grants have dropped to a
very low level since 1982. In 1981 the Parker Morris standard for council
housing was suspended, and a substantial proportion of houses built since
then – at least in the Greater London area – have fallen below that

standard. These developments go directly against the Black recommendation that local authority spending on housing improvements should be substantially increased.

In 1992, the Royal Institution of Chartered Surveyors put forward a new estimate for the 1990s. At least 100,000 new homes per year for renting would be needed for the next ten years – 60,000 more than current output.

Another major problem is that housing has to be *affordable* for people on low income, and with the rise in house prices over the last twenty years decent housing is becoming out of reach for a growing number of people. Added to this is the perverse system of mortgage interest tax relief, which by the end of the 1980s amounted to £7 billion per year: a state subsidy awarded to the more affluent sections of society, with a much smaller sum (£4.8 billion) going to people on low income in the form of 'housing benefit'.

Improving housing

The housing crisis is particularly acute in Britain, with a combination of cold climate, poor state of existing housing stock, insufficient building of new homes, and rising costs of rents and mortgages all conspiring to put decent living conditions out of reach of a substantial section of the population. There is consensus among those active in pressing for improvements that:

- ways have to be found to finance and stimulate a new building and repair programme;
- health standards need to be incorporated into building regulations for new homes;
- the problem of how low-income groups are to afford decent and safe housing needs to be addressed;
- providing healthy housing means more than providing basic amenities for each separate dwelling. It means introducing social renewal programmes as well, so that the wider environment is safer and healthier. This involves paying attention to the design of schemes; transport arrangements; and access to social amenities such as nurseries, health centres, meeting places, etc.

Several detailed proposals have been put forward on these points, but they differ in where they lay the emphasis. The Royal Institution of Chartered Surveyors, for instance, suggests that finance for the much-needed building programme could be found from two main sources: the £8 billion receipts from council house sales which councils are not allowed to spend at the moment, and the phasing out of mortgage interest tax relief. The funds generated by withdrawing this tax relief would run into billions of pounds and could be used to provide a new housing allowance on the basis of *need* – whether to owner-occupiers or tenants. The Institution also suggested a National Housing Investment Bank for loans for low-cost housing, and a National Housing Agency to monitor standards in rented and leased property. Shelter points out that building new homes is cheaper for councils than providing bed-and-breakfast accommodation at 1989 prices.

The Joseph Rowntree Foundation inquiry into British housing in 1991 also recommended the phased withdrawal of mortgage interest tax relief and housing benefit, and conversion of savings into a housing allowance related to need. The report also put forward wide-ranging measures to reverse the continuing decline in the rented sector (Joseph Rowntree Foundation, 1991). The question of how to pay for the necessary national reforms to housing is addressed in this and other reports (Merrett, 1991).

It has been pointed out that although putting the money from mortgage interest tax relief into a new form of housing allowance is a logical solution, no political party would be brave enough to do so because of the loss of mortgage-paying voters. There is obviously no easy solution to be spelt out in a few pages of this report, but the problem has grown to such an extent that a national consensus needs to be found on the best way forward.

At a more local level, a 1991 Audit Commission report made recommendations on the role of environmental health officers in promoting healthier housing. The Commission suggested several ways of improving efficiency; for example, in achieving faster rates of dealing with applications, in serving more enforcement orders on properties in a poor state of repair and in issuing more renovation grants. However, it also acknowledged that increased productivity would lead to a higher local authority expenditure and to a substantial effect on housing basic credit approvals – but that central government's housing expenditure plans showed a *fall* of nearly 30 per cent over three years. They concluded: 'Were productivity to increase, authorities would, on current plans, have difficulty funding the capital consequences of their officers' actions' (Audit Commission 1991). The funding dilemma, therefore, returns to be solved by policy at national level.

Despite the enormity of the national problem, some local councils, housing associations and voluntary bodies have for years been carrying out imaginative schemes to improve local living conditions in ways which would benefit health. Two relatively small-scale schemes are worth noting here because they are among the few that have tried to evaluate the effect on health of their improvements. They are also unusual in being stimulated by the research on damp housing and health described on p. 329, which itself was triggered by tenants' concern about the effect of damp on their children's health, rather than by some outside academic interest. Liverpool City Council's 'Better Housing, Better Health' scheme responded to evidence about damp, cold homes by initiating improvements in housing design on a single estate. Outside evaluators compared the health of groups of people living in unimproved, partially improved, and fully renovated housing. The evaluation showed that fully renovated houses were less damp, less noisy and more secure than the others, and were linked to higher levels of satisfaction with housing, fewer symptoms of ill-health and lower levels of emotional distress in the occupants (McKenna and Hunt, 1990).

Similarly, Glasgow District Council and the South of Scotland Electricity Board devised a 'Heat with Rent' scheme on a deprived housing estate which had an insufficient and expensive-to-run heating system. The residents were getting into debt with fuel bills and still had damp, cold homes. In some blocks of flats the old heating system was removed and replaced with a cheaper, more efficient system that residents could pay for by a fixed sum each week with their rent. Residents were interviewed before and after installation of the new system, and compared with people living in unimproved flats in the same estate. Evaluation showed that the children in the warmer, improved flats were protected from symptoms associated with dampness and mould (Hopton and Hunt, 1990). During the course of the evaluation, though, the extent of poverty worsened in these deprived areas, reducing the potential of the scheme to improve health.

Residents themselves have initiated some projects, when frustrated by lack of action. The European Community Solar Energy Demonstration Project in Glasgow started originally with residents in damp, cold housing getting together and requesting teach-ins on how to apply for funding to various bodies. They eventually secured funds from the local authority and the EC Social Fund for a prototype project to improve their own housing conditions. The initial project showed that the modified flats could be kept at a comfortable temperature for a tenth of the cost of unimproved flats. Further funding was then secured for a larger project making use of solar energy, and this is to be closely monitored over the period 1991–4.

Another approach has been to try to do something to ease the poor social environment in which people live in deprived housing areas – the isolation and lack of social support. The Newpin project in London, for example, began as a response to local concern at high rates of maternal depression, isolation, poor child health and child abuse in a severely deprived area. The aim was to encourage the creation of a mutually supportive community of parents with young children. The project consists of a voluntary befriending service at home and a drop-in centre which referred women were encouraged to attend by trained volunteers recruited from the local community. The centre contains an office, kitchen, sitting-room for mothers and a playroom/crèche, as well as individual counselling-rooms. Women are referred by health or social service staff, or by themselves, or by friends, usually because of depression, isolation or parenting problems. Women joining the project are carefully matched with another local mother and given a list of telephone numbers so that they can contact other mothers at night or over weekends. Once a befriender has been assigned, she visits the referred woman and together they decide what they will do together for mutual support. Befrienders are also encouraged to bring women to the drop-in centre. At the centre, women can relax, meet and talk to others in the same circumstances and see how others handle their children. They can also take part in individual and group therapy and counselling. Small-scale evaluation of the Newpin project indicated improvements in self-esteem and recovery from depression, reduction in social isolation and fewer child behaviour problems (Pound, 1991).

Barriers to living a healthier life

Some inequalities in health are linked to a higher prevalence of behavioural risk factors in disadvantaged groups – smoking, poorer diet, lack of exercise and lower uptake of preventive health care. The case of alcohol abuse is not so clear-cut, but the *effects* of abuse are often more severe in disadvantaged groups because they may have weaker networks for social and professional support and fewer resources to cushion them from poverty if they lose their jobs.

From a policy point of view there are two aspects to the problem of inequalities in this area:

1. There may be financial and structural barriers to adopting a healthier life-style. People may wish to follow a healthier way of life but cannot afford more nutritious food, or the bus fare to the clinic, or they may lack facilities or time to take more exercise.

2. Substances like tobacco and alcohol may be used to help people survive adverse conditions – a small pleasure to make depressing circumstances

bearable. In some workplaces, for example, smoking may be the only accepted reason for taking a break, and as detailed on p. 333, mothers living in cramped conditions with small children may use smoking as a way of easing stress without leaving children unattended.

Improvements in this second aspect will only occur as part of a broader strategy on improving living and working conditions and by helping people cope with stress in a less destructive way:

> While to specialists in public health the most attractive points of initial attack (for reducing inequalities in health) are health promotion initiatives to reduce risk factors such as smoking, poor diet and physical inactivity, there is a limit to the extent to which such improvements are likely to occur in the absence of a wider strategy to change the circumstances in which these risks arise, by reducing deprivation and improving the physical environment. (Acheson, 1991)

However, much can be done about the first aspect – the barriers to change – by a concerted effort on educational, social and public policy fronts involving:

– well-researched educational approaches tailored to the needs of people in difficult conditions and sensitive to the limitations they live under;
– pricing policy to ensure cheap, nutritious food in the shops and easier access to exercise facilities;
– legislation to control harmful substances and the advertising which seeks to influence vulnerable groups, including children;
– voluntary initiatives to make it easier to choose a healthier life-style in the setting in which people live and work – health-promoting schools, especially in disadvantaged areas; health-promoting workplaces, and so on.

The effectiveness of different educational approaches has recently been reviewed (Whitehead, 1989; Whitehead and Tones, 1991) and ways of approaching the issue of smoking with women on low income have been put forward (ASH, 1992; Graham, 1989). Some of the promising projects, including ones using community development techniques, are discussed in Chapter 9, along with the initiative by Oxford Regional Health Authority to take equity into consideration in its ten-year health promotion strategy (see p. 373).

On pricing policy, there is evidence that people on low income are more responsive to shifts in prices than more prosperous groups. A few pence difference between the price of a white and a brown loaf is enough to influence the decision on which type to buy, whereas for higher-income groups that sort of pricing does not matter so much. Pricing policy is therefore particularly important if the aim is to influence the consumption patterns of low-income groups. For example, policies that encourage the production of cheap, nutritious food by the use of selective subsidies and incentives to producers, where necessary, will help to remove financial barriers to healthy eating. Offering free or subsidized entrance fees to leisure facilities for certain groups will also help to encourage exercise.

Likewise, pricing policy when used to raise the price of health-damaging goods will have the greatest effects on consumption in low-income groups. This is a very sensitive area of policy, not least because some poverty campaigners argue that raising the price of cigarettes will damage the living standards of poorer people, as they will still continue to smoke to ease their stressful conditions. However, others argue that tobacco and alcohol taxes need not be regressive (Townsend, 1987; Ashton *et al.*, 1989). Analysis shows that as smokers from lower social classes are more responsive to tax changes, they are more likely to give up or cut down in response to higher cigarette taxes than their counterparts in higher social classes. From the findings of this study, it is suggested that the downward drift in the real price of cigarettes in the UK since the war has effectively increased the smoking levels of lower social class groups and children relative to classes I and II, and may have been one of the major factors in widening the gap in social class smoking (Townsend, 1987). The challenge is to couple price rises of this nature with broader policies to change the conditions in which people live, and to help them develop the skills to cope with stress in less destructive ways (ASH, 1992).

On legislation, controls on the sale and advertising of health-damaging goods can be brought in, though so far the national controls on such activities as tobacco advertising have been too weak to make a difference (Jacobson *et al.*, 1991). At a more local level, controls on advertising posters and on smoking in public places, combined with voluntary activities to encourage healthier life-styles, have been implemented in many localities. For example, Manchester City Council agreed a wide-ranging policy on smoking with the North-Western Regional Health Authority, including the designation of no-smoking areas and the setting-up of smoking cessation groups. A healthy eating policy has also been pursued in the Education and Social Services Departments, and in the catering section of the Council. This led to a review of nutrition in Manchester schools. A joint working party with the health authorities was set up to look at the question of accidents to children.

Sheffield City Council has also pushed forward with a food policy and is looking at the ways in which more nutritious food can be supplied and promoted in all the authority's outlets. Schools and residential homes for the elderly are particular priorities. Similarly, a city smoking policy has been developed to control tobacco advertising and promote non-smoking in Council-controlled sites. A mobile clinic for cervical cytology targeted on certain areas is being developed by the health authority as a result of the deficiencies in health care which showed up in the city's health profile.

By 1991, a survey of local authority policy and practice on smoking found that 53 per cent of district councils and 69 per cent of county councils had written smoking policies. Most of those had a total ban on smoking in public waiting areas and in communal office space. Half also had smoke-free staff restaurants and civic occasions (Batten and Allen, 1991).

Food policies are also beginning to spread slowly through local authorities. For example, by 1988, 7 per cent of local authorities had a food policy for civic occasions; 14 per cent for council restaurants, and 13 per cent for residential homes for children and elderly people (Ashton, 1988).

All these examples are indicative of the growing awareness of local agencies of their important role in making the choice of a healthy personal life-style easier.

Putting inequalities in health on the agenda

In discussions on what can be done about inequalities in health, two key messages stand out, and they apply to all levels of policy-making:

- It would be a great step forward if policies at all levels became more sensitive to equity issues. Increased awareness of inequalities can lead to increased monitoring of the extent of the problem, and assessments of the possible consequences of new policies when changes are planned. In this way a consideration for equity becomes a criterion for assessing policies, rather than a separate policy in its own right. At its most ambitious, this approach leads to 'health impact assessments', though we are some way from being able to carry these out in any great detail, as much more development work is needed in this area.
- Greater progress would be made if ways were found to make it easier for different agencies and sectors to work together in a co-ordinated way. A national commitment to reducing inequalities in health would open the way for many more links to be forged.

The Black Working Group stressed this need in their recommendations for interdepartmental machinery in the Cabinet Office to co-ordinate the administration of health-related policies (recommendation 36), and for equivalent local mechanisms to be developed. Although for almost ten years similar calls from public health quarters for a co-ordinated strategy for health appeared to fall on deaf ears, or were even ridiculed, attitudes have changed rapidly in the 1990s. Draft strategies have been drawn up for Wales in 1990 (Health Promotion Authority for Wales, 1990) and in England in 1991 (DoH, 1991). In the Welsh document, inequalities were clearly acknowledged and some of the detailed targets aim for reductions in inequalities. For example;

Wales residents:
. . . reduce the infant mortality rate to below 7 per 1,000 live births in all six social groups (i.e. I, II, IIIN, IIIM, IV, V).
(baseline 1981–86 = only one group met this level)
Proposed targets – three groups by 1995, all groups by 2000 (Health Promotion Authority for Wales, 1990).

The English document, issued as a Green Paper, although not containing the word 'inequalities', did discuss the existence of 'variations in health'; however, the issue was considered too complex to tackle as a priority target. This was a significant step forward from the position the Department of Health and the government had held throughout the 1980s. There was disappointment in many quarters, though, that no commitment had been given in the Green Paper to take action on inequalities in health, and many of the 2,000 responses to the consultation on the document made this point and called for a rethink of the Department's position.

When the revised document was published as a White Paper in July, 1992 (DoH, 1992), there was still no commitment to make inequalities in health a priority. But in all five of the Key Areas chosen as priorities – CHD, cancers, mental illness, sexual health and accidents – variations by region and socio-economic group were mentioned with a note that: 'the different needs of people in different socio-economic groups will need to be considered in framing action in Key Areas' (p. 122). This is something, however small, for concerned people to make use of in the development of policy, but it falls far short of a national commitment. Though welcome, it also remains to be seen whether the proposed inter-departmental committee to coordinate government policy in line with the strategy will be given the staff and resources to function effectively.

The White Paper, however, is still some way away from being a national strategy for health, as the more difficult aspect of bringing in other key sectors and putting resources where priorities lie is still underdeveloped. Even so, there is much greater potential for developing them in the 1990s than in the previous decade.

Although as yet there has been no unifying national lead on the issue, nevertheless what has been done by individuals and organizations to raise awareness and co-ordinate policy should not go unrecorded.

The medical and nursing professional bodies and health service unions have all been active in raising awareness throughout the 1980s, keeping the issue alive and under consideration. This is markedly different from the situation in some other countries, such as Sweden, where pressure has come from work-related organizations and the voice of the medical profession has been muted.

For example, the former Health Education Council and the HEA, with bodies like the BMA and TUC, have organized conferences on deprivation and ill-health, and on the community development approach to deprivation, in an attempt to inform and motivate professional action on the subject. Similarly, the Scottish Health Education Co-ordinating Committee convened a working party on multiple deprivation which has reviewed projects and action on the issue throughout Scotland, and has made recommendations for wide-ranging action (Scottish Health Education Co-ordinating Committee, 1984). Following on from this, bodies like the Royal College of Physicians and Surgeons of Glasgow held symposia on the subject in 1986 and June 1987. Various professional bodies, like the Health Visitors Association, the BMA and the Faculty of Public Health, have all addressed the issue from their own particular perspectives.

In July 1987 a new organization, the Public Health Alliance, was formed to bring together individuals from the health, local government, voluntary and consumer sectors, with the aim of making sure that the public health aspect was given priority on a wide range of national matters. These range from poverty and food policy to housing and transport. It was thought that if such an organization could raise the awareness of policy-makers to such issues, then there would be a greater chance that recommendations on reducing inequalities in health would at last be taken seriously (Smith, 1986).

Under the WHO's 'Healthy Cities' umbrella, many towns as well as city councils have joined together with health, business and voluntary agencies in the locality to draw up a local 'Health for All' strategy, and in some reducing inequalities in health has been the central theme of the strategy. Sheffield, for example, undertook a city-wide consultation in 1992 on a new public health strategy to involve the people of Sheffield in planning for co-ordinated action on health involving all these agencies, and the reduction of inequalities in health was a basic principle in it (Halliday and Adams, 1992).

Oxford adopted a city-wide health strategy in 1986 and later widened its scope to take in the 'Healthy Cities' approach. Included in the strategy were two important aims: 'to offset health inequalities related to social class, gender, ethnic origin, age and disability', and 'to secure and sustain a safe and healthy environment within the city'. Many practical initiatives stemming from the strategy are now well under way. The Environmental Health Department, for example, now has a health liaison and promotion section consisting of officers concerned with health liaison, home safety and smoking prevention. But health promotion is being introduced into other areas too, to extend the traditional work of the department. In the food hygiene section, for instance, a community dietician has been appointed to develop a healthy eating programme for the city. In the housing section an energy and heating officer has developed a programme to tackle ill-health and deaths associated with inadequate heating. Each of the Council's departments was asked to produce health targets to focus their work on the overall goals of the health strategy, and to date 100 targets have been identified and are being refined with the help of public health physicians. The Planning Department investigated ways of producing a health database for the city, ranking the neighbourhoods against a deprivation index in readiness for health profiles of the areas to be drawn up. A community development project is under way in one of the more deprived neighbourhoods, sponsored jointly with the health authority. This combines action on fitness testing, welfare benefits, health screening and home safety.

The city engineers and Recreation Department have developed safe cycle routes for school children, and a community fitness programme. As a major employer itself, the City Council is also attempting to develop a model occupational health policy, with smoke-free atmospheres in offices and workplaces, smoke cessation courses, a health screening programme and so on, with the aim of extending the policy to workplaces across the city (Fryer, 1987).

All these examples show that the potential for co-ordination of policy is beginning to be recognized at local level.

Public attitudes

Before leaving the subject, it is worth looking at what has been happening to public attitudes to social inequalities over the same period. From survey evidence there appears to be a softening of attitudes to poverty by the general public, with the poor now attracting greater sympathy. For instance, a survey of the UK in 1976 found that 43 per cent of people blamed the poor for their own plight. In 1983, the figure had dropped to 22 per cent and by 1990 only 19 per cent blamed the poor, while 40 per cent blamed 'injustice in our society' (Frayman, 1991). Both the 1983 and the 1990 'Breadline Britain' surveys found that 75 per cent of people said they would be willing to pay an extra 1p in the pound income tax to enable everyone to afford the items classed as necessities. Twenty-five per cent in 1983 and 44 per cent in 1990 said they would be willing to pay an extra 5p in the pound (Frayman, 1991).

Perhaps the community at large would now, more than ever, appreciate concerted action on inequalities in health.

Conclusions

A wider strategy to tackle inequalities in health could move forward on four broad fronts: ensuring an adequate income for all; improving living conditions and the chance to obtain housing in the first place; improving working conditions and the chance of safe and fulfilling employment; and removing barriers to the adoption of healthy personal life-styles. In addition, co-ordination of strategy at national and local levels would be of great benefit.

Some of the practical details of such a strategy are covered by this chapter, after a discussion of the current situation on these four fronts, a situation which seems to have grown worse rather than better over the last decade. There is evidence, for example, that the number of children living in poverty has increased rather than decreased, that welfare benefit policy has failed to improve the living standards of poorer people to any appreciable extent and that poor nutrition, housing and working conditions abound. As yet, there has not been a recognizable national effort to tackle inequalities in health.

Against this extremely negative picture can be set the many positive initiatives which have been taken around the country. There has been a dramatic re-awakening of interest in public health in the local authorities, a growing concern and pressure for action from the various professional associations, and numerous examples of individual health workers and health authorities doing their best to counteract the inequality in health and health care which they face in their day-to-day work.

There are also attempts to set up mechanisms for the co-ordination of relevant policy at the local level, and at last a little recognition from the government that inequality in health is a problem to be taken seriously. Prospects for building a consensus on inequalities in health in the 1990s look more hopeful than at any time in the 1980s. Action on this crucial issue is long overdue.

Summary

Background and format

The pattern of health inequalities in Britain was thoroughly documented by the Black Working Group, drawing on evidence from the early 1970s. But what does the picture on inequalities in health look like in the 1980s and at the beginning of the 1990s? How has it changed, and what progress, if any, has been made towards implementing the recommendations of the Working Group and moving forward on policy development?

These questions formed the starting-point for the present review, which summarizes the evidence on social inequalities in health published between 1980 and 1992 and draws attention to some of the recent initiatives which have been undertaken in this field. The review first considers how the experience of health of people living in Britain varies with their occupational class, employment status, gender, area of residence, ethnic origin and other social classifications. It goes on to look at whether the health gap between the occupational classes has widened or narrowed in recent years; whether health services are fair and equitable; and whether international comparisons can offer further insight. New studies investigating the causes of inequalities in health are outlined and discussed. The final chapters cover action on inequalities in health, addressing the question: 'What can be done about inequalities in health?'

The extent of the problem

The evidence presented in Chapter 2 confirms that serious social inequalities in health persisted throughout the 1980s. Whether social position is measured by occupational class, or by assets such as house and car ownership, or by employment status, a similar picture emerges. Those at the bottom of the social scale have much higher death rates than those at the top. This applies at every stage of life from birth through to adulthood and well into old age.

Neither is it just a few specific conditions which account for these higher death rates. All the major killer diseases now affect the poor more than the rich (and so do most of the less common ones). The less favoured occupational classes also experience higher rates of chronic sickness and their children tend to have lower birth-weights, shorter stature and other indicators suggesting poorer health status.

The unemployed and their families have considerably worse physical and mental health than those in work. Until recently, however, direct evidence that unemployment *caused* this poorer health was not available. Now there is substantial evidence of unemployment causing a deterioration in mental health, with improvements observed on re-employment.

The well-established pattern of women having lower death rates than men but experiencing higher sickness rates still held good in the 1980s. Recent studies have shown that the situation is far more complex, though. Women's health has been found to vary with social class, family circumstances, employment and marital status in ways which give greater insight into inequalities in health in women. The health of working-class women is particularly poor.

Striking regional disparities in health can still be observed. Death rates were highest in Scotland, followed by the North and North-West regions of England, and were lowest in the South-East of England and East Anglia, confirming the long-established North/South gradient. What is becoming increasingly clear from fresh evidence, though, is the great inequalities which exist between communities living side by side in the same region. Numerous studies at the level of local authority wards have pinpointed pockets of very poor health corresponding to areas of social and material deprivation. Alongside them, areas with much better health profiles can be detected and these exhibit more affluent characteristics. Although such deprived areas can be found throughout the country, the North has a higher concentration of them than the South and South-East.

The health of ethnic minorities presents a varied picture. Strikingly high mortality from hypertension and strokes is found among people of Afro-Caribbean origin, and high mortality rates for babies of mothers born in Pakistan. Coronary heart disease rates are high in groups of Asian origin. High death rates from accidents for all immigrant groups also cause concern. However, some ethnic minority groups have lower death rates from other major diseases like lung cancer and chronic bronchitis than people born in the UK. These findings are based on country of birth as an indicator of ethnic origin, which is not a very precise measure and which of course says nothing about the health of members of ethnic minority groups who were born in this country. As many suffer poor housing and working conditions and a high risk of unemployment, there are fears that the health of some ethnic minority groups may be very poor, but we need better information collection to help investigate this possibility.

Recent trends

Chapter 3 considers whether the health inequalities have increased or decreased in recent years. In the decade from 1971 to 1981 there was a fall in 'all cause' death rates in Britain, but these improvements in health were not experienced equally across the population. Non-manual groups experienced a much greater decline in death rates than manual groups; as a result the gap between the two groups widened. Furthermore, death rates among women from coronary heart disease and lung cancer actually rose in manual groups over the ten-year period, while showing a substantial decline for non-manual women. There was also a widening gap between manual and non-manual groups in their rates of chronic sickness from 1974 to 1984, stabilizing after that.

The more controversial issue of long-term trends is discussed and new assessments of the data reviewed in the Black Report are summarized. Some studies confirm the original conclusions of the report: that inequalities in health have widened since the 1950s for adults of working age. The exception to this trend is in relation to babies aged one month to one year. There was a dramatic decline in their death rates during the 1970s in all classes, but especially in class V, bringing about a reduction in the health gap. Although there was very little further improvement, at least until 1988, for manual or non-manual classes, the evidence does illustrate that the class differential is not inevitable. It can be reduced.

The regional differences in post-neonatal mortality disappeared by the mid 1970s, though regional differences in neonatal mortality remain. Trends in ethnic differences in infant mortality also showed encouraging improvement between 1975 and 1985, though high rates for babies with mothers born in Pakistan are still causing concern in the 1990s.

Fair and equitable health services

Chapter 4 considers access to and use of health services by different groups in the community. On the issue of the availability of services, there are still examples of poorer provision in more deprived areas, and poorer quality, though no overall picture of the extent of inequality around the country is available.

There is general agreement that semi-skilled and unskilled manual groups still make less use of preventive services than professional and managerial groups, but have higher rates of general practice consultations. Whether the rates of use of the primary care services fully match the different levels of perceived illness within each group is a vital question. Although there have been a few studies in this field since 1980, the evidence on this issue is still inconclusive. Concern is expressed about the danger of increasing inequalities in health care inherent in the latest NHS reforms, for example in the provision of primary care services in prosperous and deprived areas and in the new resource allocation arrangements and their effect on geographic access to care.

A European perspective

In Chapter 5 comparisons are made with other developed countries. The UK is certainly not alone in experiencing social inequalities in health. Every country to a greater or lesser extent experiences differences in health between regional, occupational or income groups, and in the late 1980s the extent of the health divide *between* countries in the east and west of Europe was revealed. Can we learn anything from the experiences of other countries? In this context, examples from the Nordic countries are illuminating. Policies to reduce regional differences in health care in Finland and to set up a national nutrition and food policy in Norway deserve special attention, as do developments in national policies in the Netherlands and Sweden.

Explaining health inequalities

Explanations of continuing inequalities are considered in Chapter 6. From the evidence, it is concluded that health inequalities between social groups are genuine and cannot be explained away as artefact. There is evidence of some selection, in which those in poor health move down the social scale. However, this is not sufficient to account for the large differentials in health found between social groups. On the other hand, the evidence that socio-economic circumstances have a major impact on health is now extremely strong. Fresh evidence shows that life-style and material living conditions influence health and vary with socio-economic status. Furthermore, recent in-depth studies have increased understanding of how living and working conditions can impose severe restrictions on an individual's ability to choose a healthy life-style. They provide fresh insight into the way behaviour is influenced by social conditions and argue for a policy which recognizes the link between the two, in preference to policies which focus solely on the individual.

A framework for policy-making

Chapters 7–10 deal with the questions of action on inequalities. In Chapter 7, the emerging consensus on broad policy aims is detailed. Starting with the Black Report's recommendations, it traces developments since then, stemming from the World Health Organization, various professional bodies, and the Chief Medical Officer in 1990 and 1991. A framework for thinking about policy development is outlined.

Information needs and research

For planning and evaluating policies to reduce inequalities in health, some long-term development work is needed to produce better indicators of social inequality and improved measures of health, as well as to develop sensitive resource allocation formulae and ways of auditing inequalities in the outcome of care. In the shorter term, immediate action could be taken to increase the recording of socio-economic factors in routinely collected health statistics, with a parallel injection of health information into routine economic and social statistics.

So far, progress on remedying the deficiencies in data collection high-lighted twelve years ago in the Black Report has been slow and gaps in the new information systems for the NHS have already been identified. In addition, some statistics which were previously available have become less accessible.

Despite these difficulties, notable advances have been made in data collection, for example, involving post-coding. More sensitive ways of measuring social circumstances continue to be explored to supplement the use of occupations. Measures of health are being developed which take more account of the impact of certain factors on a person's daily life, to supplement traditional measures like mortality and morbidity rates. There is intense activity in some centres to develop better tools for monitoring the situation and for allocating resources more equitably.

Policy in the caring services

Many recommendations for policy focus on what the health and social services could do to reduce inequalities in health, together with proposals for action in the wider community.

By attention to resource allocation, access and quality of care issues, people working in the health care sector can help to reduce those aspects of inequality in *health* caused by inequality in *health care*. There is also a vital task in alleviating the health damage caused by the wider determinants of inequalities in health. A plea is made to introduce a consideration for equity into every aspect of policy-making in the caring services. There are potential dangers in the current NHS reforms of increasing inequalities in health care and great vigilance is needed to avoid this outcome.

Extending the strategy

In the wider community, strategy needs to involve actions on income; on improvements in housing and working conditions; on removing barriers to the adoption of healthier life-styles; and a proper mechanism for co-ordinating health-related policy at a national and local level.

In reality what has happened over the past twelve years is a disturbing increase in the number of children growing up in poverty, and an increase in families becoming homeless. Policies deliberately designed to reduce child poverty have not been adopted, and the situation has been exacerbated by a sharp rise in the level of unemployment which has affected families with young children in particular.

A concerted effort to improve housing conditions has not been made and there is now growing concern over the shortage of houses and the poor state of repair of existing dwellings. There is no evidence, except in isolated cases, that government, employers and trades unions have come together to formulate plans for creating healthier working conditions or to monitor the working environment more effectively. Mechanisms for co-ordinating policies on health at local and national level have not been set up on a significant scale, even though it is widely acknowledged that health policies need to involve many agencies outside the health sector, such as housing, environmental control, transport, food and agriculture and – above all – the Treasury.

So far, much of this summary may have sounded very negative. It would be wrong to give the impression that no one cares about inequalities in health and that no attempts have been made to remedy them. Although a co-ordinated policy has not been set in motion, a great deal has been done by individuals and by organizations in direct response to the Black Report and World Health Organization initiatives. A selection of the many activities is described, including health and social service projects to improve the access of deprived communities and ethnic minority groups to primary health care; to explore the community development approach, and to reduce the harm done by unemployment – to name a few.

Chapters 8, 9 and 10 also note the tremendous efforts being made by some health and local government authorities to compile local 'Black Reports' and to build up health databases as well as to work out health strategies. The renewed interest in public health policy in local authorities is particularly noticeable. In addition, the report highlights the work of many professional bodies and organizations concerned about inequalities. Some have formulated policy and plans for tackling the problem of health inequalities from their own particular perspectives. In the 1990s there was at last official recognition at the national level of the seriousness of the problem of inequality in health. A first attempt at a national strategy for health has been drawn up, which was also a step in the right direction, though as yet it does not contain the necessary commitment to take action on inequalities in health. It is hoped that this situation will change and there will be a concerted effort in the 1990s on this vital issue.

References

Introduction to *Inequalities in Health*

Benzeval, M., Judge, K., and Solomon, M. (1992), 'The Health Status of Londoners', King's Fund Institute.

Black, D. (1981a), 'Inequalities in Health', *British Medical Journal*, 282, p. 1468.

Black, D. (1981b), 'Inequalities in Health', lecture in memory of Dr Christie Gordon, mimeo.

British Medical Association (1987), 'Deprivation and Ill-health', British Medical Association.

British Medical Journal (1986), 'Whatever Happened to the Black Report?', 293, pp. 91–2.

COHSE (1980), Research Bulletin, occasional series, Confederation of Health Service Employees, December.

Deitch, R. (1981), 'The Debate on the Black Report', *Lancet*, ii, pp. 158–9.

Department of Health (1991), 'The Health of the Nation: A Consultative Document on a Health Strategy for England', Department of Health/HMSO.

Department of Health (1992), 'The Health of the Nation: A Strategy for Health for England', HMSO.

Enthoven, A. C. (1991), 'Internal Market Reforms of the British National Health Service', *Health Affairs*, Fall 1991, pp. 60–86.

Gray, A. (1981), *On the Black Report: Inequalities in Health, a Summary and Comment*, Aberdeen, Health Economics Research Unit, University of Aberdeen.

Griffiths (1983), The National Health Service Management Inquiry (Griffiths) Report, Department of Health and Social Security.

Hart, N. (1987), 'The Health Divide: Class Still Reigns', *Poverty*, 67, pp. 17–19.

Health Promotion Authority for Wales (1990), 'Health for All in Wales: Health Promotion Challenges for the 1990s: Part B', Cardiff, Health Promotion Authority for Wales.

Illsley, R. (1986), 'Occupational Class, Selection and the Production of Inequalities in Health', *Quarterly Journal of Social Affairs*, 2 (2), pp. 151–65.

Illsley, R. (1987a), 'Occupational Class, Selection and Inequalities in Health – Rejoinder to Richard Wilkinson's Reply', *Quarterly Journal of Social Affairs*, 3 (3), pp. 213–23.

Illsley, R. (1987b), 'The Health Divide: Bad Welfare or Bad Statistics?', *Poverty*, 67, pp. 16–17.

Illsley, R., and LeGrand, J. (1986), *Measurement of Inequality in Health*, No. 12 in the Welfare State Programme of STICERD, London School of Economics.

Jencks, C. (1989), 'What Is the Underclass – and Is It Growing?, *Focus*, Spring and Summer, 1989.

Kilmarnock (1987), House of Lords *Hansard*, 1 April, Col. 645.

King's Fund (1992), 'London Health Care 2010', King Edward's Hospital Fund for London.

Klein, R. (1988), 'Acceptable Inequalities', in Green, D. (ed.), *Acceptable Inequalities? Essays on the Pursuit of Equality in Health Care*, Institute of Economic Affairs.

Klein, R. (1991), 'Making Sense of Inequalities: A Response to Peter Townsend', *International Journal of Health Services*, 21, pp. 175–81.

Kornblum, W. (1991), 'Who Is the Underclass? Contrasting Approaches', *Dissent*, Spring 1991.

Lancet (1987a), 'Suspicion about the New Health Education Authority', i, p. 517.

Lancet (1987b), 'The Health Education Council Goes Out with a Flourish', i, p. 816.

Lancet (1987c), 'The Health Divide: Swan-song of the Health Education Council', i, pp. 724–5.

Lancet (1990), 'The Underclass', *Lancet*, 335, pp. 1312–5.

LeGrand, J. (1985), *Inequalites in Health: the Human Capital Approach*, No. 1 in the Welfare State Programme of STICERD, London School of Economics.

LeGrand, J. (1987), 'Inequalities of Health: An International Comparison', *European Economic Review*, 31, pp. 182–91.

LeGrand, J., and Rabin, M. (1986), 'Trends in British Health Inequality, 1931–83', in A. J. Culyer and B. Jonsson (eds.), *Public and Private Health Services,* Oxford, Basil Blackwell.

Lister, R. (1990), 'The Exclusive Society: Citizenship and the Poor', Child Poverty Action Group.

Marmot, M., and McDowall, M. (1986), 'Mortality Decline and Widening Social Inequalities', *Lancet*, ii, pp. 274–6.

Mincey, R. B., *et al.* (1990), 'The Underclass: Definition and Measurement', *Science*, 248, pp. 450–53.

Morris, J. N. (1980a), 'Social Inequalities Undiminished', *Lancet*, i, pp. 87–90; *Health Visitor*, 53, pp. 361–5.

Morris, J. N. (1980b), 'Equalities and Inequalities in Health', *British Medical Journal*, 281, p. 1003.

Morris, J. N. (1980c), 'Medicine's Order of Priorities', *The Times*, 19 September.

Murray, C., *et al.* (1990), 'The Emerging British Underclass', Institute for Economic Affairs.

National Association of Health Authorities (1986), *NHS Economic Review*, Birmingham, NAHA.

Newman, B. A., and Thomson, R. J. (1989), 'Economic Growth and Social Development: A Longitudinal Analysis of Causal Priority', *Journal of World Development*, pp. 451–71.

Quick, A., and Wilkinson, R. G. (1991), 'Income and Health,' Socialist Health Association.

Radical Community Medicine (1980), 4.

Radical Statistics Health Group (1992), 'A Growing Health Service?' *Health Matters*, 11 (in press).

Scott-Samuel, A. (1992), 'Health Gain Versus Equity', *Health Visitor*, 65, p. 176.

Seear (1987), House of Lords *Hansard*, 30 March, Col. 358.

Strong, P. M. (1990), 'Black on Class and Mortality: Theory, Method and History', *Journal of Public Health Medicine*, 12, pp. 168–80.

Townsend, P. (1982), 'The Policy Implications of a Positive Approach to Health', *Health Visitor*, 55, pp. 97–101.

Townsend, P. (1990), 'Widening Inequalities of Health in Britain: A rejoinder to Rudolf Klein', *International Journal of Health Services*, 20, pp. 363–72.

Townsend, P. (1991), 'Evading the Issue of Widening Inequalities of Health in Britain: A Reply to Rudolf Klein', *International Journal of Health Services*, 21, pp. 183–9.

Townsend, P. (1992), 'Underclass and Overclass: the Widening Gulf between Social Classes in Britain in the 1980s', in Payne, G., and Cross, M. (eds.), *Sociology in Action*, Macmillan.

Townsend, P., Phillimore, P., and Beattie, A. (1986), 'Inequalities in Health in the Northern Region: an Interim Report', Northern Regional Health Authority/Bristol University.

TUC (1981), *The Unequal Health of the Nation*, a TUC summary of the Black Report, TUC.

Watkins, S., and Elton, P. (1981), 'Inequalities in Health: a Response', paper prepared for a working party of the North-West Regional Health Authority (unpublished).

Whitehead, M., and Dahlgren, G. (1991), 'What Can Be Done about Inequaltities in Health?', *Lancet*, 338, pp. 1059–63.

Whitney, R. (1987a), House of Commons *Hansard*, 6 April, Col. 53.

Whitney, R. (1987b), House of Commons *Hansard*, 6 April, Col. 54.

Wilkinson, R. G. (1986), 'Occupational Class, Selection and Inequalities in Health: a Reply to Raymond Illsley', *Quarterly Journal of Social Affairs*, 2 (4), pp. 415–22.

Wilkinson, R. G. (1987), 'A Rejoinder', *Quarterly Journal of Social Affairs*, 3 (3), pp. 225–8.

Wilson, W. J. (1987), *The Truly Disadvantaged*, University of Chicago Press.

World Bank, *World Development Report 1981*, Oxford, Oxford University Press.

The Black Report

1: Concepts of Health and Inequality

Abel-Smith, B., *The Hospitals 1800–1948*, Heinemann, 1964.

Birch, H. G., and Gussow, J. D., *Disadvantaged Children: Health, Nutrition and School Failure*, New York, Harcourt, Brace and World, 1970.

Black, D., 'The Paradox of Medical Care', *Journal of the Royal College of Physicians*, 13, 57, 1979.

Brown, G. W., and Harris, T., *Social Origins of Depression: A Study of Psychiatric Disorder in Women*, Tavistock, 1978.

Culyer, A. J., Lavers, R. J., and Williams, A., in Shonfield, A., and Shaw, S. (eds.), *Social Indicators and Social Policy*, Heinemann, 1972.

Disability Rights Handbook for 1980, Disability Alliance, 1979.

Dollery, C., *The End of an Age of Optimism*, Nuffield Provincial Hospitals Trust, 1978.

Dubos, R., *Mirage and Health*, Allen & Unwin, 1960.

Help for the Disabled, Louis Harris International, 1974.

McKeown, T., *The Role of Medicine: Dream, Mirage or Nemesis?*, Nuffield Provincial Hospitals Trust, 1976.

Marshall, W. A., *Human Growth and Its Disorders*, Academic Press, 1977.

Mechanic, D., *Medical Sociology: A Selective View*, New York, Free Press, 1968.

Morris, J. N., *Uses of Epidemiology*, 3rd edn, Churchill Livingstone, 1975.

Royal Commission on the Distribution of Income and Wealth, Reports Nos. 1, 4, 5 and 7, Cmnds 6171, 6626, 6999 and 7595, London, HMSO, 1975–9.

Sackett, D. L., Chambers, L. W., MacPherson, A. S., Goldsmith, C. H., and Macauley, R. G., 'The Development and Application of Indices of Health: General Methods and a Summary of Results', *American Journal of Public Health*, Vol. 67, No. 5, 1977.

Sigerist, H. E., *Civilization and Disease*, University of Chicago Press, Phoenix Edition, 1962 (first published Cornell University Press, 1943).

Stevenson, T. H. C., 'The Vital Statistics of Wealth and Poverty', *Journal of the Royal Statistical Society*, Vol. 91, 1928.

Susser, M. W., and Watson, W., *Sociology in Medicine*, Oxford University Press, 1971.

Tuckett, D. A. (ed.), *An Introduction to Medical Sociology*, Tavistock, 1976.

2: The Pattern of Present Health Inequalities

Gans, B., 'Health Problems and the Immigrant Child', in CIBA Foundation, *Immigration: Medical and Social Aspects*, 1966.

Hood, C., Oppé, T. E., Pless, I. B., and Apte, E., *West Indian Immigrants: A Study of One-Year-Olds in Paddington*, Institute of Race Relations, 1970.

Logan, W. P. D., and Cushion, A. A., *Morbidity Statistics from General Practice*, HMSO, 1960.

Ministry of Pensions and National Insurance, *Report of an Inquiry into the Incidence of Incapacity for Work*, HMSO, 1964.

OPCS, *Occupational Mortality 1970–72, Decennial Supplement*, HMSO, 1978.

Oppé, T. E., 'The Health of West Indian Children', *Proceedings of the Royal Society of Medicine*, 57, 1967, pp. 321–3.

Smith, D., *The Facts of Racial Disadvantage: A National Survey*, PEP, 1976.

Thomas, H. E., 'Tuberculosis in Immigrants', *Proceedings of the Royal Society of Medicine*, 61, 1968.

3: Trends in Inequality of Health

Fit for the Future: The Report of the Committee on Child Health Services (Court Report), Cmnd 6684, HMSO, 1977

McKeown, T., *The Role of Medicine*, Nuffield Provincial Hospitals Trust, 1976.

Morris, J. N., 'Health and Social Class', *Lancet*, 7 February 1959.

OPCS, *Occupational Mortality, Decennial Supplement, 1970–72, England and Wales*, HMSO, 1978.

Registrar General's Decennial Supplement England and Wales, 1961: Occupational Mortality Tables, HMSO, 1971.

4: Inequality in the Availability and Use of the Health Service

Bone, M., *Family Planning Services in England and Wales*, HMSO, 1973.

Brotherston, J., 'Inequality: Is It Inevitable?', in Carter and Peel (eds.), *Equalities and Inequalities in Health*, Academic Press, 1976.

Bulman, J. S., Richards, N. D., Slack, G. L., and Willcocks, A. J., *Demand and Need for Dental Care*, OUP, 1968.

Buxton, M. J., and Klein, R. E., 'Distribution of Hospital Provision: Policy Themes and Resource Variations', *British Medical Journal*, 1, 1976, p. 299.

Cartwright, A., *Human Relations and Hospital Care*, Routledge, 1964. *Parents and Family Planning Services*, Routledge, 1970.

Cartwright, A., and O'Brien, M., 'Social Class Variations in Health Care', in Stacey, M. (ed.), *The Sociology of the NHS*, Sociological Review Monograph 22, 1976.

Clarke, M., *Trouble with Feet*, Occasional Papers on Social Administration, Bell, 1969.

Coombe, V., 'Health and Social Services and Minority Ethnic Groups', *Journal of the Royal Society of Health*, 96, 1976.

Douglas, J. W. B., and Rowntree, G., 'Supplementary Maternal and Child Health Services', *Population Studies*, 2, 1949.

Forster, D. P., 'Social Class Differences in Sickness and General Practitioner Consultations', Health Trends, 8, 1976, p. 29.

General Household Survey Reports, 1971–7.

Gordon, I., 'Social Status and Active Prevention of Disease', *Monthly Bulletin of the Ministry of Health*, 10, 1951.

Gray, P. G., *et al., Adult Dental Health in England and Wales in 1968*, HMSO, 1970.

Jones, D. R., and Masterman, S., 'NHS Resources: Scales of Variation', *British Journal of Preventive and Social Medicine*, 30, 1976, p. 244.

Martin, D., *Social Aspects of Prescribing*, Heinemann, 1957.

Martin, J., and Morgan, M., *Prolonged Sickness and the Return to Work*, HMSO, 1975.

Martini, C. J. M., *et al.*, 'Health Indexes Sensitive to Medical Care Variation', *International Journal of Health Services*, 7, 1977, p. 293.

Morris, J. N., *The Uses of Epidemiology*, 3rd edn, Churchill Livingstone, 1975.

Noyce, J., Snaith, A. H., and Trickey, A. J., 'Regional Variations in the Allocation of Financial Resources to the Community Health Services', *Lancet*, 1974.

Rickard, J. H., 'Per Capita Expenditure of the English Area Health Authorities', *British Medical Journal*, 1, 1976, p. 299.

Sheiham, A., and Hobdell, M. H., 'Decayed, Missing and Filled Teeth in British Adult Populations', *British Dental Journal*, 126, 1969, p. 401.

Skrimshire. A., *Area Disadvantage, Social Class and the Health Service*, Department of Social and Administrative Studies, University of Oxford, 1978.

Titmuss, R. M., *Commitment to Welfare*, Allen & Unwin, 1968.

Townsend, P., *The Last Refuge*, Routledge, 1962.

Townsend. P., and Wedderburn, D., *The Aged in the Welfare State*, Bell Occasional Papers on Social Administration, 1965.

Tudor Hart, J., 'The Inverse Care Law', *Lancet*, 1, 1971.

West, R. R., and Lowe, C. R., 'Regional Variations in Need for and Provision and Use of Child Health Services in England and Wales', *British Medical Journal*, October 1976, p. 843.

5: *International Comparisons*

Anderson, O. W., *Health Care – Can There Be Equity?*, New York, Wiley, 1972.

Chase, H. C., 'Infant Mortality and Its Concomitants 1960–1972', *Medical Care*, 15, 8, August 1977, p. 662.

Denmark, *Medicinsk Fødselsstatistik*, Copenhagen, 1974.

Derrienic, F., Ducimetière, P., and Kritsikis, S., 'La mortalité cardiaque des Français actif d'âge moyen selon leur catégorie socio-professionelle et leur région de domicile', *Revue d'Épidémiologie, Médecine Sociale, et Santé Publique*, 25, 1977, p. 131.

Dinh Quang Chi, and Hemery, S., 'Disparités régionales de la mortalité infantile', *Économie et Statistiques*, 1977, 85, pp. 3–12.

Doguet, M. L., 'Les prestations familiales en France: Bilan et perspectives', *Revue Française des Affaires Sociales*, 32, 1, January-March 1978, pp. 3–48.

Geijerstam, G., 'Low Birth Weight and Perinatal Mortality', *Public Health Report*, 84, November 1969, pp. 939–48.

Germany, *Bevölkerung und Kultur*, Reiche 7: *Gesundheitswesen* 1974, Wiesbaden, Statistisches Bundesamt, 1974.

Kaminsky, M., Blondel, B., Bréart, G., Franc, M., Du Mazaubrun, C., 'Issue de la grossesse et surveillance prénatale chez les femmes migrantes. Enquête sur un échantillon représentatif des naissances en France en 1972', *Revue d'Épidémiologie, Médecine Sociale, et Santé Publique*, 26, 1, 1978, pp. 29–46.

Lerner, M., and Stutz, R. N., 'Have We Narrowed the Gap between the Poor and the Non-Poor? Narrowing the Gaps 1959–61 and 1969–71 – Mortality', *Medical Care*, 15, 8, August 1977, p. 620.

Lindgren, Gunilla, 'Height, Weight and Menarche in Swedish Urban School Children in Relation to Socio-Economic and Regional Factors', *Annals of Human Biology*, 3, 1976, 6, pp. 501–28.

Maynard, A., 'The Medical Profession and the Efficiency and Equity of Health Services', *Social and Economic Administration*, 12, 1, 1978, p. 3.

Morris, J. N., 'Scottish Hearts', *Lancet*, 3 November 1979.

Naytia, S., 'Social Group and Mortality in Finland', *British Journal of Preventive and Social Medicine*, 31, 4, 1977, p. 231.

Netherlands, *Compendium Gezondheidsstatistiek Nederland*, Centraal Bureau voor de Statistiek, 1974.

Norway, *Sosialt Utsyn 1977*, Oslo, Statistisk Sentralbyra, 1977.

Pharaoh, P. O., and Morris, J. N., 'Postneonatal Mortality', in Sartwell, P. E. (ed.), *Epidemiological Reviews* I, 1979, pp. 170–83.

Purola, T., Kalimo, E., Nyman, K., and Sievers, K., *The Utilization of the Medical Services and its Relationship to Morbidity, Health Resources and Social Factors*, Helsinki, Research Institute for Social Security, 1968.

Rona, R. J., Swan, A. V., and Altman, D. G., 'Social Factors and Height of Primary School Children in England and Scotland', *Journal of Epidemiology and Community Health*, 32, 1978, pp. 147–54.

Rumeau-Rouquette, C., *et al.*, 'Evaluation épidémiologique du programme de santé en périnatologie, I Région Rhône-Alpes 1972–1975', *Revue d'Épidémiologie, Médecine Sociale, et Santé Publique*, 25, 1977, p. 107.

Salkever, D. S., 'Economic Class and Differential Access to Care: Comparisons among Health Care Systems', *International Journal of Health Services*, 5, 1975, 3, p. 373.

Sjolin, S., 'Infant Mortality in Sweden', in Wallace, Helen M. (ed.), *Health Care of Mothers and Children in National Health Services*, Cambridge, Mass., Ballinger, 1975.

Wilson, R. W., and White, E. L., 'Changes in Morbidity, Disability and Utilization Differentials between the Poor and the Non-Poor. Data from the Health Interview Survey 1964 and 1973', *Medical Care*, 15, 8, 1977, p. 636.

Wynn, M., and A., *The Protection of Maternity and Infancy* (A Study of the Services for Pregnant Women and Young Children in Finland with Some Comparisons with Britain), Council for Children's Welfare, 1974. *Prevention of Handicap of Perinatal Origin* (An Introduction to French Policy and Legislation), Foundation for Education and Research in Childbearing, 1976.

6: *Towards an Explanation of Health Inequalities*

Abel-Smith, B., and Townsend, P., *The Poor and the Poorest*, Bell, 1965.

Baird, D., 'Epidemiology of Congenital Malformations of the Central Nervous System in (a) Aberdeen and (b) Scotland', *Journal of Biosocial Science*, 6, 1974, p. 113. 'The Epidemiology of Low Birth Weight: Changes in Incidence in Aberdeen, 1948–1972', *Journal of Biosocial Science*, 6, 1974, p. 323.

Banks, J. and O., *Feminism and Family Planning*, Routledge, 1964.

Bernstein, B., *Class, Codes and Control*, Routledge, 1971.

Birch, H. G., and Gussow, J. D., *Disadvantaged Children: Health, Nutrition and School Failure*, New York, Harcourt, Brace and World, 1970.

Brennan, M. E., 'Medical Characteristics of Children Supervised by the Local Authority Social Services Department', *Policy and Politics*, 1, 1973, 3, p. 255.

Brenner, M. H., 'Fetal, Infant, and Maternal Mortality during Periods of Economic Instability', *International Journal of Health Services*, 3, 1973, 2, p. 145. 'Estimating the Social Costs of National Economic Policy: Implications for Mental and Physical Health and Criminal Aggression', Joint Economic Committee, US Congress, US Government Printing Office, Washington DC, 1976. 'Health Costs and Benefits of Economic Policy', *International Journal of Health Services*, 7, 1977, 4.

Brown, G., and Harris, T., *Social Origins of Depression*, Tavistock, 1978.

Colley, J. R. T., and Reid, D. D., 'Urban and Social Class Origins of Childhood Bronchitis in England and Wales', *British Medical Journal*, 2, 1970, p. 213.

DHSS, *Eating for Health*, 1978.

DHSS, *Nutrition among the Elderly*, 1980.

Doll, R., Hill, A. B., and Sakula, J., *British Journal of Preventive and Social Medicine*, 1960.

Douglas, J. W. B., and Waller. R. E., 'Air Pollution and Respiratory Infection in Children', *British Journal of Preventive and Social Medicine*, 20, 1966, 1.

Eichenwald, H. F., and Fry, P. C., 'Nutrition and Learning', *Science* 163, 1949, p. 644.

Eyer, J., 'Hypertension as a Disease of Modern Society', *International Journal of Health Services*, 5, 1975, 4, p. 539. 'Prosperity as a Cause of Death', *International Journal of Health Services*, 7, 1977(a), 1, p. 125. 'Does Employment Cause the Death Rate Peak in Each Business Cycle?' *International Journal of Health Services*, 7, 1977(b), 4, p. 625.

Fuchs, V., *Who Shall Live? Health, Economics, and Social Choice*, New York, Basic Books, 1974.

Goldberg, E. M., and Morrison, S. L., 'Schizophrenia and Social Class', *British Journal of Psychiatry*, 109, 1963, p. 785.

Hellier, J., 'Perinatal Mortality 1950 and 1973', *Population Trends*, 10, Winter 1977.

Holman, R. T., *Poverty: Explanations of Social Deprivation*, Robertson, 1978.

Illsley, R., 'Social Class Selection and Class Differences in Relation to Stillbirths', *British Medical Journal*, 2, 1955, p. 1520.

Janerich, D. T., 'Maternal Age and Spina Bifida: Longitudinal Versus Cross-Sectional Analysis', *American Journal of Epidemiology*, 96, 1972, p. 389.

Lawrence, K. M., Carter, C. O., and David, P. A., 'Major CNS Malformations in South Wales II', *British Journal of Preventive and Social Medicine*, 22, 1968, p. 212.

Leeder, S. R., Corkhill, R., Irwig, L. M., Holland, W. W., and Colley, J. R. T., 'Influence of Family Factors on the Incidence of Lower Respiratory Tract Illness during the First Year of Life', *British Journal of Preventive and Social Medicine*, 30, 1976, p. 203.

Lewis, O., *The Children of Sanchez*, New York, Random House, 1967.

McKeown, T., *The Modern Use of Population*, Arnold, 1976.

Miller, F. J. W., Court, S. D. M., Knox, E. G., and Brandon, S., *The School Years in Newcastle-upon-Tyne, 1952–1962*, Oxford University Press, 1974.

Morris, J. N., *Uses of Epidemiology*, 3rd edn, Churchill Livingstone, 1975. 'Social Inequalities Undiminished', *Lancet*, 13 January 1979, 87.

Morris, J. N., and Heady, J. A., 'Social and Biological Factors in Infant Mortality: I. Objects and Methods', *Lancet*, 1955, i, p. 343.

Morris, J. N., and Titmuss, R. M., (a) 'Health and Social Change: I The Recent History of Rheumatic Heart Disease', *Medical Officer*, 26 August, 9 September 1944. (b) 'Epidemiology of Peptic Ulcer', *Lancet*, 30 December 1944, p. 841.

OPCS, *Occupational Mortality 1970–72*, HMSO, 1978. *Trends In Mortality*, HMSO, 1978.

Powles, J., 'Health and Industrialization in Britain', Proceedings First World Congress on Environmental Medicine and Biology, Paris, 1974.

Rutter, M., and Madge, N., *Cycles of Disadvantage*, Heinemann, 1976.

Stedman-Jones, G., *Outcast London*, Oxford, Clarendon Press, 1971.

Thompson, P., *The Edwardians*, Paladin, 1976.

Townsend, P., *Poverty in the United Kingdom*, Penguin Books, 1979.

Wilson, H., and Herbert, G. W., *Parents and Children in the Inner City*, Routledge, 1978.

8: Planning the Health and Personal Social Services

Acheson Report, *Primary Health Care in Inner London: A Report of a Study Group Commissioned by the London Health Planning Consortium*, 1981.

Action on Smoking and Health, *European Survey of Smoking in Public Places*, 1976.

Alberman, E. D., Morris, J. N., and Pharaoh, P. O., 'After Court', *Lancet*, 20 August 1977.

Brennan, M. E., and Lancashire, R., 'Association of Childhood Mortality with Housing Status and Unemployment', *Journal of Epidemiology and Community Health*, 32, 1978, 1.

Butler, J. R., Bevan, J. M., and Taylor, R. C., *Family Doctors and Public Policy*, Routledge, 1973.

Carstairs, V., and Morrison, M., *The Elderly in Residential Care*, Scottish Health Studies No. 19, Edinburgh, SHHD, 1972.

Department of Health and Social Security (and the Welsh Office), *The Census of Residential Accommodation 1970*, HMSO, 1975. *Priorities for Health and Personal Social Services in England: A Consultative Document*, HMSO, 1976. *Prevention and Health*, Cmnd 7047, HMSO, 1977. *The Way Forward*, HMSO, 1977. 'The DHSS Perspective', in Barnes, J., and Connelly, N., *Social Care Research*, Bedford Square Press, 1978. *A Happy Old Age*, 1978. Circular HC (78)5, *Health Services Development: Court Report on Child Health Services*, January 1978. *Local Authority Social Service Summary of Planning Returns 1976–77 to 1979–80*, HMSO, 1978. *Report of the Committee of Inquiry into Mental Handicap Nursing and Care* (Jay Report), Cmnd 7468, HMSO, 1979.

Expenditure Committee, First Report, Session 1976-7, *Preventive Medicine*, HC 169-i, HMSO, 1977. Ninth Report, Session 1976-7, Chapter V, 'Spending on the Health and Personal Social Services', HC, HMSO, 1977.

Fitzherbert, K., *Child Care Services and the Teacher*, Temple Smith, 1977.

Forster, H. D. P., Frost, B., Francis, B., and Heath, P., 'Need and Demand for Health Care', University of Sheffield.

Gardner, M. J., Crawford, M. D., and Morris, J. N., 'Patterns of Mortality in Middle and Early Old Age in the County Boroughs of England and Wales', *British Journal of Preventive and Social Medicine*, 23, 1969, 3.

Graham, H., 'Problems in Antenatal Care', unpublished paper, DHSS/CPAG conference, 'Reaching the Consumer in the Antenatal and Child Health Services' April 1978.

Kimbell, A., and Townsend, J., *Residents in Elderly Persons' Homes*, Cheshire CC Social Services Department, April 1974.

Lind, G., and Wiseman, C., 'Setting Health Priorities: A review of Concepts and Approaches', *Journal of Social Policy*, 7, 4, 1978.

Morris, J. N., 'Social Inequality Undiminished', *Health Visitor*, September 1980.

Plank, D., *Caring for the Elderly, Report of a Study of Various Means of Caring for Elderly People in Eight London Boroughs*, GLC, 1977. *Report of the Royal Commission on the National Health Service* (Merrison Report), Cmnd 7615, HMSO, 1979.

Rutter, M., Tizard, J., and Whitmore, K., *Educational Health and Behaviour*, Longman, 1970.

Rutter, M., *et al.*, 'Attainment and Adjustment in Two Geographical Areas: Some Factors Accounting for Area Differences', *British Journal of Psychology*, 126, 1975.

Scottish Home and Health Department, *Towards an Integrated Child Health Service*, Edinburgh, HMSO, 1973.

Smith, D., *The Facts of Racial Disadvantage*, PEP, 1976.

Townsend, P., *The Last Refuge*, Routledge, 1962. 'The Needs of the Elderly and the Planning of Hospitals' in Canvin, R. W., and Pearson, N. G. (eds.), *Needs of the Elderly for Health and Welfare Services*, University of Exeter, 1973.

Tuckett, D., 'Choices for Health Education: A Framework for Decision Making', Health Education Studies Unit, 1979.

9: The Wider Strategy

Baker, J. A., *et al.*, 'School Milk and Growth in Primary School Children', *Lancet*, ii, 1978, p. 575.

Benjamin, B., *Social and Economic Factors Affecting Mortality*, Mouton, The Hague and Paris, 1965.

Bone, M., *Pre-School Children and the Need for Day Care*, OPCS Social Survey Division, HMSO, 1977.

Bradshaw, J., Edwards, H., Staden, F., and Weale, J., 'Area Variations in Infant Mortality 1975/77', *Journal of Epidemiology and Community Medicine*, November 1978.

Brown, G. W., and Harris, T., *The Social Origins of Depression*, Tavistock, 1978.

Cook, J., Altman, D. G., Moore, D. M. C., Topp, S. G., Holland, W. W., and Elliott, A., 'A Study of the Nutritional Status of School Children', *British Journal of Preventive and Social Medicine*, 27, 2, 1973.

Cook, J., Altman, D. G., Jacoby, A., Holland, W. W., and Elliott, A., 'School Meals and Nutrition of School Children', *British Journal of Preventive and Social Medicine*, 29, 3 September 1975.

Cook, J., Altman, D. G., Jacoby, A., and Holland, W. W., 'The Contribution Made by School Milk to the Nutrition of Primary School Children', *British Journal of Nutrition*, 1975, 34, 91.

Cook, J., Irwig, L. M., Chinn, S., Altman, D. G., Florey, C. du V., 'The Influence of Availability of Free School Milk on the Height of Children in England and Scotland', *Journal of Epidemiology and Community Health* (in press).

Department of Education and Science, *Nutrition in Schools*, Report of the Working Party on the Nutritional Aspects of School Meals, HMSO, 1975.

DHSS, *A Nutrition Survey of Pre-School Children 1967–68*, Reports on Health and Social Subjects, No. 10, HMSO, 1975.

DHSS, *Eating for Health*, HMSO, 1978.

DHSS and DES, *Joint Circular on Co-ordination of Provision for Under-5s*, January 1978.

DHSS and Supplementary Benefits Commission, *Response of the Supplementary Benefits Commission to 'Social Assistance: A Review of the Supplementary Benefits Scheme in Great Britain'*, HMSO, 1979.

Diamond, J., *Public Expenditure in Practice*, Allen & Unwin, 1975.

Disability Alliance, *Disability Rights Handbook for 1979*, November 1978.

Field, F., *Children Worse Off under Labour?*, Poverty Pamphlet 32, London, Child Poverty Action Group, February 1978.

Field, F., and Townsend, P., *A Social Contract for Families*, Poverty Pamphlet, 19. Child Poverty Action Group, 1975.

Fox, A. J., and Adelstein, A. M., *Journal of Epidemiology and Community Health*, 23, 1978, p. 73.

Glennerster, H. (ed.), *Labour's Social Priorities*, London's Fabian Research Series 327, 1976.

The Great Child Benefit Robbery, Child Benefit Now Campaign, London Child Poverty Action Group, April 1977.

Harris, I. A., *et al., Income and Entitlement to Benefit of Impaired People in Great Britain*, Vol. 3 of *Handicap and Impairment in Great Britain*, HMSO, 1972.

Heclo, H., and Wildavsky, A., *The Private Government of Public Money*, Macmillan, 1976.

Howe, J. R., *Two-parent Families: A Study of their Resources and Needs in 1968, 1969 and 1970*, Statistical Report Series No. 14, HMSO, 1971.

Institute for Fiscal Studies, *The Structure and Reform of Direct Taxation*, Report of a Committee chaired by Professor J. E. Meade, Allen & Unwin, 1978.

Jacoby, A., Altman, D. G., Cook, J., Holland, W. W., and Elliott, A., 'Influence of Some Social and Environmental Factors on the Nutrient Intake and Nutritional Status of School Children', *British Journal of Preventive and Social Medicine*, 29, 2, June 1975.

Land, H., 'The Introduction of Family Allowances: An Act of Historic Justice?', in Hall, P., Land, H., Parker, R., and Webb, A., *Change, Choice and Conflict in Social Policy*, Heinemann, 1975.

Land, H., 'The Child Benefit Fiasco', in Brown, M., and Jones, K. (eds.), *The Yearbook of Social Policy in Britain 1977*, Routledge, 1978.

Ministry of Pensions and National Insurance, *Financial Circumstances of Retirement Pensioners*, HMSO, 1966.

Ministry of Social Security, *Circumstances of Families*, Report of an Inquiry by the Ministry of Pensions and National Insurance with the co-operation of the National Assistance Board, HMSO, 1967.

National Food Survey, *Household Food Consumption and Expenditure*, Ministry of Agriculture, Food and Fisheries Annual Report, 1977.

Plowden, W. J. L., 'Developing a Joint Approach to Social Policy', *The Yearbook of Social Policy in Britain 1976*, Routledge, 1976.

Reed, F. B., *Lancet*, 2, 1978, pp. 675–6.

Report of the Snowdon Working Party, *Integrating the Disabled*, National Fund for Research into Crippling Diseases, 1976.

Rona, R. J., Chinn, S., and Smith, A. M., 'Height of Children Receiving Free School Meals', *Lancet*, 8 September 1979, p. 534.

Royal Commission on the Distribution of Income and Wealth, *Report No. 6, Lower Incomes*, Cmnd 7175, HMSO, May 1978.

Safety and Health at Work (Robens Report), Cmnd 5034, HMSO, July 1972.

Select Committee on Tax Credit, Session 1972–3, Vol. I, *Report and Proceedings of the Committee*, Vol. II, Evidence, HMSO, 1973.

Social Trends, Cmnd 7439, HMSO, 1979.

Supplementary Benefit Report 1973, Annual Report of the SBC 1973, Cmnd 6615, HMSO, 1974.

Townsend, P., *Poverty in the United Kingdom*, Penguin Books, 1979.

Trades Union Congress, *Handbook of Safety and Health at Work*, TUC, 1978.

Wicks, M., *Old and Cold*, Heinemann, 1978.

Wilson, H., and Herbert, G. W., with Wilson, J. V., *Parents and Children in the Inner City*, Routledge, 1978.

Working Party on Housing of the Central Council for the Disabled, *Towards a Housing Policy for Disabled People*, 1976.

The Health Divide

Acheson, E. D. (1990), 'Edwin Chadwick and the World We Live In', *Lancet*, 336, pp. 1482–85.

Acheson, E. D. (1991), 'On the State of the Public Health for the Year 1990', Department of Health/HMSO.

Agius, F. (1990), 'Health and Social Inequalities in Malta', *Social Science and Medicine*, 31, pp. 313–18.

Anderson, O. (1985), 'Dodelighed og erhverv 1970–80', Danmarks Statistik, *Statistiske Undersogelser* No. 41, quoted in Valkonen (1987).

Anderson, O., *et al.* (1987), 'A Comparative Study of Occupational Mortality in the Nordic Countries 1971–80', in *Proceedings of the 4th Meeting of the UN/WHO/CICRED Network*, Zamardi, Hungary, 13–16 September 1986, Hungarian Statistical Bureau.

Arber, S. (1987), 'Social Class, Non-employment, and Chronic Illness: Continuing the Inequalities in Health Debate', *British Medical Journal*, 294, pp. 1069–73.

Arber, S. (1989), 'Gender and Class Inequalities in Health: Understanding the

Differentials', in A. J. Fox (ed.), *Inequalities in Health within Europe*, Gower Press, Aldershot.

Arber, S. (1991), 'Class, Paid Employment and Family Roles: Making Sense of Structural Disadvantage, Gender and Health Status', *Social Science and Medicine*, 32, pp. 425–36.

Arber, S., Gilbert, G. N., and Dale, A. (1985), 'Paid Employment and Women's Health: a Benefit or a Source of Role Strain?', *Sociology of Health and Illness*, 7 (3), pp. 375–400.

Archbishop of Canterbury's Commission on Urban Priority Areas (1985), *Faith in the City: a Call for Action by Church and Nation*, Church House Publishing.

ASH (1992), 'Her Share of Misfortune: Smoking, Women and Low Income', Action on Smoking and Health/Health Education Authority.

Ashton, J. (1984), 'Health in Mersey: a Review', Department of Community Health, University of Liverpool.

Ashton, J. (1986), 'Healthy Cities – a WHO Project', Department of Community Health, University of Liverpool.

Ashton, L. (1988), 'Survey of Local Authority Food Policies 1988', Health Education Authority.

Audit Commission (1986), 'Making a Reality of Community Care', HMSO.

Audit Commission (1991), 'Healthy Housing: the Role of Environmental Health Services', Audit Commission Local Government Report No. 6, HMSO.

Backett, K. C. (1990), 'Image and Reality: Health Enhancing Behaviours in Middle-class Families', *Health Education Journal*, 49, pp. 61–3.

Backett, K. C., and Alexander, H. (1991), 'Talking to Young Children about Health: Methods and Findings', *Health Education Journal*, 50, pp. 34–8.

Baker, D., and Illsley, R. (1991), 'Trends in Inequality in Health in Europe', *International Journal of Health Sciences*, 1/2, pp. 89–111.

Balarajan, R. (1991), 'Ethnic Differences in Mortality from IHD and CVD in England and Wales', *British Medical Journal*, 302, pp. 560–64.

Balarajan, R., *et al.* (1984), 'Patterns of Mortality among Immigrants in England and Wales', *British Medical Journal*, 289, pp. 1185–7.

Balarajan, R., and Yuen, P. (1986), 'British Smoking and Drinking Habits: Variations by Country of Birth', *Community Medicine*, 8 (3), pp. 237–9.

Balarajan, R., *et al.* (1992), 'Deprivation and General Practice Workload', *British Medical Journal*, 304, pp. 529–34.

Banks, M. H., and Jackson, P. R. (1982), 'Unemployment and Risk of Minor Psychiatric Disorder in Young People: Cross-sectional and Longitudinal Evidence', *Psychological Medicine*, 12, pp. 789–98.

Barker, D. J. P. (1990), 'The Fetal and Infant Origins of Adult Disease', *British Medical Journal*, 301, p. 1111.

Barker, D. J. P., Osmond, C., and Law, C. M. (1989), 'The Intrauterine and Early Postnatal Origins of Cardiovascular Disease and Chronic Bronchitis', *Journal of Epidemiology and Community Health*, 43, pp. 237–40.

Bartley, M. (1990), 'Health and Labour-force Participation "Stress", Selection and the Reproduction Costs of Labour Power', *Journal of Social Policy*, 20 (3), pp. 327–64.

Batten, E., and Allen, S. (1991), 'Towards a Smoke-free Environment: Local Authority Policies and Practice', Health Education Authority.

Battersby, S. (1991), 'Using the Law to Improve Housing Conditions', *Health Visitor*, 64, pp. 373–5.

Beale, N., and Nethercott, S. (1985), 'Job-loss and Family Morbidity: a Study of a Factory Closure', *Journal of the Royal College of General Practitioners*, 35, pp. 510–14.

Beale, N., and Nethercott, S. (1986a), 'Job-loss and Morbidity in Married Men with and without Children', *Journal of the Royal College of General Practitioners*, 36, pp. 557–9.

Beale, N., and Nethercott, S. (1986b), 'Job-loss and Morbidity: the Influence of Job Tenure and Previous Work History', *Journal of the Royal College of General Practitioners*, 36, pp. 560–63.

Becker, S. (ed.) (1991), *Windows of Opportunity*, Child Poverty Action Group.

Benzeval, M., Goodwin, S., and Judge, K. (1992), 'New Strategies for Child Health', King's Fund Institute (in press).

Berg, L., and Diderichsen, F. (1989), 'Some Examples of Inequity in Health in Sweden', *Health Promotion*, 4, pp. 151–3.

Berkman, L. F., and Breslow, L. (1983), *Health and Ways of Living: the Alameda County Study*, Oxford University Press.

Berkman, L. F., and Syme, S. L. (1979), 'Social Networks, Host Resistance and Mortality: a Nine-year Follow-up Study', *American Journal of Epidemiology*, 109, pp. 186–204.

Betts, G. (1985), 'Report of a Survey on Health in Glyndon Ward, Greenwich', Greenwich Health Rights Project.

Bhopal, R. S. (1988), 'Health Care for Asians: Conflict in Need, Demand and Provision', in *Equity: a Prerequisite for Health*, Proceedings of the 1987 Summer Conference, Geneva, WHO.

Bhopal, R. S. (1991), 'Health Education and Ethnic Minorities', *British Medical Journal*, 302, p. 1338.

Binysh, K., *et al.* (1985), 'The Health of Coventry', Department of Community Medicine, Coventry Health Authority.

Black, D. (1984), Evidence to the Scottish Health Education Co-ordinating Committee, 1984.

Black, D., and Laughlin, S. (eds.) (1985), 'Unemployment and Health: Resources, Action, Discussion, Information', Health Education Department, Greater Glasgow Health Board.

Blackburn, C. (1991), 'Family Poverty: What Can Health Visitors Do?', *Health Visitor*, 64, pp. 368–70.

Blackburn, C. (1992), *Improving Health and Welfare Practice with Families in Poverty: a Practical Guide*, Buckingham, Open University Press.

Blane, D. (1985), 'An Assessment of the Black Report's Explanations of Health Inequalities', *Sociology of Health and Illness*, 7, pp. 423–45.

Blane, D., Davey Smith, G., and Bartley, M. (1990), 'Social Class Differences in Years of Potential Life Lost: Size, Trends and Principal Causes', *British Medical Journal*, 301, pp. 429–32.

Blane, D., Davey Smith, G., and Bartley, M. (1993), 'Social Selection: What Does It Contribute to Social Class Differences in Health?', *Sociology of Health and Illness*, 15 (1) (in press).

Blaxter, M. (1983), 'Health Services as a Defence against the Consequences of Poverty in Industrialized Societies', *Social Science and Medicine*, 17, pp. 1139–1148.

Blaxter, M. (1984), 'Equity and Consultation Rates in General Practice', *British Medical Journal*, 288, pp. 1963–7.

Blaxter, M. (1985), 'Self-definition of Health Status and Consulting Rates in Primary Care', *Quarterly Journal of Social Affairs*, 1, pp. 131–71.

Blaxter, M. (1987a), 'Fifty Years On – Inequalities in Health', in J. Hobcraft and M. Murphy (eds.), *Proceedings of the British Society for Population Studies*, Oxford University Press (in press).

Blaxter, M. (1987b), 'Evidence on Inequality in Health from a National Survey', *Lancet*, ii, pp. 30–33.

Blaxter, M. (1989), 'A Comparison of Measures of Inequality in Morbidity', in A. J. Fox (ed.), *Inequalities in Health within Europe*, Gower Press, Aldershot.

Blaxter, M. (1990), *Health and Lifestyles*, Tavistock/Routledge.

Blaxter, M., and Paterson, L. (1982), *Mothers and Daughters: a Three Generational Study of Health Attitudes and Health Behaviour*, Heinemann.

Bloor, M., Samphier, M., and Prior, L. (1987), 'Artifact Explanations of Inequalities in Health: an Assessment of the Evidence', *Sociology of Health and Illness*, 9, pp. 231–64.

BMA (1986), 'All Our Tomorrows: Growing Old in Britain', report of the Board of Science and Education, British Medical Association.

BMA (1987), 'Deprivation and Ill-health', Board of Science and Education, British Medical Association.

Boardman, B. (1986), 'Seasonal Mortality and Cold Homes', paper presented to the Institute of Environmental Health Officers/Legal Research Institute conference on 'Unhealthy Housing: a Diagnosis', Warwick University, 14–16 December 1986.

Bone, M., and Meltzer, H. (1989), 'The Prevalence of Disability among Children', OPCS Surveys of Disability in Great Britain, Report 3, HMSO.

Borgan, J., and Kristofersen, L. (1986), 'Mortality by Occupation and Socio-economic Group in Norway 1978–80', Central Bureau of Statistics of Norway, *Statistiske Analyser*, 56, quoted in Valkonen (1987).

Bos, G. A. M. van den, and Lenoir, M. E. (1992), 'Socioeconomic Inequalities and Chronic Diseases', *Social Science and Medicine* (forthcoming).

Bosanquet, N., and Leese, B. (1988), 'Family Doctors and Innovation in General Practice', *British Medical Journal*, 296, pp. 157–80.

Botting, B., and Macfarlane, A. (1990), 'Geographic Variation in Infant Mortality in Relation to Birthweight 1983–85', in M. Britton (ed.), *Mortality and Geography*, OPCS series DS 9, HMSO.

Bowling, A. (1991), 'Social Support and Social Networks: their Relationship to the Successful and Unsuccessful Survival of Elderly People in the Community. An analysis of concepts and a review of the evidence', *Family Practice*, 8, pp. 68–83.

Boys, R. J., Forster, D. P., and Jojan, P. (1991), 'Mortality from Causes Amenable and Non-amenable to Medical Care: the Experience of Eastern Europe, *British Medical Journal*, 303, pp. 879–83.

Braddon, F. E. M., *et al.* (1986), 'Onset of Obesity in a 36-year Birth Cohort Study', *British Medical Journal*, 293, pp. 299–303.

Braddon, F. E. M., Wadsworth, M. E. J., Davies, J. M. C., and Cripps, H. A. (1988), 'Social and Regional Differences in Food and Alcohol Consumption and their Measurement in a National Birth Cohort', *Journal of Epidemiology and Community Health*, 42, pp. 341–9.

Brenner, M. H. (1979), 'Mortality and the National Economy: a Review and the Experience of England and Wales 1936–1976', *Lancet*, ii, pp. 568–73.

Brenner, M. H. (1983), 'Mortality and Economic Instability: Detailed Analysis for Britain and Comparative Analysis for Selected Industrial Countries', *International Journal of Health Services*, 13 (4), pp. 563–619.

British Medical Journal (1986), editorial, 'Lies, Damned Lies and Suppressed Statistics', *British Medical Journal*, 293, pp. 349–50.

Britton, M. (ed.) (1990), 'Mortality and Geography', OPCS series DS 9, HMSO.

Brown, G. W., and Harris, T. (1982), 'Social Class and Affective Disorder', in Ihsam Al-Issa (ed.), *Culture and Psychopathology*, University Park Press, Baltimore.

Bucquet, D., and Curtis, S. (1986), 'Socio-demographic Variation in Perceived Illness and the Use of Primary Care: the Value of Community Survey Data for Primary Care Service Planning', *Social Science and Medicine*, 23 (7), pp. 737–44.

Bucquet, D., Jarman, B., and White, P. (1985), 'Factors Associated with Home Visiting in an Inner London General Practice', *British Medical Journal*, 290, pp. 1480–83.

Burghes, L. (1980), 'Living from Hand to Mouth: a Study of 65 Families Living on Supplementary Benefit', Child Poverty Action Group/Family Services Unit.

Burr, M. L., St Leger, A. S., and Yarnell, J. (1981), 'Wheezing, Dampness and Coal Fires', *Community Medicine*, 3, pp. 205–9.

Butler, N. R., *et al.* (1982), 'Research Findings from the 1970 Child Health and Education Study', *Journal of the Royal Society of Medicine*, 75, pp. 781–4.

Cade, J. E., Barker, D. J. P., Martetts, B. M., and Morris, J. A. (1988), 'Diet and Inequalities in Health in Three English Towns', *British Medical Journal*, 296, pp. 1359–62.

Calnan, M., and Johnson, B. (1985), 'Health, Health Risks and Inequalities: an Exploratory Study of Women's Perceptions', *Sociology of Health and Illness*, 7, pp. 55–75.

Campbell, D. A., Radford, J. M. C., and Burton, P. (1991), 'Unemployment Rates: an Alternative to the Jarman Index?', *British Medical Journal*, 303, pp. 750–55.

Carmichael, C. L. (1985), 'Inner-city Britain: a Challenge for the Dental Profession.

A Review of Dental and Related Deprivation in Inner-City Newcastle upon Tyne', *British Dental Journal*, 159 (1), pp. 24–7.

Carr-Hill, R. (1990), 'The Measurement of Inequities in Health: Lessons from the British Experience', *Social Science and Medicine*, 31, pp. 393–404.

Carr-Hill, R., and Sheldon, T. (1991), 'Designing a Deprivation Payment for GPs: the UPA (8) Wonderland', *British Medicine Journal*, 302, pp. 393–6.

Carstairs, V. (1981a), 'Small Area Analysis and Health Service Research', *Community Medicine*, 3, pp. 131–9.

Carstairs, V. (1981b), 'Multiple Deprivation and Health State', *Community Medicine*, 3, pp. 4–13.

Carstairs, V. (1988), 'Differentials in Mortality', *Health Bulletin*, 46, pp. 226–36.

Carstairs, V., and Morris, R. (1988), 'Deprivation and Mortality: an Alternative to Social Class?', *Community Medicine*, 11, pp. 210–19.

Carstairs, V., and Morris, R. (1989), 'Deprivation: Explaining Differences in Mortality between Scotland and England and Wales', *British Medical Journal*, 299, pp. 886–9.

Carstairs, V., and Morris, R. (1990), 'Deprivation and Health in Scotland', *Health Bulletin*, 48, pp. 162–75.

Cartwright, A. (1979), *The Dignity of Labour?*, Tavistock.

Central Statistical Office (1991), 'Family Spending', HMSO.

Central Statistical Office (1992), *Social Trends*, 22, 1992 edition, HMSO.

Charles, N., and Kerr, M. (1985), 'Attitudes towards the Feeding and Nutrition of Young Children', Research Report No. 4, Health Education Council.

Charlton, J. R. H., *et al.*, (1983), 'Geographical Variation in Mortality from Conditions Amenable to Medical Intervention in England and Wales', *Lancet*, i, pp. 691–6.

Clarke, J. (1983), 'Sexism, Feminism and Medicalization – a Decade Review of Literature on Gender and Illness', *Sociology of Health and Illness*, 5, p. 62.

Cole-Hamilton, I., and Lang, T. (1986), 'Tightening Belts: a Report on the Impact of Poverty on Food', London Food Commission.

Coleman, A. (1985), *Utopia on Trial: Vision and Reality in Planned Housing*, Hilary Shipman.

Collins, E., and Klein, R. (1980), 'Equity and the NHS: Self-reported Morbidity, Access and Primary Care', *British Medical Journal*, 282, pp. 111–15.

Colver, A., *et al.* (1982), 'Promoting Children's Home Safety', *British Medical Journal*, 285, pp. 1177–80.

Connelly, J., Roderick, P., and Victor, C. (1990), 'Health Service Planning for the Homeless Population: Availability and Quality of Existing Information', *Public Health*, 104, pp. 109–116.

Connelly, J., *et. al.* (1991), 'Housing and Homelessness: a Public Health Perspective', Faculty of Public Health Medicine.

Constantinides, P., and Walker, G. (1985), 'Child Accidents and Health Inequalities in a London Borough', paper presented at 'Symposium on Accidents in Childhood', King's Fund Centre, 3 October 1985.

Cook, D. G., Bartley, M. J., Cummins, R. O., and Shaper, A. G. (1982), 'Health of Unemployed Middle-aged Men in Great Britain', *Lancet*, i, pp. 1290–94.

Cook, G. (1990), 'Health and Social Inequities in Ireland', *Social Science and Medicine*, 31, pp. 285–90.

Coronary Prevention Group (1986), 'Coronary Heart Disease and Asians in Britain', Confederation of Indian Organizations and Coronary Prevention Group.

Coulter, A. (1987), 'Lifestyles and Social Class: Implications for Primary Care', *Journal of the Royal College of General Practitioners*, 37, pp. 533–6.

Cox, B., *et al.* (1987), 'Health and Life-style Survey: Preliminary Report', Health Promotion Research Trust.

Crombie, D. L. (1984), 'Social Class and Health Status. Inequality or Difference', *Journal of the Royal College of General Practitioners*, Occasional Paper 25.

Crombie, I., Lee, A., Smith, W. C. S., Tunstall-Pedoe, H. (1990), 'Levels and Social Patterns of Self-reported Physical Activity in Scotland', *Health Education Journal*, 49, pp. 71–4.

Cubbon, J. (1986), 'The Health of Grimsby: a Review of Statistical Information on Mortality and Morbidity', Grimsby Health Authority.

Dahl, E. (1990), 'Inequalities in Health in Norway: a Review of the Evidence', Working Paper No. 4/90, Oslo, National Institute of Public Health, Unit for Health Services Research.

Dahlgren, G., and Diderichsen, F. (1986), 'Strategies for Equity in Health: Report from Sweden', *International Journal of Health Services*, 16, pp. 517–37.

Dahlgren, G., and Whitehead, M. (1992), 'Policies and Strategies to Promote Social Equity in Health', Copenhagen, World Health Organization.

Darley, C. D. (1981), 'High Density Housing: the Wirral's Experience', *Royal Society of Health Journal*, 101 (6), pp. 229–33.

Davey Smith, G. (1991), 'Second Thoughts on the Jarman Index', *British Medical Journal*, 302, pp. 359–60.

Davey Smith, G., Shipley, M. J., and Rose, G. (1990a), 'The Magnitude and Causes of Socio-economic Differentials in Mortality: Further Evidence from the Whitehall Study', *Journal of Epidemiology and Community Health*, 44, pp. 265–70.

Davey Smith, G., Bartley, M., and Blane, D. (1990b), 'The Black Report on Socioeconomic Inequalities in Health Ten Years On', *British Medical Journal*, 301, pp. 373–7.

Davey Smith, G., Leon, D., Shipley, M. J., and Rose, G. (1991), 'Socioeconomic Differentials in Cancer among Men', *International Journal of Epidemiology*, 20, pp. 339–45.

Davey Smith, G., Blane, D., and Bartley, M. (1992), 'Explanations for Socioeconomic Differentials in Mortality', *Social Science and Medicine* (in press).

Dekker, E. (1992), 'Reorientation of Health Care in Europe and Health for All', Copenhagen, World Health Organization Regional Office for Europe.

Delamothe, T. (1991), 'Social Inequalities in Health', *British Medical Journal*, 303, pp. 1046–50.

Department of Health (1991), 'The Health of the Nation: a Consultative Document on a Health Strategy for England', Department of Health/HMSO.

Department of Health (1992), 'The Health of the Nation: A Strategy for Health in England', HMSO.

Department of the Environment (1981a), 'An Investigation of "Difficult to Let" Housing', HMSO.

Department of the Environment (1981b), *Families in Flats*, HMSO.

Department of the Environment (1983), 'Urban Deprivation: Information Note No. 2 from the Inner Cities Directorate', Department of the Environment.

Department of the Environment (1988), 'English House Condition Survey 1986', HMSO.

Department of Social Security (1992), 'Households below average income: 1979–1988/89', HMSO.

Desplanques, G. (1984), 'L'Inégalité devant la mort', *Économie et Statistiques* No. 162, quoted in Valkonen (1987).

Dhooge, Y., and Dooris, M. (1988), 'Working with Unemployment and Poverty: a Training Manual for Health Promotion', South Bank Polytechnic.

DHSS (1976a), 'Prevention and Health: Everybody's Business', HMSO.

DHSS (1976b), 'Priorities for the Health and Personal Social Services in England', HMSO.

DHSS (1980), 'Inequalities in Health: Report of a Research Working Group Chaired by Sir Douglas Black', DHSS.

DHSS (1986a), 'Low Income Families 1983', DHSS.

DHSS (1986b), 'On the State of the Public Health: 1985', HMSO.

DHSS (1986c), 'The Diets of British Schoolchildren', DHSS.

DHSS (1988), 'Low Income Families', DHSS.

Diderichsen, F. (1990), 'Health and Social Inequities in Sweden', *Social Science and Medicine*, 31, pp. 359–67.

Diderichsen, F. (1991), 'Widening Social Inequities – Trends in Occupational Cardiovascular Mortality among Swedish Men 1961–86', mimeo.

Diderichsen, F., Bostrom, G., and Norman, A. (1990), 'Public Health in Stockholm 1990: Can There Be Efficiency and Equity in Health Policy?', Report to the Annual Healthy Cities Symposium, Stockholm, 23–27 September.

Donaldson, L. J., and Odell, A. (1984), 'Planning and Providing Services for the Asian Population: a Survey of DHAs', *Journal of the Royal Society of Health*, 104 (6), pp. 199–202.

Donovan, J. (1984), 'Ethnicity and Health: a Research Review', *Social Science and Medicine*, 19 (7), pp. 663–70.

Dowding, V. M. (1981), 'New Assessment of the Effects of Birth Order and Socio-economic Status on Birth Weight', *British Medical Journal*, 282, pp. 683–6.

Dowding, V. M., and Barry, C. (1990), 'Cerebral Palsy: Social Class Differences in Prevalence in Relation to Birthweight and Severity of Disability', *Journal of Community Health*, 44, pp. 191–5.

Dowling, S. (1983), *Health for a Change: the Provision of Preventive Health Care in Pregnancy and Early Childhood*, Child Poverty Action Group/National Extension College.

Dunnell, K. (1991), 'Deaths among 15–44-year-olds', *Population Trends*, No. 64, Spring, pp. 38–43.

Durward, L. (1984), 'Poverty in Pregnancy', Maternity Alliance.

Eales, M. J. (1989), 'Shame among Unemployed Men', *Social Science and Medicine*, 28, pp. 783–9.

Eddie, S., and Davies, J. A. (1985), 'The Effect of Social Class on Attendance Frequency and Dental Treatment Received in the General Dental Service in Scotland', *British Dental Journal*, 159, pp. 370–72.

Egger, M., Minder, C. E., and Davey Smith, G. (1990), 'Health Inequalities and Migrant Workers in Switzerland', *Lancet*, 336, p. 816.

Elliott, K. (1992), 'Working with Black and Ethnic Minority Groups', in P. Webb (ed.), '*Health Promotion and Patient Education: a Professional's Guide*' (forthcoming).

Ensinger, M., and Celentano, D. (1988), 'Unemployment and Psychiatric Distress: Social Resources and Coping', *Social Science and Medicine*, 27, pp. 239–47.

Ericson, A., *et al.* (1984), 'Pregnancy Outcome and Social Indicators in Sweden', *Acta Paediatrica Scandinavica*, 73, pp. 69–74, quoted in Valkonen (1987).

Faculty of Community Medicine (1986), 'Health for All by the Year 2000. Charter for Action', Faculty of Community Medicine.

Fagin, L., and Little, M. (1984), *The Forsaken Families*, Penguin Books.

Fallowfield, L. (1990),'Quality of Life: the Missing Dimension in Health Care', Souvenir Press.

Farrant, W. (1986), 'Health for All in the Inner City: a Proposed Framework for Health Promotion Policy Development within Paddington and North Kensington Health Authority', Paddington and North Kensington Health Authority.

Findley, I. N., *et al.* (1991), 'Coronary Angiography in Glasgow: Relation to CHD and Social Class', *British Heart Journal*, 66, p. 70.

Fisher, M. J., *et al.* (1983), 'Patterns of Attendance at Developmental Assessment Clinics', *Journal of the Royal College of General Practitioners*, 33 (249), pp. 213–18.

Fogelman, K., Fox, J., and Power, C. (1987), 'Class and Tenure Mobility. Do They Explain the Social Inequalities in Health among Young Adults in Britain?', National Child Development Study Working Paper No. 21, Social Statistics Research Unit, City University, London.

Forwell, G. (1991), 'Annual Report of the Director of Public Health 1990', Glasgow, Greater Glasgow Health Board.

Fox, A. J., and Goldblatt, P. O. (1982), 'Socio-demographic Mortality Differentials: Longitudinal Study 1971–75', Series L.S. No. 1, HMSO.

Fox, A. J., Goldblatt, P. O., and Jones, D. R. (1986), 'Social Class Mortality Differentials: Artefact, Selection, or Life Circumstances?', in R. G. Wilkinson (ed.), *Class and Health*, Tavistock.

Fox, A. J., Jones, D. R., and Goldblatt, P. O. (1984), 'Approaches to Studying the Effect of Socio-economic Circumstances on Geographic Differences in Mortality in England and Wales', *British Medical Bulletin*, 40 (4), pp. 309–14.

Fox, A. J., and Shewry, M. C. (1988), 'New Longitudinal Insights into Relationships between Unemployment and Mortality', *Stress Medicine*, 4, pp. 11–19.

Frayman, H. (1991), 'Breadline Britain in the 1990s: the Findings of the Television Series (booklet), Domino Films/LWT Community Education Office.

Fryer, P. (1987), 'Oxford's Aim of Health for All', *Health Service Journal*, 5 March 1987, pp. 274–5.

Gillies, D. R. N., *et al.* (1984), 'Analysis of Ethnic Influences on Stillbirths', *Journal of Epidemiology and Community Health*, 38 (3), pp. 214–17.

Ginnety, P., Kelly, K., and Black, M. (1985), 'Moyard: a Health Profile', Parts 1 and 2, Eastern Health and Social Services Board, Belfast.

Gillam, S. (1992), 'Provision of Health Promotion Clinics in Relation to Population Need: Another Example of the Inverse Care Law', *British Journal of General Practice*, 42, pp. 54–6.

Giraldes, M. (1988), 'The Equity Principle in the Allocation of Health Care Expenditure in Portugal', *International Journal of Health Planning and Management*, 3, pp. 167–83.

Goldblatt, P. (1988), 'Changes in Social Class between 1971 and 1981: Could These Affect Mortality Differentials among Men of Working Age?', *Population Trends*, 51, pp. 9–17.

Goldblatt, P. (1989), 'Mortality by Social Class, 1971–85', *Population Trends*, 56, pp. 6–15.

Goldblatt, P. (1990a), 'Social Class Mortality Differences', in N. M. Mascie-Taylor (ed.), *Bio-social Aspects of Social Class*, Oxford, Oxford University Press.

Goldblatt, P. (1990b) 'Mortality and Alternative Social Classifications', in P. Goldblatt (ed.), *Longitudinal Study 1971–81: Mortality and Social Organisation*, OPCS LS series No. 6, HMSO.

Goldthorpe, J. H. (1980), *Social Mobility and Class Structure in Modern Britain*, Oxford, Clarendon Press.

Goodwin, S. (1991), 'Breaking the Links between Social Deprivation and Poor Child Health', *Health Visitor*, 64, pp. 376–80.

Goodwin, S. (1992), 'Community Nursing and the New Public Health', *Health Visitor*, 65, pp. 78–80.

Government Statistical Service (1990), 'Households below Average Income – a Statistical Analysis 1981–87', HMSO.

Graham, H. (1976), 'Smoking in Pregnancy: the Attitudes of Expectant Mothers', *Social Science and Medicine*, 10, pp. 399–405.

Graham, H. (1979), 'Problems in Antenatal Care', Department of Sociology, University of York.

Graham, H. (1980), 'Family Influences in Early Years on the Eating Habits of Children', in M. Turner (ed.), *Nutrition and Lifestyles*, Applied Science Publishers.

Graham, H. (1984), *Women, Health and Family*, Wheatsheaf Books, Brighton.

Graham, H. (1986), 'Caring for the Family', Research Report No. 1, Health Education Council.

Graham, H. (1989), 'Women and Smoking in the UK: the Implications for Health Promotion', *Health Promotion*, 3, pp. 371–82.

Graham, H., and McKee, L. (1980), 'The First Months of Motherhood', Research Monograph No. 3, Health Education Council.

Greater Glasgow Health Board (1984), 'Ten Year Report, 1974–1983', Greater Glasgow Health Board.

Gregory, J., Foster, K., Tyler, H., and Wiseman, M. (1990), 'Dietary and Nutritional Survey of British Adults', HMSO.

Griffiths, J., Pollock, R., Grice, D., Glasson, J., and Dunkley, R. (1991), 'Lessons in Class', *Health Service Journal*, 22 August, pp. 20–21.

Grimsley, M., and Bhat, A. (1988), 'Health', in A. Bhat, R. Carr-Hill, and S. Ohri, *Britain's Black Population: a New Perspective*, Aldershot, Gower.

Gunning-Schepers, L. J. (1989), 'How to Put Equity and Health on the Political Agenda', *Health Promotion*, 4, pp. 149–50.

Gunning-Schepers, L. J. (1991), 'A Policy Response to Socioeconomic Differentials in Health', paper presented to EC workshop on 'Socioeconomic factors in health and health care', Lisbon, 23–25 May.

Haan, M., Kaplan, G., and Camacho, T. (1987), 'Prospective Evidence from the Alameda County Study', *American Journal of Epidemiology*, 125, pp. 989–98.

Haavio-Mannila, E. (1986), 'Inequalities in Health and Gender', *Social Science and Medicine*, 22 (2), pp. 141–9.

Haberman, M. A., and Bloomfield, D. S. F. (1988), 'Social Class Differentials in Mortality in Great Britain around 1981', *Journal of the Institute of Actuaries*, 115, pp. 495–517.

Haines, F. A., and de Looy, A. E. (1986), 'Can I Afford the Diet? The Effect of Low Income on People's Eating Habits with Particular Reference to Groups at Risk', British Dietetic Association, Birmingham.

Halliday, M., and Adams, L. (1992), 'Healthy Sheffield: the Consultation Experiment', *Health Education Journal*, 51, 43–6.

Halsey, A. H. (1987), 'Social Trends Since World War II', in Central Statistical Office *Social Trends*, 17, pp. 11–19, 1987 edition, HMSO.

Halsey, A. H., Heath, A. F., and Ridge, J. M. (1980), *Origins and Destinations: Family Class and Education in Modern Britain*, Oxford, Clarendon Press.

Hammerstrom, A., Janler, U., and Theorell, T. (1988), 'Youth Unemployment and Ill-health: Results from a Two-year Follow-up Study', *Social Science and Medicine*, 26, pp. 1025–33.

Hansard (1991), 'Income Support: Child Recipients', House of Lords *Hansard*, WA 140, 22 October 1991.

Harris, C., and Smith, R. (1987), 'What Are Health Authorities Doing about the Health Problems Caused by Unemployment?', *British Medical Journal*, 294, pp. 1076–9.

Hart, J. T. (1971), 'The Inverse Care Law', *Lancet*, i, pp. 405–12.

Hart, J. T., Thomas, C., Gibbons, B., Edwards, C., Hart, M., Jones, J., *et al.* (1991), 'Twenty-five Years of Case Finding and Audit in a Socially Deprived Community,' *British Medical Journal*, 302, pp. 1509–13.

Hart, N. (1991), 'The Social and Economic Environment and Human Health', in Holland, Detels and Knox (eds.), *Oxford Textbook of Public Health*, 2nd edition.

Hawton, K., and Rose, N. (1986), 'Unemployment and Attempted Suicide among Men in Oxford', *Health Trends*, 8, pp. 29–32.

Haynes, R. (1991), 'Inequalities in Health and Health Service Use: Evidence from the General Household Survey', *Social Science and Medicine*, 33, pp. 361–8.

Heady, P., and Smyth, M. (1989), 'Living Standards during Unemployment: the Results', OPCS SS190, HMSO.

Health Education Authority (1990), 'Food and Health Policies in the UK: District Health Authorities and Health Boards National Study Interim Report', Health Education Authority.

Health Promotion Authority for Wales (1990), 'Health for All in Wales: Health Promotion Challenges for the 1990s: Part B', Cardiff, Health Promotion Authority for Wales.

Health Visitors Association (1991), 'Project Health: Health Promotion and the Role of the School Nurse in the School Community', Health Visitors Association.

Heyman, B., Bell, B., Kingham, M., and Handyside, E. (1990), 'Social Class and the Prevalence of Handicapping Conditions', *Disability, Handicap and Society*, 5, pp. 167–84.

Hibbard, J., and Pope, C. (1991), 'Effect of Domestic and Occupational Roles on Morbidity and Mortality', *Social Science and Medicine*, 32, pp. 805–11.

Hills, J. (1988), 'Changing Tax: How the Tax System Works and How to Change It', Child Poverty Action Group.

Holden, J., *et al*, (1989), 'Counselling in a General Practice Setting: Controlled Study of Health Visitor Intervention in the Treatment of Postnatal Depression', *British Medical Journal*, 298, pp. 223–6.

Holland, W. W. (1986), 'The RAWP Review: Pious Hopes', *Lancet*, ii, pp. 1087–90.

Holstein, B. (1985), 'Denmark Country Paper', in *Inequalities in Health and Health Care*, Nordic School of Public Health, NHV Report 1985:5, Göteborg, Sweden.

Hopton, J., and Hunt, S. (1990), 'Changing Housing Conditions in Relation to Health and Wellbeing', Manchester, Galen Research and Consultancy.

House, J., Landis, K., and Umberson, D. (1988), 'Social Relationships and Health', *Science*, 241, pp. 540–45.

Huhne, C. (1986), 'Share Boom Halts Equality Trend', *Guardian*, 23 September 1986.

Hunt, S., and McEwen, J. (1980), 'The Development of a Subjective Health Indicator', *Sociology of Health and Illness*, 2, pp. 231–46.

Hunt, S., McEwen, J., and McKenna, S. P. (1985), 'Social Inequalities in Perceived Health', *Effective Health Care*, 2 (4), pp. 151–60.

Huntington, J., and Killoran, A. (1991), 'Winning at the Primaries', *Health Service Journal*, 21 November, pp. 24–5.

HVA/BMA (1989), *Homeless Families and their Health*, Health Visitors Association/British Medical Association.

Illsley, R. (1986), 'Occupational Class, Selection and the Production of Inequalities in Health', *Quarterly Journal of Social Affairs*, 2 (2), pp. 151–65.

Illsley, R., and Baker, D. (1991), 'Contextual Variations in the Meaning of Health Inequality', *Social Science and Medicine*, 32, pp. 359–65.

Illsley, R., and LeGrand, J. (1987), 'The Measurement of Inequality in Health', in A. Williams (ed.), *Health and Economics*, Macmillan.

Inland Revenue Board (1986), 'Inland Revenue Statistics', HMSO.

Iversen, L. (1989), 'Unemployment and Mortality', *Stress Medicine*, 5, pp. 85–92.

Jacobson, B. (1988), *Beating the Ladykillers: Women and Smoking*, Gollancz.

Jacobson, B., Smith, A., and Whitehead, M. (1991), 'The Nation's Health: a Strategy for the 1990s', second edition, King's Fund.

James, J., Oakhill, A., and Evans, J. (1989), 'Preventing Iron Deficiency in Preschool Children by Implementing an Educational and Screening Programme in an Inner City Practice', *British Medical Journal*, 299, pp. 838–40.

James, J., Brown, J., and Douglas, M. (1991), 'Promoting Healthy Nutrition in the Inner City: the True Cost', *Lancet*, 338, p. 58.

Jamrozik, K., *et al.* (1984), 'Controlled Trials of Three Different Anti-smoking Interventions in General Practice', *British Medical Journal*, 288, pp. 1499–503.

Jarman, B. (1983), 'Identification of Underprivileged Areas', *British Medical Journal*, 286, pp. 1705–9.

Jarman, B. (1984), 'Under-privileged Areas: Validation and Distribution of Scores', *British Medical Journal*, 289, pp. 1587–92. For critical response to the Jarman Score, *see* A. Scott-Samuel, 'Identification of Underprivileged Areas', *British Medical Journal*, 287 (1983), p. 130; J. R. H. Charlton and A. Lakhani, 'Is the Jarman Underprivileged Area Score Valid?', *British Medical Journal*, 290 (1985), pp. 1714–16; R. Leavey and J. Wood, 'Does the Underprivileged Area Index Work?', *British Medical Journal*, 291 (1985), pp. 709–11.

Jarman, B. (1991), 'General Practice, the NHS Review and Social Deprivation', *British Journal of General Practice*, 41, pp. 76–9.

Jarman, B. (1991), 'Unemployment Rates: an Alternative to the Jarman Index?', *British Medical Journal*, 303, p. 1136.

Jarman, B., Townsend, P., and Carstairs, V. (1991), 'Deprivation Indices', *British Medical Journal*, 303, p. 523.

Jedrychowski, W., Becher, H., Wahrendorf, J., and Basa-Cierpialek, Z. (1990), 'A Case-control Study of Lung Cancer with Special Reference to the Effect of Air Pollution in Poland', *Journal of Epidemiology and Community Health*, 44, pp. 114–20.

Jenkins, P. M., *et al.* (1984), 'The Effect of Social Factors on Referrals for Orthodontic Advice and Treatment', *British Journal of Orthodontics*, 11 (1), pp. 24–6.

Joffe, M. (1989), 'Social Inequalities in Low Birthweight: Timing of Effects and Selective Mobility', *Social Science and Medicine*, 28, pp. 613–19.

Johnson, M. R. D. (1984), 'Ethnic Minorities and Health', *Journal of the Royal College of Physicians of London*, 18 (4), pp. 228–30.

Jones, I. G., and Cameron, D. (1984), 'Social Class: an Embarrassment to Epidemiology?', *Community Medicine*, 6, pp. 37–46.

Joseph, K., and Sumption, J. (1979), *Equality*, John Murray.

Joseph Rowntree Foundation (1991), 'Inquiry into British Housing: Second Report, June 1991', York, Joseph Rowntree Foundation.

Kaplan, G. A. (1985), 'Twenty Years of Health in Alameda County: the Human Population Laboratory Analyses', paper presented to the Society for Prospective Medicine, Annual Meeting, San Francisco, 24 November 1985.

Kaplan, G., and Salonen, J. (1990), 'Socioeconomic Conditions in Childhood and IHD during Middle-age', *British Medical Journal*, 301, pp. 1121–3.

Keithley, J., Byrne, D., Harrison, S., and McCarthy, P. (1984), 'Health and Housing Conditions in Public Sector Housing Estates', *Public Health*, 98, pp. 344–53.

Klepp, K., and Forster, J. L. (1985), 'The Norwegian Nutrition and Food Policy: an Integrated Policy Approach to a Public Health Problem', *Journal of Public Health Policy*, 6, pp. 447–63.

Knight, I. (1984), 'The Height and Weight of Adults in Great Britain', OPCS/HMSO.

Knox, P. L. (1979), 'The Accessibility of Primary Care to Urban Patients: a Geographical Analysis', *Journal of the Royal College of General Practitioners*, 29 (220), pp. 160–68.

Kogevinas, M., Marmot, M., Fox, A. J., and Goldblatt, P. (1991), 'Socioeconomic Differences in Cancer Survival', *Journal of Epidemiology and Community Health*, 45, pp. 216–19.

Kohler, L., and Martin, J. (eds.) (1985), 'Inequalities in Health and Health Care', Gothenberg, WHO/Nordic School of Public Health.

Koskinen, S. (1985), 'Time-trends in Cause-specific Mortality by Occupational Class in England and Wales', International Union for the Scientific Study of Population Conference, Florence, June 1985.

Koskinen, S., Melkas, T., and Vienonen, M. (1985), 'Finland Country Paper', in *Inequalities in Health and Health Care*, Nordic School of Public Health, NHV Report, 1985:5, Göteborg, Sweden.

Kreitman, N., and Platt, S. (1984), 'Suicide, Unemployment and Domestic Gas Detoxification in Great Britain', *Journal of Epidemiology and Community Health*, 38, pp. 1–6.

Kunst, A. (1990), 'Socio-economic Mortality Differences in the Netherlands in 1950–84: a Regional Study of Cause-Specific Mortality', *Social Science and Medicine*, 31, pp. 141–52.

Lagasse, R., Humblet, P., *et al.* (1990), 'Health and Social Inequities in Belgium', *Social Science and Medicine*, 31, pp. 237–48.

Lang, T., *et al.* (1984), 'Jam Tomorrow?', Food Policy Unit, Manchester Polytechnic.

Larbie, J., and Mares, P. (1986), *A Training Handbook for Multiracial Health Care*, National Extension College, Cambridge.

Lee, A. J., Crombie, I., Smith, W. C. S., and Tunstall-Pedoe, H. (1990), 'Alcohol Consumption and Unemployment among Men: the Scottish Heart Health Study', *British Journal of Addiction*, 85, pp. 1165–70.

Leese, B., and Bosanquet, E. N. (1989), 'High and Low Incomes in General Practice', *British Medical Journal*, 298, pp. 932–4.

LeGrand, J., and Illsley, R. (1986), 'The Measurement of Inequality in Health', paper presented to a meeting of the British Association for the Advancement of Science, Bristol, 1–5 September 1986.

LeGrand, J., and Rabin, M. (1986), 'Trends in British Health Inequality: 1931–83', in A. J. Culyer and B. Jonsson (eds.), *Public and Private Health Services*, Oxford, Blackwell.

Lehelma, E., and Valkonen, T. (1990), 'Health and Social Inequities in Finland and Elsewhere', *Social Science and Medicine*, 31, pp. 257–65.

Lehmann, P., Mamboury, C., and Minder, C. E. (1990), 'Health and Social Inequities in Switzerland', *Social Science and Medicine*, 31, pp. 369–86.

Leon, D., and Wilkinson, R. G. (1989), 'Inequalities in Prognosis: Socio-economic Differences in Cancer and Heart Disease Survival', in A. J. Fox (ed.), *Inequalities in Health within Europe*, Gower Press, Aldershot.

Leon, D. A., Vågerö, D., and Olausson, P. (1992), 'Social Class Differences in Infant Mortality in Sweden: a Comparison with England and Wales', *British Medical Journal*, 305 (in press).

Leviatan, U., and Cohen, J. (1985), 'Gender Differences in Life Expectancy among Kibbutz Members', *Social Science and Medicine*, 21, pp. 545–51.

Littlewood, R., and Cross, S. (1980), 'Ethnic Minorities and Psychiatric Services', *Sociology of Health and Illness*, 2, pp. 194–201.

Lopez, A. D. (1984), 'Sex Differentials in Mortality', WHO Chronicle, 38 (5), pp. 217–24.

Lowry, S. (1989), 'Housing and Health: Temperature and Humidity', *British Medical Journal*, 299, pp. 1326–8.

Lowry, S. (1990), 'Health and Homelessness', *British Medical Journal*, 300, pp. 32–4.

Lumb, K. M., *et al.* (1981), 'Perinatal Mortality in British Asians', *Journal of Epidemiology and Community Health*, 35, pp. 106–9.

Lundberg, B. (1991a), 'The LO Health Project: Trade Union Health Promotion in Sweden', paper presented to the European Conference on Health Promotion in the Workplace, Barcelona, April 1991.

Lundberg, B., and Starrin, B. (1990), 'Fighting Health Hazards at Work', Research Report No. 1, Centre for Public Health Research, Karlstad, Sweden.

Lundberg, O. (1986), 'Class and Health: Comparing Britain and Sweden', *Social Science and Medicine*, 23, pp. 511–17.

Lundberg, O. (1991b), 'Causal Explanations for Class Inequality in Health: an Empirical Analysis', *Social Science and Medicine*, 32, pp. 385–93.

Lunt, B. (1985), 'Terminal Cancer Care Services: Recent Changes in Regional Inequalities in Great Britain', *Social Science and Medicine*, 20 (7), pp. 753–8.

Lynch, P., and Oelman, B. J. (1981), 'Mortality from CHD in the British Army Compared with the Civil Population', *British Medical Journal*, 283, pp. 405–7.

Lynge, E. (1984), 'Experiences in Estimating Differentials in Mortality in Developed Countries – Achievements and Shortcomings of the Various Approaches', in UN Department of International Economic and Social Affairs (ed.), *Data Bases for Mortality Measurement, Population Studies* No. 84, New York.

Macfarlane, A. (1986), letter to the *British Medical Journal*, 293, p. 504.

Macfarlane, A., and Cole, T. (1985), 'From Depression to Recession – Evidence about the Effects of Unemployment on Mothers' and Babies' Health', in L. Durward (ed.), 'Born Unequal: Perspectives on Pregnancy and Childrearing in Unemployed Families', Maternity Alliance.

Macfarlane, A., and Mugford, M. (1984), 'Birth Counts: Statistics of Pregnancy and Childbirth', National Perinatal Epidemiology Unit in collaboration wih OPCS, HMSO.

Macintyre, S. (1986a), 'Health and Illness', in R. Burgess (ed.), *Key Variables in Social Investigation*, Routledge & Kegan Paul.

Macintyre, S. (1986b), 'The Patterning of Health by Social Position in Contemporary Britain: Directions for Sociological Research', *Social Science and Medicine*, 23 (4), pp. 393–415.

Macintyre, S. (1989), 'The Role of Health Services in Relation to Inequalities in Health in Europe', in A. J. Fox (ed.), *Inequalities in Health within Europe*, Gower Press, Aldershot.

Macintyre, S., and West, P. (1991), 'Lack of Class Variation in Health in Adolescence: an Artifact of an Occupational Measure of Social Class?', *Social Science and Medicine*, 32, pp. 395–402.

Maclure, A., and Stewart, G. T. (1984), 'Admission of Children to Hospital in Glasgow: Relation to Unemployment and Other Deprivation Variables', *Lancet*, ii, pp. 682–8.

McAvoy, B. R., and Raza, R. (1991), 'Can Health Education Increase Uptake of Cervical Smear Testing among Asian Women', *British Medical Journal*, 302, pp. 833–6.

McCarthy, P., *et al.* (1985), 'Respiratory Conditions: Effects of Housing and Other Factors', *Journal of Epidemiology and Community Health*, 39, pp. 15–19.

McCormick, A., Rosenbaum, M., and Flemming, D. (1990), 'Socio-economic Characteristics of People Who Consult their GP', *Population Trends*, No. 59, pp. 8–10.

McDowall, M. (1983), 'Measuring Women's Occupational Mortality', *Population Trends*, 34, pp. 25–9.

McKechnie, S., and Wilson, D. (1986), 'Homes Above All: Housing in Britain, the Facts, the Failures, the Future', Shelter.

McKenna, S. P., and Payne, R. L. (1989), 'Comparison of the General Health Questionnaire and the Nottingham Health Profile in a Study of Unemployed and Re-employed Men', *Family Practice*, 6, pp. 3–8.

McKenna, S. P., and Hunt, S. (1990), 'Better Housing Better Health: Health and Housing in Croxteth/Gilmoss Action Areas', Manchester, Galen Research and Consultancy.

McNaught, A. (1985), 'Race and Health Care in the UK', Occasional Paper No. 2, Health Education Council.

Mack, J., and Lansley, S. (1985), *Poor Britain*, Allen & Unwin.

Mackenbach, J. P., Bouvier-Colle, M., and Jougle, E. (1990), '"Avoidable" Mortality and Health Services; a Review of Aggregate Data Studies', *Journal of Epidemiology and Community Health*, 44, pp. 106–11.

Mackenbach, J. P. (1992), 'Socioeconomic Health Differences in the Netherlands: a Review of Recent Empirical Findings', *Social Science and Medicine*, 34, pp. 213–26.

Madeley, R. J. (1982), 'Positive Discrimination in Child Health', *Public Health*, 96 (6), pp. 358–64.

Madhok, R., Bhopal, R., and Ramaiah, R. (1992),'Quality of Hospital Service: an "Asian" Perspective', *Journal of Public Health Medicine*, 14, issue 3 (in press).

MAFF (1991), 'Household Food Consumption and Expenditure 1990', HMSO.

Manchester (1985), Joint Consultative Committee (Health), 'Health Inequalities and Manchester', Manchester City Council/Health Authority.

Manchester City Council (1986), 'Poverty in Manchester', Manchester City Council.

Marin, R. (1986), 'Occupational Mortality 1971–80', *Central Statistical Office of Finland Studies No. 129*, quoted in Valkonen (1987).

Marmot, M. G., Adelstein, A. M., and Bulusu, L. (1984a), 'Immigrant Mortality in England and Wales 1970–78', OPCS Studies on Medical and Population Subjects No. 47, HMSO.

Marmot, M. G., *et al.* (1981), 'Changes in Heart Disease Mortality in England and Wales and Other Countries, *Health Trends*, 13, pp. 33–8.

Marmot, M. G., and McDowall, M. E. (1986), 'Mortality Decline and Widening Social Inequalities', *Lancet*, ii, pp. 274–6.

Marmot, M. G., Shipley, M. J., and Rose, G. (1984b), 'Inequalities in Death – Specific Explanations of a General Pattern?, *Lancet*, i, pp. 1003–6.

Marmot, M. G., Davey Smith, G., Stansfield, S., Patel, C., North, F., Head, J., *et al.* (1991), 'Health Inequalities among British Civil Servants: the Whitehall II Study', *Lancet*, 337, pp. 1387–93.

Marsh, G. N. (1988), 'Clinical Medicine and the Health Divide', *Journal of the Royal College of General Practitioners*, 38, pp. 5–9.

Marsh, G. N., and Channing, D. M. (1986), 'Deprivation and Health in One General Practice', *British Medical Journal*, 292, pp. 1173–6.

Marsh, G. N., and Channing, D. (1988), 'Narrowing the Gap between a Deprived and an Endowed Community', *British Medical Journal*, 296, pp. 173–6.

Martin, C., Platt, S., and Hunt, S. (1987), 'Housing Conditions and Ill-health', *British Medical Journal*, 294, pp. 1125–7.

Måseide, P. (1985), 'Norway Country Paper', in *Inequalities in Health and Health Care*, Nordic School of Public Health, NHV Report 1985:5, Göteborg, Sweden.

Mattiasson, I., Lindgarde, F., Nilsson, J., and Theorell, T. (1990), 'Threat of Unemployment and Cardiovascular Risk Factors: Longitudinal Study of Quality of Sleep and Serum Cholesterol Concentrations in Men Threatened by Redundancy', *British Medical Journal*, 301, pp. 461–6.

Mays, N., and Chinn, S. (1989), 'Relation between All Cause SMRs and Two Indices of Deprivation at Regional and District Level in England', *Journal of Epidemiology and Community Health*, 43, pp. 191–9.

Merrett, S. (1991), 'Quality and Choice in Housing', Economic Studies No. 10, Institute for Public Policy Research.

Mezentseva, E., and Rimachevskaya, N. (1990), 'The Soviet Country Profile: Health in the USSR Population in the 1970s and 1980s – an Approach to Comprehensive Analysis', *Social Science and Medicine*, 31, pp. 867–77.

Mielck, A. (1992), 'Inequalities in Health between Two Countries: East and West Germany', *Social Science and Medicine* (forthcoming).

Minev, D., Dermendjieva, B., and Mileva, N. (1990), 'The Bulgarian Country Profile: the Dynamics of Some Inequalities in Health', *Social Science and Medicine*, 31, pp. 837–46.

Mizrahi, A., and Mizrahi, A. (1992), 'Socio-economic Factors in Health and Health Care', *Social Science and Medicine* (forthcoming).

Moran, G. (1986), 'Health Promotion in Local Government: a British Experience', *Health Promotion*, 1, pp. 191–200.

Morgan, M. (1983), 'Measuring Social Inequalities: Occupational Classifications and their Alternatives', *Community Medicine*, 5, pp. 116–24.

Morgan, M., and Chinn, S. (1983), 'ACORN, Social Class and Child Health', *Journal of Epidemiology and Community Health*, 37, pp. 196–203.

Morgan, M., Heller, R. F., and Swerdlow, A. (1989), 'Change in Diet and CHD Mortality among Social Classes in Great Britain', *Journal of Epidemiology and Community Health*, 43, pp. 162–7.

Morris, J. N. (1979), 'Social Inequalities Undiminished', *Lancet*, i, pp. 87–90.

Morris, J. N. (1981), 'Coronary Heart Disease: a Tract for the Times', *Update*, 1 August 1981, pp. 323–31.

Morris, J. N. (1986), 'Inequality, Poverty and Health', *Lancet*, ii, p. 662.

Morris, J. N. (1990), 'Inequality in Health: Ten Years and Little Further On', *Lancet*, 336, pp. 491–3.

Morris, R., and Carstairs, V. (1991), 'Which Deprivation? A Comparison of Selected Deprivation Indexes', *Journal of Public Health Medicine*, 13, pp. 318–26.

Moser, K. A., Fox, A. J., and Jones, D. R. (1984), 'Unemployment and Mortality in the OPCS Longitudinal Study', *Lancet*, ii, pp. 1324–8.

Moser, K., Goldblatt, P., Fox, A. J., and Jones, D. R (1987), 'Unemployment and Mortality: Comparison of the 1971 and 1981 Longitudinal Study Census Samples', *British Medical Journal*, 294, pp. 86–90.

Moser, K., Pugh, H., and Goldblatt, P. (1988), 'Inequalities in Women's Health: Looking at Mortality Differentials Using an Alternative Approach', *British Medical Journal*, 296, pp. 1221–4.

Moser, K., Pugh, H., and Goldblatt, P. (1990a), *Inequalities in Women's Health in England and Wales: Mortality among Women according to Social Circumstances, Employment Characteristics and Life-cycle Stage*, Genus.

Moser, K., Pugh, H., and Goldblatt, P. (1990b), 'Mortality and the Social Classification of Women', in P. Goldblatt (ed.), *Longitudinal Study 1971–81: Mortality and Social Organisation*, OPCS LS series No. 6, HMSO.

Moser, K., Goldblatt, P., Fox, J., and Jones, D. (1990c), 'Unemployment and Mortality', in P. Goldblatt (ed.), *Longitudinal Study 1971–81: Mortality and Social Organisation*, OPCS LS series No. 6, HMSO.

Moser, K., and Goldblatt, P. (1991), 'Occupational Mortality of Women aged 15–59 Years at Death in England and Wales', *Journal of Epidemiology and Community Health*, 45, pp. 117–24.

Moylan, S., Millar, J., and Davis, R. (1984), *For Richer, for Poorer? DHSS Study of Unemployed Men*, HMSO.

Murphy, M., Goldblatt, P., Thornton-Jones, H., and Silcocks, P. (1990), 'Survival among Women with Cancer of the Uterine Cervix: Influence of Marital Status and Social Class', *Journal of Epidemiology and Community Health*, 44, pp. 293–6.

NACNE (1983), 'Proposals for Nutritional Guidelines for Health Education in Britain', Health Education Council.

National Children's Bureau (1987), 'Investing in the Future: Child Health Ten Years after the Court Report', National Children's Bureau.

National Children's Homes (1991), 'Poverty and Nutrition Survey 1991', National Children's Homes.

National Extension College (1984), 'Providing Effective Health Care in a Multiracial Society', National Extension College, Cambridge.

National Extension College (1986), 'NHS Training Needs Survey', National Extension College, Cambridge.

Nelson, M., and Naismith, D. (1979), 'The Nutritional Status of Poor Children in London', *Journal of Human Nutrition*, 33 (1), pp. 33–46.

Nichols, T. (1986), 'Industrial Injuries in British Manufacturing in the 1980s – a Commentary on Wright's Article', *Sociological Review*, 34, pp. 290–306.

Nicoll, A. (1986), 'The Child Health Clinic: Results of a New Strategy of Community Care in a Deprived Area', *Lancet*, i, pp. 606–8.

Norska-Borowka, I. (1990), 'Poland: Environmental Pollution and Health in Katowice', *Lancet*, 335, pp. 1392–3.

NUPE (1987), 'Equality in Health: a Strategy for Change', National Union of Public Employees.

Nutbeam, D., Catford, J. *et al.* (1987), 'Pulse of Wales Social Survey Supplement', Heartbeat Report No. 7, Heartbeat Wales, Cardiff.

Olausson, P. O. (1991), 'Mortality among the Elderly in Sweden by Social Class', *Social Science and Medicine*, 32, pp. 437–40.

OPCS (1985), 'General Household Survey for 1983', HMSO.

OPCS (1986a), 'Mortality Statistics, Perinatal and Infant: Social and Biological Factors for 1984', Series DH3, No. 17, HMSO.

OPCS (1986b), 'Registrar General's Decennial Supplement on Occupational Mortality 1979–83', HMSO.

OPCS (1986c), 'Longitudinal Study 1981–83, SMRs for Men of Working Ages, England and Wales'. Data provided by Baroness Trumpington, Parliamentary Under-Secretary of State, DHSS, in a parliamentary written reply, quoted in *Population Trends*, 45, Autumn, pp. 2–4.

OPCS (1986d), 'General Household Survey for 1984', HMSO.

OPCS (1988), 'Occupational Mortality: Childhood Supplement 1979–80, 1982–83', Series DS. No. 8, HMSO.

OPCS (1990a), 'Mortality Statistics: Perinatal and Infant Mortality: Social and Biological Factors, 1987', HMSO.

OPCS (1990b), 'General Household Survey for 1988', No. 19, HMSO.

OPCS (1991a), 'Mortality Statistics: Perinatal and Infant Mortality: Social and Biological Factors, 1988', HMSO.

OPCS (1991b), 'General Household Survey for 1989', No. 20, HMSO.

OPCS (1991c), 'Adult Dental Health Survey 1988: UK', HMSO.

OPCS (1992), 'Mortality Statistics: Perinatal and Infant: Social and Biological Factors, 1989 and 1990', HMSO.

Orosz, E. (1990), 'The Hungarian Country Profile: Inequalities in Health and Health Care in Hungary', *Social Science and Medicine*, 31, pp. 847–57.

Osborn, A. F., and Morris, A. C. (1979), 'The Rationale for a Composite Index of Social Class and its Evaluation', *British Journal of Sociology*, 30 (1), pp. 39–60.

Östberg, V., and Vågerö, D. (1990), 'Socio-economic Differences in Mortality among Children. Do They Persist into Adulthood?', *Social Science and Medicine*.

Ostrowska, A. (1980), *The Elements of Health Culture of the Polish Society*, Warsaw, OBOP.

Pamuk, E. R. (1985), 'Social Class Inequality in Mortality from 1921–1972 in England and Wales', *Population Studies*, 39, pp. 17–31.

Pamuk, E. R. (1988), 'Social Class Inequality in Infant Mortality in England and Wales from 1921–1980', *European Journal of Population*, 4, pp. 1–21.

Parker, H. (1989), *Instead of the Dole: an Enquiry into Integration of the Tax and Benefit System*, Routledge.

Parsons, L., and Day, S. (1992), 'Improving Obstetric Outcomes in Ethnic Minorities: an Evaluation of Health Advocacy in Hackney', *Journal of Public Health Medicine*, 14 (2) (in press).

Pearson, M. (1985), 'Racial Equality and Good Practice – Maternity Care', National Extension College, Cambridge.

Pendleton, D. A., and Bochner, S. (1980), 'The Communication of Medical Information in General Practice Consultations as a Function of Patients' Social Class', *Social Science and Medicine*, 14, pp. 669–73.

Pharaoh, P., and Morris, J. N. (1979), 'Postneonatal Mortality', *Epidemiologic Reviews*, 1, pp. 170–83.

Phillimore, P. (1989), 'Shortened Lives: Premature Death in North Tyneside', Bristol Papers in Applied Social Studies, No. 12, University of Bristol.

Piachaud, D. (1987), 'The Growth of Poverty', in A. Walker and C. Walker (eds.), *The Growing Divide*, Child Poverty Action Group.

Piachaud, D. (1991), Revitalizing Social Policy', *Political Quarterly*, 62, p. 221.

Pill, R., and Stott, N. C. (1985a), 'Choice or Chance: Further Evidence on Ideas of Illness and Responsibility for Health', *Social Science and Medicine*, 20 (10), pp. 981–91.

Pill, R., and Stott, N. C. (1985b), 'Preventive Procedures and Practices among Working Class Women: New Data and Fresh Insights', *Social Science and Medicine*, 21 (9), pp. 975–83.

Pill, R., French, J., Harding, K., and Stott, N. (1988), 'Invitation to Attend a Health Check in a General Practice Setting: Comparison of Attenders and Non-attenders', *Journal of the Royal College of General Practitioners*, 38, pp. 53–6.

Piperno, A., and Orio, F. D. (1990), 'Social Differences in Health and Utilization of Health Services in Italy', *Social Science and Medicine*, 31, pp. 305–12.

Platt, S. (1984), 'Unemployment and Suicidal Behaviour: a Review of the Literature', *Social Science and Medicine*, 19, pp. 93–115.

Platt, S., and Kreitman, N. (1984), 'Unemployment and Parasuicide in Edinburgh 1968–1982', *British Medical Journal*, 289, pp. 1029–32.

Platt, S., Hawton, K., Kreitman, N., Fagg, J., and Foster, J. (1988), 'Recent Clinical and Epidemiological Trends in Parasuicide in Edinburgh and Oxford: a Tale of Two Cities', *Psychological Medicine*, 18, pp. 405–18.

Platt, S., Martin, C., Hunt, S., and Lewis, C. (1989), 'Damp Housing, Mould Growth, and Symptomatic Health State', *British Medical Journal*, 298, pp. 1673–8.

Popay, J., Dhooge, Y., and Shipman, C. (1986), 'Unemployment and Health: What Role for Health and Social Services?', Research Report No. 3, Health Education Council.

Pound, A. (1991), 'Newpin and Child Abuse', *Child Abuse Review*, 5, pp. 7–10.

Power, C. (1991), 'Social and Economic Background and Class Inequalities in Health among Young Adults', *Social Science and Medicine*, 32, pp. 411–17.

Power, C., Fogelman, K., and Fox, A. J. (1986), 'Health and Social Mobility During the Early Years of Life', National Child Development Study Working Paper No. 8, May 1986, Social Statistics Research Unit, City University, London.

Power, C., and Peckham, C. (1990), 'Childhood Morbidity and Adulthood Ill-health', *Journal of Epidemiology and Community Health*, 44, pp. 69–74.

Preston, S., Haines, M., and Pamuk, E. (1981), 'Effects of Industrialisation on Mortality in Developed Countries', in *Solicited Papers*, Vol. 2, IUSSP 19th International Population Conference, Manila, Part 2, Liegei Imprimerce Derouaux, pp. 233–54.

Pringle, M. (1989), 'The Quality Divide in Primary Care', *British Medical Journal*, 299, pp. 470–71.

Pugh, H., and Moser, K. (1990), 'Measuring Women's Mortality Differences', in H. Roberts (ed.), *Women's Health Counts*, Routledge.

Pugh, H., Power, C., Goldblatt, P., and Arber, S. (1991), 'Women's Lung Cancer Mortality, Socioeconomic Status and Changing Smoking Patterns', *Social Science and Medicine*, 32, pp. 1105–10.

Quick, A., and Wilkinson, R. (1991), 'Income and health', Socialist Health Association.

Radical Statistics Health Group (1987), 'Facing the Facts: What Really Is Happening to the NHS?', Radical Statistics Health Group.

Reading, R. F., Openshaw, S., Jarvis, S. N. (1990), 'Measuring Child Health Inequalities Using Aggregations of Enumeration Districts', *Journal of Public Health Medicine*, 12, 160–67.

Reich, M., and Goldman, R. (1984), 'Italian Occupational Health: Concepts, Conflicts and Implications', *American Journal of Public Health*, 74, pp. 1031–41.

Richards, D. (1990), 'Benefits to Health', *Social Work Today*, 26 July, pp. 18–19.

Richie, J., Jacoby, A., and Bone, M. (1981), 'Access to Primary Health Care', OPCS/HMSO.

Roberts, H. (ed.) (1990), *Women's Health Counts*, Routledge.

Roberts, J. L., and Graveling, P. A. (eds.) (1985), 'The Big Kill: Smoking Epidemic in England and Wales', published for the Health Education Council and the British Medical Association by the North West Regional Health Authority.

Robine, J. M., and Ritchie, K. (1991), 'Healthy Life Expectancy: Evaluation of a Global Indicator of Change in Population Health', *British Medical Journal*, 302, pp. 457–60.

Rocheron, Y., and Dickinson, R. (1990), 'The Asian Mother and Baby Campaign: a Way Forward in Health Promotion for Asian Women?', *Health Education Journal*, 49, pp. 128–33.

Roderick, P., Victor, C., and Connelly, J. (1991), 'Is Housing a Public Health Issue? A Survey of Directors of Public Health', *British Medical Journal*, 302, pp. 157–60.

Rodriguez, J., and Lemkow, L. (1990), 'Health and Social Inequities in Spain', *Social Science and Medicine*, 31, pp. 351–8.

Roll, J. (1985), 'Poverty and Food', *Poverty* No. 6, Spring 1985.

Rose, G., and Marmot, M. G. (1981), 'Social Class and Coronary Heart Disease', *British Medical Journal*, 45, pp. 13–19.

Ross, E., and Begg, N. (1991), 'Child Health Computing: a Springboard for a Community Health Register', *British Medical Journal*, 302, pp. 5–6.

RUHBC (1989), *Changing the Public Health*, Research Unit in Health and Behavioural Change, Chichester, John Wiley and Sons.

Ryan, M., and Birch, S. (1991), 'Charging for Health Care: Evidence on the Utilisation of NHS Prescribed Drugs', *Social Science and Medicine*, 33, pp. 681–7.

Scottish Health Education Co-ordinating Committee (1984), 'Health Education in Areas of Multiple Deprivation', a report by the Scottish Health Education Coordinating Committee, Edinburgh.

Scott-Samuel, A. (1981), 'Social Class Inequality in Access to Primary Care: a Critique of Recent Research', *British Medical Journal*, 283, pp. 510–11.

Scott-Samuel, A. (1984), 'Need for Primary Health Care: an Objective Indicator', *British Medical Journal*, 288, pp. 457–8.

Scott-Samuel, A., and Blackburn, P. (1988), 'Crossing the Health Divide – Mortality Attributable to Social Inequality in Great Britain', *Health Promotion*, 2, pp. 243–5.

Sheffield City Council (1987), 'Good Health for All', Central Policy Unit, Sheffield.

Sheffield Health Authority (1986), 'Health Care and Disease – a Profile of Sheffield', Sheffield Health Authority.

Shuval, J. (1990), 'Health in Israel: Patterns of Equality and Inequality', *Social Science and Medicine*, 31, pp. 291–303.

Smith, R. (1986), 'The Need for a Public Health Alliance', *British Medical Journal*, 293, pp. 346–7.

Smith, R. (1987a), *Unemployment and Health*, Oxford University Press.

Smith, R. (1987b), 'Medical News', *British Medical Journal*, 294, p. 1358.

Social Security Committee (1991), 'Low Income Statistics: Households Below Average Income Tables 1988', HMSO.

Starrin, B., Svensson, P-G., and Wintersberger, H. (1989), 'Unemployment, Poverty and the Quality of Working Life: Some European Experiences', Berlin, European Centre for Social Welfare, Training and Research/World Health Organization Regional Office for Europe.

Stern, J. (1983), 'Social Mobility and the Interpretation of Social Class Mortality Differentials' *Journal of Social Policy*, 12, pp. 27–49.

Stirland, H. (1985), 'Risk Factors in Childhood Accidents', paper presented to a symposium on 'Accidents in Childhood', King's Fund Centre, London, 3 October 1985.

Strachan, D. (1988), 'Damp Housing and Childhood Asthma: Validation of Reporting of Symptoms', *British Medical Journal*, 297, pp. 1223–6.

Strachan, D., and Elton, R. (1986), 'Relationship between Respiratory Morbidity in Children and the Home Environment', *Family Practice*, 3, pp. 137–42.

Strachan, D. P., and Sanders, C. H. (1989), 'Damp Housing and Childhood Asthma: Respiratory Effects of Indoor Air Temperature and Relative Humidity', *Journal of Epidemiology and Community Health*, 43, pp. 7–14.

Strathclyde Regional Council (1990), 'Strathclyde Anti-poverty Strategy and Initiatives for 1990/91', Glasgow, Strathclyde Regional Council.

Strong, P. M. (1990), 'Black on Class and Mortality: Theory, Method and History', *Journal of Public Health Medicine*, 12, pp. 168–80.

Terry, P. B., *et al.* (1980), 'Analysis of Ethnic Differences in Perinatal Statistics', *British Medical Journal*, 281, pp. 1307–8.

Thomas, L. (1988), 'Winter's Tale', *Geriatric Nursing and Home Care*, November 1988, pp. 10–11.

Thompson, N. F. (1990), 'Inviting Infrequent Attenders to Attend for a Health Check: Cost and Benefits', *British Journal of General Practice*, 40, pp. 16–18.

Thunhurst, C. (1985a), 'Poverty and Health in the City of Sheffield', Environmental Health Department, Sheffield City Council.

Thunhurst, C. (1985b), 'The Analysis of Small Area Statistics and Planning for Health', *Statistician*, 34, pp. 93–106.

Thunhurst, C. (1989), 'Core Health Measures for UK Cities', Liverpool, UK Healthy Cities Network.

Thunhurst, C., and Postma, S. (1989), 'Health Profile of the City of Stoke-on-Trent', Stoke-on-Trent District Council/North Staffordshire District Health Authority.

Thunhurst, C., and Macfarlane, A. (1992), 'Monitoring the Health of Urban Populations: What Statistics Do We Need?', *Journal of the Royal Statistical Society*, A, 155 (9), (in press).

Todd, J. E., and Dodd, T. (1985), 'Children's Dental Health in the UK, 1983', OPCS/HMSO.

Townsend, J. (1987), 'Cigarette Tax, Economic Welfare and Social Class Patterns of Smoking', *Applied Economics*, 19, pp. 355–65.

Townsend, P. (1987), 'Deprivation', *Journal of Social Policy*, 16, pp. 125–46.

Townsend, P. (1988a), personal communication, from secondary analysis of Registrar General's Decennial Supplement on Occupational Mortality, 1979–83.

Townsend, P. (1988b), 'Inner City Deprivation and Premature Death in Greater Manchester', Tameside Metropolitan Borough.

Townsend, P. (1990), 'Individual or Social Responsibility for Premature Death – Current Controversies in the British Debate about Health', *International Journal of Health Services*, 20, pp. 373–92.

Townsend, P. (1991), 'The Poor Are Poorer: a Statistical Report on Changes in the Living Standards of Rich and Poor in the UK 1979–1989', Bristol, Statistical Monitoring Unit, Department of Social Policy and Social Planning, University of Bristol.

Townsend, P., Corrigan, P., and Kowarzik, O. (1986a), 'Poverty and the London Labour Market: an Interim Report', Low Pay Unit.

Townsend, P., and Davidson, N. (1982), *Inequalities in Health: the Black Report*, 1982 edition, Penguin Books, Harmondsworth, p. 24.

Townsend, P., Phillimore, P., and Beattie, A. (1986b), 'Inequalities in Health in the Northern Region: an Interim Report', Northern Regional Health Authority/Bristol University.

Townsend, P., Phillimore, P., and Beattie, A. (1988a), *Health and Deprivation: Inequality and the North*, Croom Helm.

Townsend, P., Simpson, D., and Tibbs, N. (1985), 'Inequalities in Health in the City of Bristol: a Preliminary Review of Statistical Evidence', *International Journal of Health Services*, 15 (4), pp. 637–63.

Unemployment and Health Study Group (1986), 'Unemployment: a Challenge to Public Health', Occasional Paper No. 10, Centre for Professional Development, Department of Community Medicine, University of Manchester.

Vågerö, D. (1991), 'Inequality in Health – Some Theoretical and Empirical Problems', *Social Science and Medicine*, 32, pp. 367–71.

Vågerö, D., and Lundberg, O. (1989), 'Health inequalities in Britain and Sweden', *Lancet*, ii, pp. 35–6.

Vågerö, D., and Norell, S. (1989), 'Mortality and Social Class in Sweden – Exploring a New Epidemiological Tool', *Scandinavian Journal of Social Medicine*, 17, pp. 49–58.

Vågerö, D., and Östberg, V. (1989), 'Mortality among Children and Young Persons in Sweden in relation to Childhood Socio-economic Group', *Journal of Epidemiology and Community Health*, 43, pp. 280–84.

Vågerö, D., and Persson, G. (1987), 'Cancer Survival and Social Class in Sweden', *Journal of Epidemiology and Community Health*, 41, pp. 204–9.

Valkonen, T. (1987), 'Social Inequality in the Face of Death', paper presented to the European Population Conference, Central Statistical Office of Finland.

Valkonen, T. (1989), 'Adult Mortality and Level of Education: a Comparison of Six Countries', in A. J. Fox (ed.), *Inequalities in Health within Europe*, Gower Press, Aldershot.

Valkonen, T., Martelin, T., and Rimpelä, A. (1991), 'Socio-economic Differences in Finland 1971–85', Central Statistical Office of Finland, Studies 176, Helsinki.

Victor, C. R., and Vetter, N. (1986), 'Poverty, Disability and Use of Services by the Elderly: Analysis of the 1980 General Household Survey', *Social Science and Medicine*, 22 (10), pp. 1087–91.

Wadsworth, M. E. J. (1986), 'Serious Illness in Childhood and its Association with Later-life Achievement', in R. G. Wilkinson (ed.), *Class and Health: Research and Longitudinal Data*, Tavistock.

Wagstaff, A., Paci, P., and Doorslaer, E. (1991), 'On the Measurement of Inequalities in Health', *Social Science and Medicine*, 33, pp. 545–57.

Waldron, I. (1976), 'Why Do Women Live Longer than Men?', *Social Science and Medicine*, 10, pp. 349–62.

Waldron, I. (1983), 'Sex Differences in Illness Incidence, Prognosis and Mortality: Issues and Evidence', *Social Science and Medicine*, 17, pp. 1107–23.

Walker, A., and Walker, C. (eds.) (1987), *The Growing Divide: a Social Audit 1979– 1987*, Child Poverty Action Group.

Wall, P. (1991), 'Health and Homelessness', *Health Service Journal*, 11 April, pp. 16–17.

Waller, D., Agass, M., Mant, D., Coulter, A., Fuller, A., and Jones, L. (1990), 'Health Checks in General Practice: Another Example of Inverse Care?', *British Medical Journal*, 300, pp. 1115–18.

Walsh, J., *et al.* (1985), 'Access to Primary Health Care: a Study of East Ward, Bury', Bury Community Health Council.

Warr, P. (1985), 'Twelve Questions about Unemployment and Health', in B. Roberts, R. Finnegan and D. Gallie (eds.), *New Approaches to Economic Life*, Manchester University Press.

Webb, T., Schilling, R., Babb, P., and Jacobson, B. (1987), 'Health at Work?', a report on Health Promotion in the Workplace, Health Education Council.

West, P. (1988), 'Inequalities? Social Class Differentials in Health in British Youth', *Social Science and Medicine*, 27, pp. 291–6.

West, P. (1991), 'Rethinking the Health Selection Explanation for Health Inequalities', *Social Science and Medicine*, 32, pp. 373–84.

West, P., Macintyre, S., Annandale, E., and Hunt, K. (1990), 'Social Class and Health in Youth: Findings from the West of Scotland Twenty-07 Study', *Social Science and Medicine*, 30, pp. 665–73.

Westcott, G. (1987), 'The Effects of Unemployment on Health in Scunthorpe and Related Health Risk Factors', *Public Health*, 101, pp. 399–416.

White, P. (1986), ASH, personal communication.

White, P. (1990), 'A Question on Ethnic Group for the Census: Findings from the 1989 Census Test Post-enumeration Survey', *Population Trends*, No. 59, pp. 11–20.

Whitehead, M. (1988a), 'Deaths Foretold', *Guardian*, 7 December.

Whitehead, M. (1988b), 'National Health Success', Association of Community Health Councils for England and Wales/South Birmingham Health Authority, Birmingham.

Whitehead, M. (1989a), 'Swimming Upstream: Trends and Prospects in Education for Health', Research Report No. 5, King's Fund Institute.

Whitehead, M. (1989b), 'The Way We Live: Lifestyle, Behaviour, the Individual and Health', Health Studies in Nurse Education, Edinburgh, Health Education Board for Scotland.

Whitehead, M. (1990), 'Concepts and Principles of Equity and Health', Copenhagen, World Health Organization Regional Office for Europe. Also reprinted in *Health Promotion International* (1991), 6, pp. 217–27.

Whitehead, M., and Dahlgren, G. (1991), 'What Can Be Done about Inequalities in Health?', *Lancet*, 338, pp. 1059–63.

Whitehead, M., and Tones, B.K. (1991), 'Avoiding the Pitfalls: Notes on the Planning and Implementation of Health Education Strategies', Health Education Authority.

Whitehouse, C. R. (1985), 'Effect of Distance from Surgery on Consultation Rates in an Urban Practice', *British Medical Journal*, 290, pp. 359–62.

WHO (1984), 'Report of the Working Group on Concepts and Principles of Health Promotion', Copenhagen, 9–13 July 1984, World Health Organization.

WHO (1985), 'Targets for Health for All: Targets in Support of the European Regional Strategy for Health for All by the Year 2000', World Health Organization Regional Office for Europe, Copenhagen.

WHO (1991a), Health for All Statistical Database', September 1991 edition, WHO Regional Office for Europe, Copenhagen.

WHO (1991b), 'Health for All Policy in Finland: WHO Health Policy Review', Copenhagen, World Health Organization Regional Office for Europe.

Wilkinson, R. G. (1986a), 'Socio-economic Differences in Mortality: Interpreting the Data on their Size and Trends', in R. G. Wilkinson (ed.), *Class and Health: Research and Longitudinal Data*, Tavistock.

Wilkinson, R. G. (1986b), 'Occupational Class, Selection and Inequalities in Health: a Reply to Raymond Illsley', *Quarterly Journal of Social Affairs*, 2 (4), pp. 415–22.

Wilkinson, R. G. (1986c), 'Income and Mortality', in R. G. Wilkinson (ed.), *Class and Health: Research and Longitudinal Data*, Tavistock.

Wilkinson, R. G. (1989), 'Class Mortality Differentials and Trends in Poverty 1921–81', *Journal of Social Policy*, 18, pp. 307–35.

Wilkinson, R. G. (1990), 'Income Distribution and Mortality: a Natural Experiment', *Sociology of Health and Illness*, 12, pp. 391–412.

Wilkinson, R. G. (1992), 'Income Distribution and Life Expectancy', *British Medical Journal*, 304, pp. 165–8.

Winkler, J. T. (1987), 'Nurturing Nutrition the Norwegian Way', *Guardian*, 2 May 1987.

Wnuk-Lipinski, E. (1990), 'The Polish Country Profile: Economic Crisis and Inequalities in Health', *Social Science and Medicine*, 31, pp. 859–66.

Wnuk-Lipinski, E., and Illsley, R. (eds.) (1990), 'Social Equity in Health in Non-market Economies', *Social Science and Medicine*, 31, pp. 833–89 and 879–89.

Wood, J. (1991), 'A Review of Antenatal Care Initiatives in Primary Care Settings', *British Journal of General Practice*, 41, pp. 26–30.

WRR (1991), 'Socio-economic Inequity in Health and Health Policy', WRR-V72, SDU, The Hague (in Dutch: English summary available from Ministry of Welfare, Health and Cultural Affairs).

Youd, L., and Jayne, L. (1986), 'Salford Community Health Project: the First Three Years', Salford, Salford Community Health Project.

Young, B. (1980), 'Health and Housing: Infestation', *Roof*, July/August 1980, pp. 111–12.

Index